Soma in Yoga and Ayurveda

The Power of Rejuvenation and Immortality

By David Frawley

(Pandit Vamadeva Shastri)

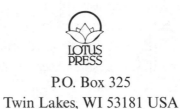

P.O. Box 325
Twin Lakes, WI 53181 USA

Disclaimer

Author: David Frawley

Copyright © 2012 by David Frawley

All Sanskrit translations cited in the book by the author unless otherwise indicated.

Illustrations by courtesy of Hinduism Today, including cover.

www.vedanet.com
pvshastri@aol.com

First Edition 2012

Printed in the United States of America
ISBN: 978-0-9406-7621-3
Library of Congress Catalog Number: 2012932154

LOTUS
PRESS

Published by:
Lotus Press, P.O. Box 325, Twin Lakes, WI53181 USA
web:www.lotuspress.com
Email:lotuspress@lotuspress.com
800.824.6396

TABLE OF CONTENTS

Appendix

FOREWORD

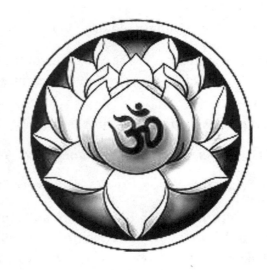

By this praise unto thee, O Soma,
May we enter the secret caves of intuitive wisdoms;
Do reveal unto us the luminosities that are thine,
The earthly ones and the heavenly ones.
By this power and sacrament thine, Oh Soma,
May we wander freely in the secret contemplative revelations;
Do kindle unto us the fires that are thine,
The earthly ones and the heavenly ones.[1]

Soma is one of the key words in the ancient traditions of India. It stands for all that is gentle, beautiful, delicate, and sweet of temperament. It is also a synonym for the Moon. A person is complimented by calling him/her *saumya*, moon-like. A *saumya* face, *saumya* mien is what one looks for in choosing a friend. When one looks at a *saumya* person, it generates the kind delight, the feeling of soft light that looking at the moon generates. This is a common idiom in all the languages of India.

Soma is part of the eternal pair of *Agni-Soma*. Agni is the fire element; Soma is the water element, moonlike. This pair is the Vedic equivalent of the Taoist yin-yang principle, balancing of the female and the male, energizer (female) and the energized (male). We read in *Rigveda* that this fire wears the ocean as a robe:

Agnim samudra-vāsasam...Rigveda VIII.102.6

In the daily fire sacrament of the Vedic-Hindu tradition, one of the offerings is made to this biune principle. The mantra for that offering is simple:

Agnī-ṣomābhyām svāhā; Idam Agnī-ṣomābhyām, idam na mama

Unto Agni and Soma, this sincere, truthful, beautiful offering.

This is unto Agni and Soma; [I seek] nothing [in] this as mine.[2]

The purpose of this offering is to balance and unite within oneself what appear to be opposites but are in truth complementary principles. This balancing and uniting reaches a point where Soma is itself called *Agni*; moon that is water is called 'immortal fire' in the mantra:

Abhi vahnir amartyaḥ... Rigveda IX.9.6

This very gentle feminine power is identified with the mind as:

Candramā manaso jātaḥ

[Universal] mind is born from the moon... Rigveda X.90.13

This moon is the same that is "in the waters":

Candramā apsv antarā ...Rigveda I.105.1

This mind of the waters and the moon blows towards us eternal peace:

Naḥ pavasva śam... Rigveda IX.11.3

In the mystic poetry of all spiritual traditions we hear about a state of divine inebriation. This wine is drunk not from the mouth but in the heart.[3] The wine of the Sufi mystic is well known. When Omar Khayyam sings of the wine of dawn he extols the intoxication of enlightenment. In the Vedic lore it is the Soma juice that plays the same part. "Dripping the intoxication, Soma resorts in the divine feminine"[4]

This is not the inebriation that renders a mind crazy, but the bliss that makes us masters of the mind, the nectar that grants us spiritual immortality. "This Soma finds the world, knows the world; it is the lord of the mind."[5] Thus it enters our minds free and we discover and proclaim: "Mind itself is the lord of the mind."[6]

It is no longer an enslaved mind, for Soma has rendered it free. Thus this Soma is the one that moves with the subtlest intuitive wisdom, sends forth inspired speech, guards the Perennial Poem and with the same Perennial Contemplation, races in diverse ways to the luminous heaven.[7]

It is not intended here to summarize all the 114 paeans to Soma sung in the ninth book of *Rigveda*, and many more elsewhere. The above references are just to give a glimpse of how deep spiritual realizations are sung of in the Vedic lore.

Shri Vamadeva Shastri (Dr. David Frawley) has brought out the core knowledge of Soma in the present volume. With his *Dhī* (intuitive wisdom and insight) and *manman* (contemplation), he has revealed the manifold connections of Soma with centers of consciousness and vitality, secrets of immortality, diet and herbs, Ayurvedic theory, Yoga practices and meditation, with Vedic astrology, Vastu and many other profound regions of the deeper knowledge not easily accessible today.

The Vedic lore teaches us to see connections everywhere in the expanse from the subtlest to the grossest, from the most minute to the most all-pervasive. Just to look at the book's Contents page awakens in us an awareness of the vast scale of connections from the earth of our physical identities to the highest heavens of our inner lights that Soma encompasses with beauty and grace. Dr. Frawley shows us in this wonderful book his ability to see such wide and varied connections with Soma and also provide us with the practical tools for working with them to transform our lives.

With these myriad insights presented by him, may we seek to enjoy an unending friendship and companionship with this immortal nectar of the Moon-Soma:

Indo sakhitvam uśmasi...Rigveda IX.66.14

Swami Veda Bharati

Mahamandaleshwar Swami Veda Bharati

Swami Rama Sadhaka Grama, Rishikesh, India

Author's Preface

Today as most of us are living longer, we must be concerned about the quality of our lives. Longevity is not a simple matter of having more chronological years, but should include physical, mental and spiritual well-being. It is not merely the quantity of our lifespan that matters but the joy, freedom, love and awareness that we can experience along the way.

Curiously, in spite of a greater physical longevity overall today, we seem to be suffering from more psychological malaise, depression, unhappiness, and sorrow. Greater longevity is certainly possible but to really benefit us, it must be linked with life of greater meaning, creativity and consciousness. This requires an ability to connect with the immortal essence of our being.

The pursuit of longevity should be part of an inner quest for eternal truth and bliss. Seeking to live longer physically should be connected with an endeavor to grow and evolve in intelligence and awareness. Our lives must become a spiritual search, not simply a running after sensory enjoyments and worldly possessions that change from moment to moment. Certainly the spiritual life – particularly the yogic life of meditation – can improve our health and longevity as well as our emotional state. Yet it can offer us something far more, an inner immortality, taking our awareness beyond the limitations of time and circumstances. In fact, if we discover this inner immortality, how long we may actually live physically may lose its importance. We will be able to drop the body at any moment without a sense of loss to embrace a greater existence in consciousness itself.

The following book, *Soma in Yoga and Ayurveda*, weaves together the outer and inner search for immortality and transcendence of death and sorrow. It shows that an immortality in consciousness is our very nature – and that it is possible to prolong our outer lives by aligning ourselves to it. The orientation of the book is practical, presenting comprehensive knowledge and special methods to heal and rejuvenate body and mind – and to resurrect the immortal spirit within us. Yet the

11

book does require that we look at ourselves, examining our nature not simply as human beings, but as immortal souls. The book rests upon a yogic view of who we are, what our greater existence is, the nature of mind and consciousness, and the place of our physical life within the context of many lives and incarnations.

Soma in Yoga and Ayurveda explores different tools for prolonging our physical lives according to Ayurveda, India's traditional natural healing system, particularly special foods and herbs. It adds to these yogic methods of asana and pranayama that improve our physical energy and flexibility. In addition, it examines rejuvenation of the mind, bringing in special yogic practices of mantra, pranayama and meditation. Yet most importantly, the book connects rejuvenation of the body and mind with our inherent immortality in pure consciousness that is their origin and support. It does not promote a blind seeking of a long life for the body, but asks us to open ourselves to an inner bliss, the immortality of the spirit.

The book rests upon the terminology of Ayurvedic medicine, which has an entire system of rejuvenation (*rasayana*) therapies for healing and revitalizing body and mind as one of its eight traditional branches. The book looks to Raja or classical Yoga and its eight limbs for its practices of Yoga and meditation, placing these in the context of the related system of *Vedanta* or Upanishadic knowledge for its background theory and world view. Rejuvenation is an important concern of traditional Yoga in both Tantric and Vedic lines. Tantric Yoga in particular contains special practices that both promote longevity and awaken our higher energies. Vedic rituals have as one of the fruits of their performance a long and healthy life, which Vedic mantras set in motion at a powerful way. The book, therefore, is a study of Ayurvedic medicine and classical Yoga as a means of awakening our inner faculties, along with their background philosophies, worldviews and related systems.

As the title suggests, *Soma in Yoga and Ayurveda* develops the ancient Vedic theme of Soma, the nectar of immortality, but relative to all aspects of its symbolism and application, not simply the search for the original Soma plant. It does explore the identity of Soma as a plant, but comes to the conclusion that the real Soma was not a single plant but a type of rejuvenative plants and their preparations, which can be found to some extent in all geographical regions. Even that outer plant or botanical Soma is only one aspect of the universal reality of Soma, which also lies within us.

The key to physical, psychological and spiritual well-being lies in our Soma, which can perhaps best be defined as the essence of bliss or *Ananda* arising from the core of our being. This is not an outer Soma only, but an 'inner Soma' or 'nectar of immortality' in our own deeper awareness. We must access this inner Soma if we wish to discover lasting happiness and joy. The book teaches us how to uncover, perceive, and work with the many Somas of our lives from foods, prana and sensory impressions to art, mantra, meditation and the very delight of existence itself.

The gaining of immortality is the main concern of all spiritual, religious and occult traditions from throughout the world. Some groups attempt this through faith and devotion, others through knowledge and perception, yet others through inner practices involving speech, breath and mind, like pranayama, mantra and meditation. All such methods are examined in the book, as all can be found in the Vedic tradition in various forms.

Soma in Yoga and Ayurveda complements my other books on Ayurveda, Yoga and Vedic astrology, which can serve as a reference for what is presented here. I have focused the discussion on the Vedic and India based tradition, bringing other forms of traditional medicine or modern medicine, only in a secondary manner. This is because the aim is to bring out the Vedic view in more detail, which unlike the others is not so commonly represented. This is not to say that other traditions and disciplines do not have a lot to offer on this important subject. In fact, traditional and natural systems of medicine overall have much knowledge about rejuvenation and afford it a greater place than modern medicine.

The book rests upon my own years of experience from reciting, chanting and meditating on the Soma hymns of the *Rigveda*, to working with a variety of herbs, to exploring the different paths of Yoga, mantra and Tantra. Initially I was drawn more to the Agni and Surya principles of light and fire in the *Vedas* and to the greater science of Prana. Yet in recent years the Soma hymns and their inner principles have come to life for me. This inner Soma has begun to speak to me and hopefully the book is a manifestation of its voice as well. The book, therefore, reflects more inner explorations than outer studies, though it is rooted in classical Vedic principles applied in life and discovered through nature.

Please note that the book is meant to be complex and many sided, as per the nature of the subject – a detailed presentation, not simply introductory in orientation. It is not meant to be a simple study of physical longevity but to draw the connection between physical longevity and our greater inner immortality.

Relative to Ayurvedic herbs, I have introduced a few important rejuvenative herbs used in Ayurveda, recognizing the limited accessibility these currently have in the West. In the Indian context much more could be said. The purpose of my herbal presentation is to encourage the reader to explore this angle further, not to produce a definitive herbal text.

Relative to the Sanskrit, I have used a Unicode font for the diacritical marks helpful to pronounce mantras, as it does not require any special Sanskrit fonts in order to read. However, Sanskrit terms that have already entered into the English language like Shiva or Shakti, or those of more general usage, I have rendered without any diacritical marks.

I am most happy to have a foreword from Swami Veda Bharati. Swamiji is, first of all, one of the greatest living authorities on the *Yoga Sutras,* providing an extensive study of the text according to both traditional sources. Yet, more importantly for this Soma book, he is one of the greatest living authorities on the *Rigveda*, which his name as Veda Bharati or 'Voice of the *Vedas*' indicates. Swami Veda has included in his foreword to the book some of his own Vedic verses, of which he has many more. Since a child he has been able to spontaneously compose Sanskrit verses in the Vedic style and has a profound understanding of the Vedic Yoga.

Soma is a very rich Vedic theme, like Agni (the sacred fire), and deserves much more attention. It unlocks the highest secrets of life and consciousness and offers an important field for further research both in meditation and in mind-body healing. I hope that others will examine this theme as well and bring in their own insights by the inspiration of their own Soma.

It is my heartfelt wish that the book awakens an inner flow of Soma, allowing the reader to connect with the supreme essence of happiness and immortality – as well aiding in a longer and more fruitful life for all.

May the supreme Soma, the eternal and universal energy of peace, bliss and delight, flow both within and around you for the benefit of all!

Om Īm Śrīm Somāya Namaḥ!

Acharya David Frawley (Pandit Vamadeva Shastri)

Santa Fe NM, March 2012

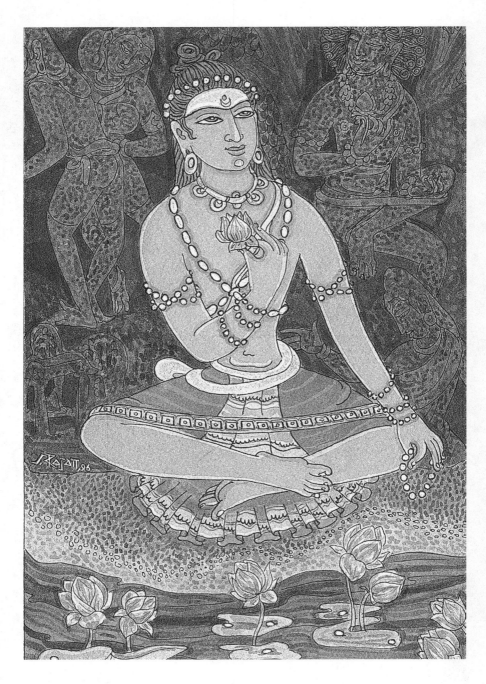

Soma as the Principle of Inner Unfoldment

PART I

The Search for Bliss, Longevity and Immortality

We have drunk the Soma. We have become immortal. We have reached the Gods. We have entered the realm of heavenly light. What now can the ungrateful do to us, what harm of the mortal, O immortal Soma?

Grant peace to our hearts when drunk, O drop. Gracious as a father to his son, as a friend to a friend, wise and of good counsel, O Soma extend our lives for our souls.

Rigveda VIII.48.3-4

THE QUEST FOR IMMORTALITY

From the unreal lead us to the real.
From darkness lead us to light.
From death lead us to immortality.

Soma Chant from the Brihadaranyaka Upanishad I.3.28

The quest for immortality has been the ultimate concern of all human beings since the beginning of time. We all naturally want to live forever and never die. Whatever may be our other pursuits in life for wealth, fame, knowledge or happiness, whether we attain them or not, a greater seeking for immortality remains in the background waiting for us to take it up as our highest goal.

This desire for deathlessness, however, is no mere hope, fantasy or delusion. It reflects the innate urge of the immortal soul hidden within us, which itself is never born and never dies. In our inmost being, we are one with the eternal and infinite and maintain a deep wish to return to it as our true home. Our physical life journey must eventually cause us to recognize this greater spiritual origin and goal. Our longing for immortality is an indication of our deeper Self and essence that we can never forget, which dwells far beyond the travails of this mortal realm.

At the same time as much as we wish for immortality, we have an equally deep fear of death. Death appears as the great barrier for all things in our lives, the end of all that we can do in this world and all that we hold dear within it. We innately sense that there is something unnecessary about death, which holds the tragedy of human existence, and calls into question our entire outer reality. We cannot accept death as final, and sense something greater within us beyond its grasp.

Yet we observe that each creature that is born grows old and eventually dies in the inevitable course of time. Infancy turns into youth, then into maturity, decline, debility and finally complete cessation of life for all creatures. We watch our pets and our parents grow old and die, and then experience it for those of our own generation and for ourselves. The aging process appears as the great leveler in life, affecting equally the rich and the poor, the famous and the ordinary. The relentless ticking of our biological clock seems to rule over all else that we do with an imperial and unbending force.

Certainly, we see people who live longer and age better than others, maintaining health, intelligence and happiness well into their later years. Such long-lived individuals represent another desirable goal of life, which is longevity, but they still stand on this side of death, compared to which even a long life is but a short episode in the enduring world of eternity. Longevity, however helpful, is not enough to take us beyond death.

Realizing the inevitability of death, we have sought to create or to discover another life beyond the demise of the body. Most of what we call religion has arisen to deal with the issue of death and offers some continued existence beyond the limitations of our earthly life. Religion has envisioned an afterlife in various forms; sometimes a resurrection of the physical body in a heavenly world where it will not die again, or gaining an immortal subtle body of light or energy that unlike the physical body does not need to die. Religion tells us that through faith, belief and good works that we can be led to such a greater life after death, as a reward for our good thoughts and actions here.

On the other hand, deeper spiritual and mystical teachings, particularly the great meditation traditions of Asia, emphasize an immortality of consciousness not only beyond the mortality of the physical body, but beyond any type of creaturely existence in this or in subtler realms. They teach that our own inner essence exists not only beyond death but also beyond birth, ever free of limitation to body or form in this world or another. We can take birth in any number of bodies and, more importantly, we can reach a state in which we no longer dwell in time and its limitations and are under no compulsion to be born again.

Yet whatever our spiritual background or our religious views, we all want to live longer, if not go beyond death altogether. The quest for immortality therefore has two levels, outer and inner, physical and spiritual.

- The first or outer aspect of the quest for immortality is

rejuvenation of the body and mind, which includes the promotion of physical longevity.

- The second or inner aspect is immortality of the spirit or consciousness, which can include the continued existence of a subtle mind or astral body.

However, we must recognize that the quest for immortality is part of a greater seeking for perfect happiness. The longing for immortality is linked with a greater quest for an end to all suffering. It is not simply an unending existence that we wish for but an immortal bliss.

Physical Immortality, Rejuvenation and Longevity

The question then arises: "Is physical immortality at all possible?" There are indications in the Yoga tradition of India that a few rare individuals have achieved if not physical immortality, at least great longevity extending through many ordinary human lifetimes. Various mystical and esoteric traditions suggest the same, such as the long-lived prophets of the Bible or the Taoist immortals of ancient China. The Vedic rishis of India were said to have lived for very long periods of time, extending into the centuries, through accessing the power of *Soma*, a special energy connected with the healing forces of nature and the inner powers of the psyche arising from special Yoga and meditation practices. Hindu thought mentions various *chiranjivas* or 'long lived sages', some who are said to be still alive. There are other traditions of immortal ascended masters, though sometimes their immortality is said to be in a subtle, not a physical body, or only accessible to those of a certain purity of mind and heart. While there are often a number of fantasies and illusions associated with such ideas, there seems to be a core of truth behind them as well.

Classical Tantric Yoga – which teaches us to work with the secret energies of nature like the Kundalini – has developed special outer methods of extending physical longevity, including the use of powerful herbs, minerals, gems, and elixirs, much like other alchemical traditions worldwide. These are combined with special inner Tantric Yoga practices of pranayama, mantra, and yantra and working with the deities and powers of nature in a precise spiritual science of inner transformation to take us beyond our ordinary human limitations.

Probably the most famous yogic case of physical immortality is that of Mahavatar Babaji, the immortal Himalayan Yogi introduced to the world by Paramahamsa Yogananda, one of his disciples, in Paramahamsa Yogananda's classic *Autobiography of a Yogi*.[9] Babaji and his female companion Mataji are said to live in yogically energized immortal physical bodies in special retreat areas of the high Himalayas above Badrinath along with a select group of disciples, some of which have also taken on undying physical bodies themselves.

However, such yogic achievements of physical immortality are so extremely rare as to be for all practical purposes impossible for the ordinary human being. They rest upon a special birth in yogic families in the Himalayas after an exalted spiritual birth that took one to the highest spiritual realization already, not on any ordinary human birth. They involve a pure diet and environment, and special yogic practices from birth along with these great masters - nothing like an ordinary, much less stressful modern human life in a toxic urban environment. There is no reason for us to think that such a physical immortality is possible for us or even desirable for the type of mentality that we have in the world today.

It is mainly in the Integral Yoga of Sri Aurobindo – one of the greatest spiritual masters and visionaries of modern India – that one finds a clear and specific discipline designed to develop physical immortality, which is addressed in great depth and detail in his voluminous and profound writings.[10] However, in Sri Aurobindo's Integral Yoga, physical immortality is not the prime concern but only the ultimate highlight, following a comprehensive yogic development of a deeper devotion and awareness within us. Moreover, Aurobindo approaches the immortalization of the physical body not as a personal achievement for furthering our mundane desires, but as part of a long-term evolutionary process for developing a higher type of human being, if not a higher species altogether. It is not physical immortality for the ordinary person that Aurobindo seeks but that of the realized soul, who has transformed the mind and emotional nature. He realizes that the current human being with its various negative karmic and genetic

influences requires a considerable recasting before it is worthy of a prolonged existence or can naturally hold a higher consciousness.

Aurobindo aims at a long-term, if not millennial creation of a new
spiritual being on Earth, not just making we existing humans live longer or avoid physical death such as we are in our current undeveloped
states of awareness and intelligence. It is an evolutionary goal of the
species that he seeks, which we can individually help prepare the way
for, but are quite unlikely to attain personally. His disciples seek the
development of a new humanity, not simply their own longer physical existence.[11] Moreover, his Integral Yoga seeks this transformation
of the human being through a new descent of Divine grace or Shakti
– the force of the Divine Mother – not simply through outer methods of diet, herbs or yoga techniques, much less scientific or genetic
breakthroughs. It rests upon awakening to and surrendering to that
descent of grace from above, which has its own powers and processes.
Aurobindo puts us in contact with this higher evolutionary Shakti that
is a powerful Divine force already present in the spiritual atmosphere
of the planet.

*Yet while physical immortality is nearly impossible, physical rejuve-
nation is something attainable to some degree for everyone.* One can
undergo special Yogic and Ayurvedic rejuvenative regimens that can
remove years off of one's biological age and effectively prolong one's
life beyond what would otherwise be achievable. This doesn't mean
that such methods can turn an eighty year old into a forty year old, but
it is possible to be happier, healthier and more aware far beyond one's
ordinary age! The body is always rejuvenating itself and replacing its
old cells with new. New pranas are ever moving through us with every
sunrise and sunset. Rejuvenation aims at speeding up this natural process of revitalization, which ordinarily declines with age.

A physical longevity of a hundred years should be the norm for human beings if we live a healthy natural life in a clean natural environment, even longer if we are doing Yoga practices. The fact that we
do not have such longevity is a sign of an unhealthy life-style on our
own parts or an unhealthy culture. The added complication for any
personal pursuit of longevity today is that it is difficult for we as mere

individuals to prolong our lives, if our environment and way of life collectively is toxic and unhealthy, which is now the case almost everywhere on the planet. It can be hard to live long and healthy in a world that is polluted, disturbed and full of conflict, even if the individual is otherwise well informed as to what to do to prolong their existence.

The pursuit of longevity, therefore, is not merely a personal issue but an ecological concern today. We are beginning to see declining longevities in the western world along with the artificial life styles that are part of the high tech media age. Prolonging our own lives and protecting the life of the planet cannot be turned into separate issues. Indeed we may need to sacrifice some of our own personal time to ensure the health of the planet for future generations.

Physical longevity also has important spiritual implications. Longevity is very desirable for those on the spiritual path because having made the great effort necessary to awaken to one's higher purpose in life – which is very difficult in any age – one wants a full life in order to progress along it as much as possible. *The right pursuit of physical longevity can be a helpful aid to the deeper pursuit of the immortality of the spirit.* This is probably its most important value, as long life without spirituality not only has no real value but also removes us from the soul that is the very source of life. Otherwise, we are only seeking immortality for our ego and desire nature that inevitably leads to suffering and confusion. We are merely seeking more time to enmesh ourselves further in the karmic complications of the earthly realm that end in sorrow.

Immortality and Rejuvenation of the Mind

If immortality of the body is nearly impossible, the further question arises whether immortality of the mind is possible? Certainly it is easier to keep the mind young than it is to stop the body from aging. In fact, as we age in our bodies, we often feel younger in our minds – and usually hold a youthful image of ourselves in our minds that no longer corresponds to our outer appearance.

It is possible to have a fresh, clear and youthful mind even in an old and decaying body. We see many elderly people even above eighty years of age with active, creative and cheerful minds, able to excel the young in expression, logic or insight. All of us have encountered such individuals who surprise us by their age. For them age has helped them mature in mind and spirit, the effect of which is more energy and vitality for their inner being. This should be normal for humanity, with those older in years becoming elders in wisdom by developing clarity and vitality of mind and heart.

While the body matures and ceases to grow around the age of twenty-five, the mind usually does not fully mature until around the age of fifty, and can keep growing as long as one is alive. One of the great sorrows of many older people – particularly in this culture that rarely honor its elders – is that though their minds are not old, they are treated according to the condition of their bodies, and their advice accordingly is not heeded. Their wisdom seems lost on the younger generation that does not want to look at inner realities but remains enmeshed in outer sensations.

It is possible to rejuvenate the mind so that a seventy, eighty or ninety year old person can have a youthful and creative mind. However, it is difficult to make the mind young if the mind has already been made old by years of mindless and thoughtless living, in which there is no cultivation of creativity or inner awareness. Yet those who have developed a creative and spiritual mind in their youth can easily maintain it to the end of their lives, and leave this world with full consciousness and no regrets!

Besides maintaining a youthful mind into old age, there is also a search for immortality of the mind, or at least its continuity, beyond the death of the physical body. Many spiritual teachings contain methods to prepare the mind to continue beyond death. The mind's ability to transcend death is reflected in the phenomenon of rebirth, which depends upon the mind being able to survive death and take on a new body. In the case of ordinary rebirth, the mind falls into a deep slumber and its memories of the previous life are almost entirely lost before awakening in the new life. Yet after following higher Yoga practices, one can carry much of one's mind and intelligence into the next birth and maintain a continuity of awareness after death.

According to yogic thought, the mind is by nature undying, though it does go through phases of manifestation and rest. The mind does not die with the death of the physical body. It simply undergoes a period of withdrawal, followed by a new active phase after awakening in a new body. The inner core mind carries the samskaras or karmic tendencies that propel us from one birth to another. That inner mind survives the death of the body and its tendencies take it on to a new body.

Yet it is only the core of the mind that has this immortality, not our ordinary outer mind and ego, with its personal thoughts, emotions and memories bound to the outer world of the current birth. At the time of death the mind is reduced to its core tendencies, much like the latent state of the mind in the state of deep sleep. The outer aspect of the mind is dissolved and only the inner core of the mind goes on to another birth. *This means that the immortality of the mind is limited and broken by the death of the body*, hidden by an ignorance that prevents the ordinary person benefiting from it, and making it difficult for them to access past life skills and wisdom. Most of us cannot experience our mind's greater existence beyond the body because we cannot sustain our awareness after death from one life to another. But it is something that we can learn to develop.

Higher Yoga practices allow us to contact the hidden immortality at the core of the mind and gradually spread it to the rest of the mind, making it eventually into a conscious possession of our daily awareness. Great yogis carry their personalities and minds into successive births. We see this also in the concept of tulkus and the reincarnation of the Dalai Lamas of Tibetan yoga. The more evolved a soul becomes, the more it holds its mind and intelligence through the reincarnation process, not losing it at death. For such exalted souls, death and rebirth are like going to sleep at night and waking up in the morning, not any real end or beginning of existence.

Immortality of the Spirit or Higher Self (Atman or Purusha)

Yet besides this 'broken' immortality of the mind, there is a deeper unbroken immortality within each one of us. *Our spirit or inner Being is immortal by nature and exists beyond the phases of withdrawal and manifestation of the mind from birth to birth.* Our true Self consists of pure unmodified awareness, immutable, changeless and serene. Our true nature resides in pure consciousness beyond all the shifting currents of time, space and action that we experience through the mind. We can always access this immortality of our inner Being even when the body is dying.

The fact is that in our true nature we are not born and do not die, we do not suffer and are ever beyond gain and loss, pleasure and pain, advance and retreat. Death is an illusion of our outer experience through the mind, not an enduring truth of our inmost Self. Death is perhaps the ultimate illusion, whose veil we must rend asunder to find our true reality. It is the body that dies, not we ourselves as the masters of the body. This immortality of the Spirit should rule over our entire existence; we should not be mere victims of the ups and downs of the body, mind and senses. We should not be victims of death but use death to take us to yet a greater awareness.

This immortality of the spirit is absolute, without qualification or diminution. It is there for everyone to experience. It is the ground of experience itself. The mind has only a relative immortality, enduring at its core but undergoing death and withdrawal in its outer layers. Its immortality is enshrouded in ignorance and is not a fact of experience in our lives.

Yet this immortality of the spirit is not without its relevance for the body. *The inner immortality of consciousness contains the power to rejuvenate body and mind,* should we aim to do that. It is the wellspring of immortal Prana or undying life-energy that is ever accessible within our deepest hearts. We all have the power of immortality within us already as the most intimate layer of all that we are. The issue is how to access our immortal consciousness and connect it with our outer nature, particularly to the surface mind where most of us experience life.

In this regard, our pursuit of immortality is something of a joke that we play upon ourselves. The problem is not that we unfairly die, and the solution is not to learn how to preserve our existing personality beyond death. The problem is that we have forgotten our natural immortality, which resides in our inner awareness, and are looking for it where it does not exist, in the physical body and outer personality bound by time. We confine ourselves to the mortal outer aspect of our

27

being, which must eventually die whatever we may do. We are trying to make lasting that which is inherently impermanent and fleeting, which only leads to frustration, failure and sorrow. The solution is to give up our attachment to what dies and merge back into our immortal nature beyond death. This is the real going beyond death.

Death only affects the body and the mind, which are but the instruments of the spirit, and like any instrument are subject to friction, decay and ultimate destruction. The body is our outer instrument somewhat like our automobile, necessary to take us places in the material world that is the main focus of our outer existence. But the body is not who we really are and its fulfillment is not our true fulfillment. The mind is our inner instrument, something like our computer, necessary for us to deal with information, particularly about the external world. It is crucial for our outer functioning but its fulfillment is also not that of our true nature either. Our spirit or consciousness is the being or person who operates these two instruments and is not limited by their functioning, like the person who operates the car or the computer.

When our car breaks down, we don't say, "I am dead". When our computer crashes, we similarly don't feel that we are no more. Yet because of our deep-seated attachment to the physical body that occurs through the mind, we feel that physical death is the end of who we are as well. This is only because we do not understand ourselves. Death is merely the end of the limited outer personality but does not touch the real person within us. Death is just a moment in time in which we transition from one realm of experience to another, nothing more than a doorway. For our inner being, death can be a release from the ego and its endless desires. It is a means of purifying our outer nature so that we can grow more spiritually in another life. As the *Bhagavad Gita* so eloquently states: "Of that which is real, there is no non-existence. Of that which is unreal, there is no existence."[12] What is bound by death never truly exists and what is not bound by death can never be killed.

The surest means to go beyond death and gain immortality is simply to rest in our own immortal Self, the core consciousness within us that is the detached witness of all the movements of the body and mind. You are immortal as you are in your inner being and can never fall prey to death or dissolution. This is an eternal truth, not any mere hope or speculation. It is the most enduring and powerful of all truths. It does not require belief or salvation but merely the awakening of an inner knowing.

We can all breathe a big sigh of relief here, if we wish, and accept the immortality, peace and transcendence of our inner being, letting go of the entire realm of death. There is nothing holding us back from this except our own reluctance to do so based upon our identification with our surface ego. However, such letting go is very difficult to do owing to our deep-seated attachment to the body and mind extending over many lifetimes. Yet there are many tools to help us through Yoga and meditation to make the task easier and quicker.

The Three Key Points

- Mortality of the Body

- Relative Immortality of the Mind

- Absolute Immortality of the Consciousness

These are the three aspects of death, rejuvenation and immortality to reflect deeply upon. The body is mortal and akin to death as it is a limited material structure. Its existence can be prolonged but must eventually come to an end.

1. The mind has a relative immortality, broken up into segments by the birth and death of one body as it moves on to another. The mind continues until it is merged into the pure consciousness beyond time and space of which it is but the reflection.

2. Our inner consciousness alone has an absolute immortality regardless of what happens to the body or mind. But we must detach from body and mind in order to realize it.

The crucial issue, therefore, is how we can access and realize the natural immortality of our inner being? The prime means to do this can be described simply. It requires aligning the mind with our inner being. This means merging our outer mind into pure consciousness, and extending the unconscious immortality of the mind into the conscious immortality of the spirit. To do this is a matter of *sadhana* or spiritual practice covering many decades, in fact many lifetimes. It is not a quick fix or the result of a special therapy, retreat or technique. It is the essence of our striving as an immortal soul.

Deep meditation aligned with Self-inquiry is the ultimate means of gaining immortality, merging into the immortal Self in the heart.[13] This is the main approach of *Advaita or Non-dualistic Vedanta* and the related Yoga of Knowledge. Other yogic practices can be powerful aids, particular a deep love and devotion for the Divine within us along the path of Bhakti Yoga. In fact, Yoga in the classical sense was originally devised as a science of consciousness devised to bring us to our higher immortality called the *Atman* or *Purusha*, the true Self. Traditional Kundalini Yoga, as found in the Hindu *Tantras,* is formulated to bring about the opening of the crown chakra or lotus of the head, which carries our deeper immortal consciousness and energy, the Shiva and Shakti principles of Tantric thought.[14]

Yet to merge the minds into our immortal Self is aided by bringing harmony and purity to the physical body, which means to rejuvenate the body as well. For the pursuit of inner immortality, physical longevity is a great aid as it is a process that cannot be easily achieved in a short span of time. But physical longevity is not an end-in-itself or a means of prolonging mere outer enjoyments.

The Vision of Heaven and the Subtle Body

As death and suffering seem part of this physical world, many people have longed for some heavenly world or paradise in which death and suffering do not occur. Such higher worlds do exist, though not always in the way we might imagine them to be.

Some of our imagined heavens are little more than glorified physical worlds in which a resurrected physical body, much like our earthly flesh body, continues, hosted by a personality much like our flawed earthly personality, perhaps indulging in continued sensory pleasures. Such heavens are but earth in disguise and appeal to the wishful thinking of the human ego that does not want to face its own mortality or discover the real immortality of the soul that is not physical or form based.

Other heavens are portrayed as realms of a subtle or astral body, in appearance much like our physical body but made of light or life-energy, radiant and blissful, able to fly or transform itself in various ways, beyond the travails of physical matter and its impermanence, even having wings like an angel! Such subtle bodies are akin to our dream body as the subtle worlds are also the dream worlds. These are more genuine heavens in which the soul can enjoy refined impressions much like great art or beautiful music, along with a deeper love and devotion. Yet even these subtle realms are still bound by time and desire, located on this side of death.

Beyond these heavens of subtle energy and pure form are formless heavens and higher realms of space in which we have no form body but exist in mind alone, with vast powers of thought, vision, perception and awareness. This formless body is called a 'causal body', as it holds the causal power behind all that we can become in the form-based worlds. In it we stand at the heart of creation above any specific manifest worlds, a truly exalted state like a divine co-creator.[15]

However, even these causal realms are beneath the realm of pure immortality which is beyond all manifestation, form or formless. All worlds of embodied existence, physical, subtle or causal, are limited by karma and rebirth. One must eventually leave even the highest heavenly worlds for another birth until all ones karmas are worked out.

Many yogis and occultists work to develop their subtle bodies in order to access these subtle or astral realms after death or even during life. Some occultists aim to live in the subtle body with its greater powers and enjoyments after the death of the physical body. Yogis also can develop the subtle body as a vehicle for deeper practices of devotion or meditation, even if they do not pursue the subtle realms as the final goal of their journey. Yet other yogis strive to develop the causal body as the prime instrument to reach our true nature as pure consciousness, as the higher mind is but one step removed from pure awareness. In this way a development of these more refined vestures of the soul can serve as important steps in a higher realization of immortality.

However, regeneration of the physical body, particularly the brain and nervous system, can help us energize the subtle body as well. A rejuvenated subtle body, with our inner prana and senses revitalized, helps rejuvenate the physical body as well. So developing the subtle body and a greater pursuit of rejuvenation and immortality can be linked together in various ways. The subtle body, on one level at least, can also be defined as our 'Soma body' or body of enjoyment, which represents the fruit of our actions in the gross of physical body, as well as the essence of the energies and motivations that we put forth in our physical lives.

Karma, Death and Destiny

Our lives are limited by the karma and destiny of our souls. Karma consists of the results of our actions and their energetic residues, stemming back to distant previous lives. Destiny could be best defined as a karmic inevitability, a fixed karma that it is very difficult, if not impossible to change. The Vedic astrology chart is a good index of our karmas, as we will discuss later in the book.

Yet if our lives are based upon karma, including a certain 'karmic longevity' or lifespan that we may be born with, we might ask: "Of what use is the seeking of rejuvenation or greater longevity?" The answer to this question is that karma as a result of our habitual actions can be changed, though we cannot likely change all of our karmas in a single life. We can improve, modify or shape our karmas for the future. There are special yogic means of altering and transcending karma through mantra, ritual, service and offerings, which come into play here. Yogic methods of rejuvenation, properly employed, can reduce the negative inertia of our karmas, as well as project a more positive karma into life.

This does not mean that all karmas, including disease, injury or premature death, can be overcome for everyone. But karma is something we do, something we are constantly creating and, therefore, something we can alter. It is not something imposed upon us from the outside. If we work to create a karma of well-being in body, mind and spirit, it will help neutralize any corresponding negative karmas of suffering, death and disease.

The seeking of rejuvenation begins with 'karmic rectification' as it were, which means seeing what karmas we have set in motion in life and where they are likely to lead us. It implies assuming 'karmic responsibility' for who we are, accepting that we are the result of our own actions, which means giving up any blaming of others for our condition in life. We must first face the fact of our karmas in life and acknowledge that we have created them, including the type of circumstances, vocation and community setting that we find ourselves dwelling in. We can observe the karmas that we have set forth in our bodies and minds by how we live and what our daily routine has become. Only after we have taken responsibility for our karmas can we really begin to change them. Once we have accepted the 'wisdom of karma', then we can begin to free ourselves from the negative effects of karma, including any premature aging or loss of mental acuity, by developing higher spiritual and healing practices.

Yet we must always remember: our inner being exists beyond karma, which is only the mechanism that unfolds the connection of cause and effect operative in the body and mind. If we reside in our inner core awareness, death cannot touch us, regardless of what happens to the body or when. Our immortal inner being is the matrix for proper energization and rejuvenation of body and mind as it holds the power of eternity.

Death and Immortality

All great spiritual teachings tell us that the path to immortality lies through death, not by avoiding it. Death itself can be used as a doorway to take us beyond time. As we examine how to go beyond death, we must remember this key principle: *That which is immortal can never truly become mortal and that which is mortal can never truly become immortal.*[16] Nothing can change its nature. What can die must die and cannot continue on forever, whatever we may try. Only what is by nature deathless will never die. If we can die to what is mortal or death bound in this life, we gain access to the immortal and deathless reality even while alive. As the great poet Rabindranath Tagore so eloquently stated "Let me carry death in life that I might know life in death."

In this regard, we must discriminate between the soul's wish for immortality and the urge of the ego to never die. The soul seeks an inner immortality in consciousness that involves going beyond the form-based body and thought-based mind. The ego seeks to continue its worldly drives and ambitions by renewing the body. The soul seeks for true immortality beyond the body. The ego wants to make immortal that which is inherently mortal and wants to prolong the body as long as it can, often even if unwell. The ego is rooted in the fear of death.

The soul meanwhile is not afraid of death but only of ignorance or lack of awareness. The soul is happy to discard the body if the body is too old or unwell and can no longer serve as a useful vehicle for its inner growth. For the soul the loss of the physical body is just a change of clothes, not a loss of its essence. Even if we are pursuing longevity and rejuvenation, we should not fear the inevitable death of the body. We should use the life of the body to pursue the immortality of the soul, which as eternal life is the source of all real healing as well. This immortality of the soul does not consist of long lasting physical existence but of realizing that our true nature of pure awareness never dies.

More important than learning how to live longer is learning how to reconcile ourselves with the inevitability of our own death. If we learn to die every day to the ego, then our entire lives will be rooted in immortality. We cannot make what is inherently mortal, namely our ego and desire based life and identity, immortal, though this is precisely what most of us want and are seeking in our so-called pursuit of immortality. We want our physical personality to continue beyond its normal time range, even if we have not properly cared for our bodies. What we need to discover for real immortality is the higher awareness within us that never takes birth, which is unborn and without form or desire. This exists on the other side of death, not on this side!

We should ask ourselves the fundamental question: *Are we worthy of immortality or even greater longevity as we currently are?* What is our desire to continue based upon? Is it a seeking of a higher truth or more time to pursue what are ego-based drives, personal desires and worldly acclaim? Are we hoping that our unenlightened life-style can continue as long as we want, with outer affluence and pleasure and no karmic side effects?

The key to both inner immortality and outer rejuvenation rests in letting go of desire based seeking, to die to our ordinary urges in the realm of time and circumstances. Death is not an enemy or an obstacle that we must fear for our greater existence, but an opportunity for inner growth that we must honor. The phenomenon of death is not just our own physical death, which we naturally fear, but the ability to die, forget or let go of what has no enduring value, the outer surface appearances of our lives.

One can only know the immortal Self by dying to the mortal self and ego. One can only enter into the pure consciousness beyond death by letting go of the mind and its attachments in the field of time. To think that we can make our ordinary personality immortal is but wishful thinking, an attempt to prolong a shadow into light. Note the experience of the great sage, Ramana Maharshi, who as a mere lad of sixteen went into a deep meditation on death and moved beyond it to a realization of the immortal Self that remained throughout his life.[17] This is what is required.

The key to immortality is to die willingly while alive, which is to die to the ego or bodily identity even while the body persists. Through dying inwardly while alive, one gains an immortality even beyond death. We must learn to die daily to the known and limited, accepting our outer lives are but an offering to the inner spirit. Then everyday will be a new birth into eternity.

The spiritual journey is from death to immortality, combining a preliminary phase of death to the outer world in order to lead us to an inner immortality. Death is the great teacher and giver of immortality, not the denier of it. That is why in many Yogic teachings like the *Katha Upanishad*,[18] death is the guru, or why great deities of Yoga like Lord Shiva also personify death. Yet this mystic death requires not the mere outer death of the body but an inner state of silence, stillness, and quiescence. Only that within us that dwells in a state of perfect peace can go beyond death and gain immortality.

Death, in fact, is an illusion, perhaps the greatest of all illusions. No one has ever really died and no one ever will really die. Death is but a change of clothes for the immortal soul that cannot be diminished by any external action or agency.[19] Our true being, the *Atman* or *Purusha*, is inherently beyond all death and suffering. It is only because of our false identification with the body and mind that we fall under the illusion of death. This means that we need not fear death, which is but a moment in time, but should lift our sense of who we are beyond any outer time based identities to immutable consciousness itself. It is only on the basis of an inner sense of deathlessness that any lasting rejuvenation can be possible, not out of a fear of death or an attempt to avoid death. In affirming the deathlessness of our inner being, we can access its powers of immortality.

Purification and Renewal

All rejuvenation practices require preliminary purification, which can be described as a kind of voluntary dissolution or death. These purification procedures have some kinship with death in the sense that they involve rest, reduction of movement, silence and stillness. They involve various forms of fire purification, whether promoting sweating as in the use of saunas, fiery spicy herbs to purify the body, fiery breathing practices or fire based forms of meditation. As such, they are called *tapas* in Sanskrit, meaning generation of transforming heat.

This inner purification is aided by external fire rituals, like Vedic *yajnas* or fire sacrifices to purify our home and environment.[20] Purification practices are allied with fasting, withdrawing from sensory activity, solitude and various factors that are like a simulated death or return to the womb. In this way, we can turn withdrawal and death into a creative force to generate new life and awareness within us. Such practices are usually part of *pratyahara* or the yogic phase of internalization of the prana, senses and mind.[21]

After such an inner death, one has a second birth while living. The body, mind and senses are renewed. One experiences life as one did as a child, as though each day was the first day of creation. True rejuvenation is a second birth for body, mind and spirit that lifts us into a higher order of existence that can transcend our actual physical death. Through the spiritual death of the ego, one can enter into the immortal life of the spirit. There are many symbols of this mystic death process in world spiritual literature, such as Shiva, Osiris, Adonis, or Jesus. True resurrection is not of the body but the awakening of the immortal

Self of pure awareness within us.

This mystic death and rebirth can also be achieved through Divine love, as love has the power to endure beyond death. It can be gained through deep meditation, through immortal wisdom. It usually involves working with the healing powers of nature through the plants, rocks, waters, air and fire, as nature is ever renewing itself. It is the essence of the inner alchemy of Yoga and Tantra.

Such a second birth perhaps best occurs at the time of one's midlife or aging crisis, in the period from ages forty-five to seventy, when one has the greatest wisdom in life and the body is still capable of producing new energy. Many traditional cultures have special rituals and social events that support such a change of life. Yoga and Ayurveda have turned this inner rejuvenation into a precise science and art.

Realization of our immortal Self is possible for all of us, though likely to be attained by very few, as it requires going beyond the ordinary human mind, emotions and attachments. Rejuvenation of the mind, at least to some degree, is not difficult for all of us if we but seriously take up Yoga and meditation practices. Rejuvenation of the body, similarly, is something that we are all capable of at least to some degree. Yet for all of these to be truly beneficial and efficacious, our mindset must change. We must look within. We must work on ourselves. We must connect with the greater universe of consciousness and also look into our inner being and its treasures of the unknown, the great mystery that is both life and death, and which carries and unites both together in an ongoing transformative process of cosmic existence.

Yet even if you are not interested in the issue of immortality at the current stage of your life, particularly if you are young, you should note that the practices that promote longevity are helpful to promote general well-being and improve the quality of our awareness as well. They allow us to develop a positive joy, happiness and bliss within regardless of what may happens to us externally. They are the essence of Yoga as a means of Self-realization, which is ultimately the realization of our immortal Self.

HIGH TECH SOMAS OR
INNER SPIRITUAL SOMAS?

King Soma, your manifestations that are in Heaven, on Earth, in the mountains, in the plants and in the waters; with all those happy in mind, free of anger, welcome our offering.

Rigveda I.80.4

Soma originally refers to the nectar of immortality in Vedic thought which goes back to the most ancient period of India's great civilization.[22] It has echoes in ancient Persian, Greek and Celtic cultures and their sacred plants and trees,[23] as well as to similar traditions from throughout the world. Soma in the *Vedas* is called *Amrita*, which means both nectar and immortality (a-mrita, also meaning 'non-dying') and is one of the most important Vedic deities and symbols. Soma is said to be the king, the progenitor and ruler of all.

Soma remains a subject of great fascination in world literature and speculation extending to modern times, as in Aldous Huxley's *Brave New World*, a world dominated by the mind control through high tech drugs called Somas. The question is whether we will seek an inner spiritual Soma that liberates the mind and heart or will rest content with a high tech outer Soma that makes our lives increasingly artificial and chemically controlled?

Soma as a Great Symbol

Soma is perhaps the most universal metaphor for the human quest for immortality, not only at a physical level but also at mental and spiritual levels. It symbolizes our quest for renewal and for immortality much like the Holy Grail, which itself conceals a Soma symbolism of the mystic beverage. It is indicated by the search for the fountain of youth or fountain of immortality, the sacred waters that restore our vitality. A similar symbolism occurs in stories from all over the world of sacred plants and their healing powers.

Yet the Vedic and yogic Soma, is not simply a powerful botanical agent; it is part of a greater cosmic vision extending from healing plants and waters on Earth to the supreme bliss of the eternal Ananda in the highest heaven from which the entire universe arises as an outer expression. Soma is usually described as a special substance or elixir that once imbibed or awakened has the ability to transform body, mind and heart. We are all seeking such a magic potion, pill or nectar to bring a greater meaning and happiness into our lives.

Soma is the symbol of a deeper knowledge and awareness and of the spiritual quest overall.[24] Soma is said to be the essence of all the Vedic teachings, the aim of which is to make us immortal. The *Rigveda*, the oldest Vedic text, contains an entire book or mandala, the ninth, devoted to the subject of Soma with cryptic chants, esoteric mantras and powerful meters that even today the world's greatest minds are not able to entirely comprehend.[25] These Soma hymns are among the greatest writings in all Sanskrit or world literature, and are worthy of deep examination for unfolding all the mysteries of existence. Yet Soma also refers to poetry, mantra and chant of the highest order –wherever and whenever it may occur – which itself can evoke the flow of divine grace within us.

Soma, which also means 'bliss', reflects our lifelong seeking for happiness, which is intimately related to our seeking of immortality as the highest form of happiness. This 'search for our bliss in life' has become a bit of cliché in New Age thought but retains a deeper significance that each one of us needs to examine. Even if we are not on the spiritual path, we are seeking some form of Soma or bliss as our highest goal. And we want that Soma to last or for ourselves to become immortal in it.

Each one of us should ask ourselves at a deep level of the heart: "Have I found my bliss or Soma in life or is my search continuing? Is my current Soma or source of happiness and enjoyment enough, or will I need to move on to something more meaningful in the course of time? What is the highest Soma that I can aspire to and how can I reach it?"

Yet Soma, like happiness, is something elusive and hidden. It cannot be given to us quickly, easily or from the outside. We have to look deeply within ourselves in order to discover it. Soma is an inner essence, not an outer form or object. Soma indicates the juice, the *rasa* in Sanskrit, the essence of beauty and delight hidden in things, which requires a special process of extraction in order to bring out and appreciate it.

This process of extracting the Soma is symbolized by the plant stalk that must be ground down with a mortar and pestle in order to remove its sweet juice. Yet everything that we take into our bodies and minds – whether food, beverages or sensory impressions – possesses a certain taste. This taste notifies us of the quality of the substance that we are imbibing and helps us understand how it may affect us after we have digested it. We naturally gravitate towards those items that have a taste and essence that is pleasant and promotes a sense of well-being, from the sugars in food and drinks, to beautiful sounds and colors, to sweet emotions like love and joy. These all reflect how the pursuit of Soma is programmed into our nervous systems.

Soma and Art

To approach the subject of Soma at a deeper level, it is helpful to look into the realm of art, which has a special Soma of its own, as well as a connection to immortality. As the great German poet Goethe said, "Life is short but art is long." In this regard, art as a refined pursuit of sensation is another pursuit of Soma at an intellectual level. The aesthetic experience involves extracting an essence of delight from the outer forms and shapes that we perceive through the senses. For example, for the painter, a still life is not simply a bowl of fruit on a table to eat, but colors, forms and patterns of delight for the inner eye to imbibe and appreciate. The artist finds enjoyment in the light behind things, not in the actual objects, which recede in the background and merely become staging devices to reveal that enduring light of beauty, which most of us, in our outer pursuits in life, fail to recognize.

There are Somas or powers of beauty and delight everywhere in the universe, which itself is structured by the light of consciousness. Each thing that we encounter in nature possesses a certain beauty, energy or characteristic quality that communicates some truth or delight of the universe to us, whether it is the texture of a rock or the patterns of clouds in the sky. This 'Soma of nature' has a natural healing and calming quality for us that we all know of whether in beautiful sunrises or sunsets or the gentle luminosity of the Moon.

There are beautiful and healing Somas in the various forms of light, in the waters, the air, the cosmic spaces, and in the Earth itself down into its deepest caverns. Our lives can benefit immensely from learning how to access all these natural Somas or sacred powers of life. Unfortunately, we usually prefer to remain at the surface level of our human experience, running after the human Somas of our social and technologically based lives that are often artificial, dulling and disturbing to our deeper aspirations. Yet all of us have experienced this beauty or Soma of nature, whether in a sunset, sunrise, mountain or ocean vista, and can cultivate it more deeply if we wish. We can all appreciate the art of Soma behind the movement of life.

Soma, Yoga and Tantra

The *Upanishads* describe the Self as the rasa or essence of all, which in turn is connected to space.[26] Our own inner being is an essence, not a body, form or instrument. Beyond the artistic rasas or essences of beauty and delight, are the spiritual or yogic rasas, which lead us to the bliss or Ananda behind all existence. The Yogi seeks to develop this deeper level of rasa beyond even art, though he may use artistic tools like chanting, music or visualization in the process.

The Yogi takes his vision from the outer forms of objects to the underlying essential qualities of the five great elements of earth, water, fire, air and ether. These in turn he takes back to their subtle sensory essences as the root energies of smell, taste, sight, touch and sound. These in turn he resolves into the actions of the five sense organs (ear, skin, eye, tongue, nose) and five motor organs (voice, hand, feet, urogenital, excretory). These in turn he resolves into the mind, ego, intelligence and nature itself (Prakriti), which is all ultimately resolved into the seer or Purusha, the immortal Self. This is the movement of the 25 tattvas or cosmic principles in the philosophy of Yoga and Samkhya.[27]

Tantric Yoga, in its traditional form, is itself a science of extracting the essence of delight and awareness from the whole of life. It works with the forms of art and deeper yogic examination, following out the movement of rasas back to the essential powers of Shiva and Shakti as cosmic consciousness and its creative power. Even the left handed Tantra that at times used sacred rituals involving sexual practices or the use of intoxicants, was part of a seeking of rasas or essences beyond the outer forms employed.

The Legendary Soma Plant

In one of its prime Vedic symbolisms, Soma is described as a magical plant or herbal preparation that rejuvenates the body and mind, promoting healing and granting ecstasy and immortality. Though the Soma plant is described in various ways in early Vedic texts, it recedes into myth and legend in later Hindu teachings. There continues to be much debate in the scholarly world as to the identity of the original Soma plant, if indeed it was an actual particular plant at all.

Based upon my own research in Vedic texts going back forty years, including thirty years of published writings,[28] I do not think that Soma was ever regarded as a single plant or species. The Vedic Soma is referred to as a type of plants and as various plant preparations, including using milk, honey, ghee and yogurt. Soma appears to refer to rejuvenative plants in general, not one species, and can also refer to the juice or essence of any plant. Soma is ultimately the healing essence of all the plants and beyond that even the essence of all healing, joy and well-being.

Plant Somas do exist and their usage will be discussed in the herbal chapters of this book. The appendix also contains an examination of the possible identity of Vedic Soma plants in its "Search for the Original Soma Plant." Special Soma herbs can indeed bring about marvelous changes to our nervous and endocrine systems, if we are prepared properly to take them. Stories of sacred and powerful herbs can be found throughout the world and form an important component of mystical, yogic and shamanic traditions worldwide. They are part of our inner quest.

Yet the plant form or botanical aspect is only one side of Soma symbolism and should not be taken literally. The plant also has a deeper meaning. The *Vedas* speak of the universal tree, the immortal fig or banyan tree, whose branches are below and whose root is above.[29] The cosmic fig tree in the *Rigveda* is lauded foremost among the plants, which are described as abounding with Soma.[30] Soma is the cosmic plant, which can be symbolized as a tree, such as we find in many mystical traditions. Yet the cosmic plant is often regarded as a flower like the even more common lotus in Vedic thought, or the mystic rose of European thought.

This cosmic plant moreover exists inside of us. It is our own nervous system at a physical level, which resembles a tree with various branches. In Vedic symbolism, the spine is sometimes symbolized also as a reed or bamboo.[31] This mystic plant is also the subtle body with its system of subtle currents called *nadis* and energy centers called *chakras*, which are symbolized by flowers or lotuses. Later Tantric Yoga texts abound in such symbolisms and recognize an inner Soma or nectar through which bliss and immortality is gained.

Some scholars may argue that this yogic symbolism was added at a later point of time to an earlier Vedic nature worship. However, given the deep symbolism of early ancient teachings from the *Vedas* of India to the *Egyptian Book of the Dead*, it is clear that a spiritual and yogic indication was part of the meaning of Soma, if not its most important implication, from the very beginning. The Vedic chants themselves are said to be types of Somas, which is also related to poetic or seer inspiration. Somas are not simply plants or beverages taken in the physical body, but ecstatic experiences in meditative states, other altered states of consciousness, or even in dreams and visions. Such an 'inner drinking of the Soma' is likely the real absorption of this sacred essence that Soma implies in its Vedic symbolism as the creative power behind the entire universe.

The yogic quest for Soma is part of an inner alchemy of Self-realization, not simply an outer seeking of intoxication or use of powerful healing plants. This Vedic 'Soma alchemy' does consider the role of plants and minerals, not only as rejuvenating substances outwardly, but also as indications of inner processes and energies of the deeper psyche. We can compare the Vedic pursuit of Soma with how the great psychologist Carl Jung explained medieval European alchemy, which appeared to the modern mind as little more than a confused superstition based upon a misunderstanding of how chemicals really work but at a deeper examination could be seen to contain a symbolism of psychological regeneration, a sophisticated system of self-integration. It is this inner alchemy of Soma that is its real secret and true power. To discover it we must expand our examination of Soma from a botanical level to all aspects of life and consciousness.

All our life processes yield various types of Soma, enjoyment or vitality, whether it is eating, breathing, sensing, feeling or thinking. There is a rasa or essence of delight in all things that we can access through a higher awareness. Life itself should be an experience of Soma or lasting joy extending to all that we do. Soma reflects the ultimate movement of life as it seeks unification, integration, expansion and immortality. The Vedic Soma is part of a greater set of symbolisms than its botanical implications. Such inner types of Soma occur throughout Vedic and Tantric teachings as mantra, pranayama, devotion and meditation. In fact, we could say that the practice of Yoga in its classical sense, which is a pursuit of samadhi or a lasting state of bliss, is the ultimate quest for Soma – that Yoga is the supreme science of Soma for healing body and mind and taking us beyond all death and suffering.

The Pursuit of Soma: the Alchemy of Happiness

Soma is ultimately the bliss of our own existence that we must pursue by our very nature. We are all seeking our bliss or looking for our Soma in one form or another. We are all striving to get high, to transcend, to experience something greater, to go beyond, to achieve a peak experience, to gain lasting fame, to get into the zone, and so on, seeking happiness according to many different formulas and perspectives. Behind these diverse pursuits is an aspiration for the bliss at the core of our being that does not diminish or die, which is lastingly satisfying and refreshing. Most of our Soma-seeking, as it were, may begin as crude or gross, running after sensory stimulations, but we ultimately must refine our pursuit of happiness through the higher pursuits of art, mysticism and spirituality if we wish to gain the immortal bliss that is the real goal of our heart's wishes. If we do not consciously search out this eternal bliss, we will only consign ourselves to transient happiness that ends in lasting sorrow.

What provides us our happiness, bliss and Soma in life – or what we think does so – becomes our passion, inspiration or addiction that becomes the prime focus of our striving. Soma can be whatever exhilarates the senses, prana, mind and heart, in which all our worries and problems are forgotten. We should choose our Somas in life carefully because once we have become accustomed to a particular form of Soma, delight or pleasure, even if it is limited, we will find it difficult to give up. External Somas, the pleasure that arises through the body and the senses in particular, easily breed dependency. Only the internal Somas of the deeper mind and heart, our deeper inspirations, are truly liberating.

Look at your own life and begin to observe the happiness, Somas, rasas or essences that you are cultivating on a daily basis. What are the Somas or prime forms of enjoyment that you seek in your food, exercise, sensory impressions, associations, work or spiritual practice? What are your favorite items, events or interests, and what is it that attracts you to them? What essences are you imbibing in life from the various flowers of experience that you visit on a daily basis? Will their honey or nectar prove sweet and enduring, or end bitter or sour?

All of our life experience is a cultivation of Soma, as it were, a taking in of various essences that become deposited in our memory, which leave us with a residual sense of happiness or sorrow, fulfillment or lack, success or failure. What kind of body of Soma or inner essence of experience are we building up in life? This will reflect our karma and destiny as well as the flow of grace within us.

Once we have become aware of the pitfalls of the outer pursuit of enjoyment or become exhausted by its limitations, the following questions arise: Can one pursue a higher and more refined Soma that resides within oneself, so that one need not seek happiness on the outside? What is the alchemy of our own happiness, the chemistry of our own bliss that we need to develop? How can we reach that essence of immortality that is the highest energization of all our potentials? After all, the pleasure and happiness that we seek externally remains elusive, expensive, unreliable and unpredictable.

Our primary outer Somas are our sensory pleasures through taste, touch, sound, sight and smell. Most of our lives consist of a pursuit of new or more powerful sensations, which can be gross and noisy or subtle and refined. This sensate seeking keeps our Soma focused in the outer world where it easily becomes lost and dispersed. We end up as consumers rather than as creators, shopping for what we have been told we should have, rather than bringing into existence what is for the good of all and for our own greater well-being.

To evolve in consciousness and in happiness, we need to follow a deeper search for Soma that looks to the hidden essence of life, ultimately to the ground of Being-Consciousness-Bliss itself, what the great Yogis call *Sat-Chit-Ananda*. This is the supreme Soma beyond name, form, number and action, above all desire, seeking, imagination, gain and loss. This supreme Soma is difficult to understand but can be best approached with an honoring of the sacred. Our inner life or spiritual quest begins when we initiate this search for the mystic Soma.

The religious pursuit of heaven is another kind of seeking of Soma or bliss. Heaven is often described as flowing with healing waters, nectars, milk and honey or Soma. Yet it is easier to access Soma, or the love-bliss energies of the universe, in subtle realms of pure thought, deep feeling, and devotion beyond the physical body, through the more refined instrument of the subtle astral body made of light and prana. Such Somas of the heavenly worlds reflect the essence of our experience in life, particularly our good karmas and spiritual striving, which grant us a taste of Soma after death. Yet even these subtle realms of Soma are inferior to the bliss of pure consciousness beyond all form and should not be regarded as the ultimate. Once we have experienced such astral Somas, we must return to physical life for further inner growth.

Soma and Enjoyment

Soma at the most basic level is whatever allows us to feel good in life, starting at an outer level of what we can call 'outer Somas' that include sensory enjoyments, sexual pleasures, athletic accomplishments, monetary gains, worldly successes and achievements of all kinds. We gain a sense of Soma or contentment from listening to music, from being entertained, from any significant particularly unexpected gains, from social recognition, by becoming famous, and so on. This outer pursuit of enjoyment is our main Soma quest in life. Whatever free time or extra resources have, we use it for everything from eating good food, to searching out the latest new equipment, seeking out new partners or friends, or taking special vacations, in which we pursue our outer Soma.

Yet the outer Somas that we seek are not always good, healthy or without side effects. On the negative side, outer Somas include junk food, sugar, alcohol, tobacco, stimulants, and recreational and medicinal drugs of all types.[32] We even gain a strange delight in perversions, negative emotions, anger, hatred, the unhappiness of others, or even in our own unhappiness in life, much like the pleasure in watching war or horror movies. In these diverse phenomena, there is a strong or intense experience that we merge into: an absorption, intoxication, self-forgetting or self-transcendence, a touch of if not ecstasy, at least fascination.

These peak experiences of our outer lives do not just involve expanded external experiences. They cause our brains to secrete more positive chemicals, the famous endorphins, which bring a sense of contentment to our entire body and nervous system. It is this internal counterpart of our outer gains that hides the mystery of the deeper Somas that we can learn to experience directly inside ourselves.

Apart from these outer Somas, there is an entire range of inner Somas. These include all aspects of creativity and spirituality, in which our focus is within. The key to our inner growth is to move from lower Somas to higher Somas, which grant us peace and contentment, connecting us to our inner bliss and immortality, rather than wearing ourselves out in the external pursuit of happiness that is largely an escape from our internal emptiness and sorrow.

The outer seeking of Soma that our pursuit of enjoyment reflects, we should note, is not a quest for immortality – which requires discipline, austerity and deep search – but an indulgence in mortality, which hastens our aging process and causes disease. It is a running after the outer world rather than discovering the universe inside ourselves. This outer pursuit of desire and pleasure dissipates the senses, weakens the will, causes us to lose our independence, and eventually exhausts our vitality. It makes us lose our inner peace, happiness and contentment. As long as we are caught in the outer pursuit of enjoyment, we must remain trapped in mortality and cannot find the immortal.

This outer pursuit of happiness is called *bhoga* or enjoyment in Sanskrit, which is said to lead to *roga* or disease. The inner pursuit of happiness is *yoga*, which requires forgoing short-term enjoyment to achieve lasting bliss. If we are serious about our quest for immortality, the pursuit of transient sensory, emotional and intellectual stimulation cannot be our main preoccupation in life. We must face the mortality of our outer enjoyments in order to approach the reality of immortal bliss, which cannot be shaken by the pleasures and pains, gains and losses of the outer life. Our outer enjoyments or outer Somas become inner poisons, as it were, if we do not bring a deeper search into our lives.

The Allure of High Tech Somas – the Soma of the Media

In our commercial and high tech era today, we are ever seeking new and more sophisticated outer Somas, particularly as dished out through the entertainment realm and the mass media. In all these, the main thing is the sophistication of the equipment, bigger screens with better colors and better sounds. They do not actually change us internally or give us more control over how we think and feel. We are becoming largely inert spectators, letting other people run our lives and being content to form the audience and rate the performers and pay for their performance.

Yet while our media equipment has improved in radical ways over time from crude radios to sophisticated home entertainment systems, the content that we are witnessing has seldom changed from the same old sex, aggression and violence. In fact, the content of our entertainment has arguably gotten worse. We have better camera shots, but of a world that is egoistic, self-promoting, rude and bombastic, not at all subtle and refined. We have highlighted physical reality and bodily movement, and any refinement of feeling seems receding in the distance. We are giving up living our own lives and instead living by proxy through our entertainers, or withdrawing into our own fantasy reality.

We are now trying to create a virtual reality, including an ideal powerful or beautiful self through our computer screens that we can access at any time. We can find our Soma in and get dependent on the media, without leaving our rooms, much less doing anything to improve our lives. Even when we travel, we must take the computer with us as our primary companion, to sustain our virtual reality. We put little television screens on the backseats of our automobiles to keep our children preoccupied with the media reality as they find the world of nature to be boring. While this technology may make our lives easier and communication better on some levels, it carries a background inertia to remove us from our own minds and from the world of nature – and place our sense of identity, purpose and value in the media realm and its judgments that remain superficial and blind to the greater reality.

Through its powerful sensory displays of light, color, sound and rapid movement the mass media produces a very powerful kind of Soma in our nervous system that draws our attention and makes us passive both to ourselves and to the world around us. The mass media hooks into our brains and changes their chemistry, creating an artificial appetite and an addiction to entertainment and the news. We can become addicted to media impressions as effectively as to drugs – and without knowing it. Look at the behavior of people when any major media attraction is going on, an important sports event, for example. They literally shut off from their own bodies and minds and become glued to the screen. What happens on the screen elicits strong mental, emotional and physical reactions within their own nervous systems, like being plugged into an energy current, even though such events rarely concern them personally.

Note that most of our media fascination is with the negative or painful in life. Our movies predominate in violence and have numerous scenes of destruction and death. Our poor heroes and heroines go from one life threatening event or attack to another, experiencing various traumas or picking up various injuries along the way. Our news is mainly of crime, war, disasters, scandals or impending catastrophes. We let people into our minds that we would never let into our homes. We are addicted to negative sensations or violent Somas because these are more emotionally engaging to us, better distracting us from our own internal emptiness. We must remember that whatever information or enjoyment that we are receiving through the mass media has been selected, programmed and filtered by various vested interests, planned to make us to react one way or another, generally in an unthinking manner. We are not simply being entertained but are being conditioned and controlled, which means having the movement of our own prana and our own internal chemistry altered.

Often when I notice someone I know watching a television program, I ask him or her, "What are you looking at?" They quickly reply with the nature or name of the particular program. To this, I respond, "What you are really looking at is a screen." One of the prime laws of how the mind works is that the mind tends to imitate its environment. This means that in the media world today, we also look at the world and ourselves like a screen. We become reactive, programmed, almost two dimensional in our responses. The screen gains a greater reality than the impressions in the life around us, which we lose our sensitivity to. We live from media event to media event, in media time far removed from the rhythms of nature or the currents of our own physiology. Our own personal lives lose both their value and their interest for us, as what happens to us in daily life from sunrise and sunset cannot compare to the rapid drama and sensation that happens on the screen in a few minutes. The result is that we stop living our own lives or even having our own lives apart from the media. Our Facebook image can become our real life or main preoccupation in life.

The rapid flow of media impressions easily addicts us, stimulating the nervous system much more than nature's gentle flow of subtle light. The media has programmed our minds and nervous system to require its sensory input as a kind of food or drug. Without our daily meal, bath or inundation of media images, we feel empty and can undergo withdrawal symptoms like an addict without his drug. Our computer and television screens, our 3D movies, which are but an indication of more technology to come, create an exhilaration and a fascination, but also reed a deep dependency down to the subconscious level that is insidious in its effects. It starts in our childhood when we do not have any spiritual self-defense of wisdom or awareness. Then we become consumers for life.

Yet the side effects of our virtual reality lives are now becoming obvious. Boredom and depression are increasing rapidly throughout our high tech society, and new forms of entertainment seem to be just preparing a greater malaise for our world in the decades to come. We forget that external stimulation breeds internal emptiness and inertia, which must catch up with us in the end. It also can adversely affect our health causing immune system disorders, hormonal and nervous system problems.[33]

Without our media highs, sometimes even with them, we must face our emotional lows. We are progressively unable to be alone, to be in silence, to appreciate nature, or to experience life as it is without a camera somewhere. At the same time we are becoming progressively incapable of deep or lasting relationships as we become more used to relating to the images of people rather than to actual individuals. Rapid media sensations are like speed or cocaine, pumping us up outwardly but eventually leaving us depleted within. They destroy our contentment and detachment in life and make us hypersensitive, viscerally reactive to the fluctuations of political, economic or social events in the outer world, the on-going turbulence from throughout the world that the media blares as the daily news.

New High Tech Drug Somas: Brave New World

Our culture has become increasingly drug oriented both in terms of recreational and medicinal drugs. Nearly thirty percent of our children take medications every day, while over fifty percent of teenagers experiment with recreational drugs. Over ninety percent of our seniors take at least ten different drugs daily to sustain their health. It seems rare to find a person whose blood stream and nervous system is not in some way chemically altered or contaminated.

Modern medicine has created a new Soma of high tech designer drugs including special anti-depressants, sedatives and pain relieving agents to make us feel better. Some of these Soma drugs exist to counter the dullness or wearing out of our nervous system caused by our media addictions. All tend to be expensive and have significant side effects that we are only beginning to discover. Our medicine now prescribes powerful drugs first, and only recommends natural healing after the drugs have failed or damaged our nervous system. We rarely seek out the cause of disease in wrong diet, lack of exercise or emotional disharmonies, but quickly embrace soothing drugs to cover over the symptoms of our lives out of balance. The use of anti-depressants has become so rampant that it is becoming the norm, rather than the exception for our psychological issues.

There is also a new range and availability of recreational drugs, narcotics and psychedelics, from old standards like heroin or cannabis, to a whole new set of designer drugs that can be mixed together in various new and powerful combinations. We can easily find a bewildering diversity of drugs to choose from, as often can our own children, a smorgasbord of intoxicants to choose from. Meanwhile the war on drugs has expanded to a literal war that makes our borders unsafe, as well as provoking overseas conflicts.

On top of these overt drugs, our foods and beverages contain many chemical additives of different types. Our food industry has created its new high tech Somas of junk food, with high fructose corn syrup augmenting our sugar cravings. People take as their main beverages soft drinks that have little natural within them. We have new Somas of Coke and Pepsi that are nutritionally of little value but easily addict the nervous system, using media entertainers to sell them, connecting one artificial Soma with another. More people are drinking alcohol as well, not simply as a sidelight but as their prime beverage, their main Soma in life. Even natural foods stores now abound with large alcohol sections that seem to be the most rapidly growing sections of the stores.

We can add to these artificial food and drink Somas, the chemicals in our air, water and soil, the pollutants that seem to be everywhere around us. These also contaminate our nervous systems and make us prone to other drug or media addictions. The artificial chemicals that have come into our bodies cause us to crave more from the outside as well. As we become more chemically dependent our lives become more mechanical as well, losing the freshness of prana and awareness.

Along with high tech Soma drugs we are trying to remake the physical body at a high tech level as well. Genetic manipulation, still in its initial phases, is part of this process. It includes plastic surgery, Botox and other ways to make our bodily appearance more attractive, without actually improving our internal energy or state of awareness. This high tech body remaking is a dangerous process that can leave us progressively artificial inwardly and outwardly. Besides artificial chemicals, we have plastic in our bodies as part of our own self-image.

These Somas of the modern media and high tech realms resemble the Somas of Aldous Huxley's *Brave New World*, and it is possible that they will remain the dominant cultural force for decades to come. Clearly our culture has become more adept in producing outer Somas, in stimulating and distracting ourselves externally, but we have not gained lasting happiness in the process, much less internal peace or peace in our society. Faced with the obvious limitations and dangers of these high tech Somas, we need to develop an alternative; a return to nature to find the real essence of Soma, beauty and delight that does not depend upon external stimulation or artificial equipment. We need the inner Soma that no one can give to us, that cannot be bought, that does not require any equipment or change our natural chemistry.

These high tech Somas, including the many new drugs, can provide much entertainment and be of medical benefit in acute conditions, but they can reduce the quality of our life and awareness. They tend to remove us from our own direct experience of reality and make us dependent upon the media and the medical establishment for our well-being. We remain spectators and consumers, in a world where others run our lives and occupy our minds and hearts with their own secret agendas. These outer Somas, however high tech in nature, cannot bring fulfillment to our inner being. They can only stimulate our senses and push our emotional buttons so that we do not develop the power of attention to look within. The way to inner rejuvenation is along a different route, not through the outer stimulation of the nervous system but through its inner calming and quiescence through Yoga and meditation. While we can use the media and computer worlds to enhance our outer lives, we should not allow them to substitute for our deeper inner search or become our dominant reality.

The Transformative Power of the Inner Soma

Though we have access to many new forms of enjoyment in this media age, we are getting progressively agitated, bored and depleted. We fail to realize in our outer pursuit of enjoyment that true happiness or Soma comes from the inside. It can never be bought, much less produced externally. True happiness is a positive energy and contentment within our own hearts, minds and nervous systems. Real Soma comes from within, not from the outside. It is not a dramatic external sensation but a subtle internal flow of grace. It heightens our awareness and independence; it does not breed addiction or dependency, though it remains ever fascinating, engaging and uplifting in its effects.

The outer factors that appear to provide us with happiness are simply triggering our own inner current of happiness or inner Soma to flow, but in a distorted manner that we ourselves do not control. Entertaining media impressions or mood elevating drugs irritate our nervous systems to release the same chemicals of contentment that are the natural products of our inner well-being, depleting them in the process. The problem is that we identify this feeling of well-being or Soma with the outer factors that cause it to arise. We confuse the external factors that stimulate our Soma with the Soma itself, thinking that our actual happiness and well-being depends upon them. We then lose our inner Soma and get addicted and dependent on these outer forms of enjoyment, losing our inner integrity in the process.

All outer forms of Soma – to the extent that they become our primary focus in life – weaken or agitate our inner Soma. They promote inertia, decay and death, particularly of the mind. Some outer drug based Somas can keep the body alive artificially a bit longer, but cannot vitalize us from within. They cause us to lose our real Soma or happiness and become hostage to some external agency to make us happy or to take care of us. The result is that we are not happy or content in ourselves or in our own lives, relationships or occupations. We go from entertainment to therapy and back again, not connecting with the flow of grace inherent in the natural movement of life.

We need to recognize that the inner Soma is much more important than the outer, which is at best an external complement. While not having the same external hype, allure and drama, this inner Soma has a much deeper transformative power. The inner Soma invigorates and vitalizes us in an organic manner, just as the outer Soma can take away our energy and motivation. When we begin to awaken spiritually and enter into a life of conscious awareness, we gradually turn away from the outer Somas and begin to seek the Soma or nectar of bliss within. There are inner Somas, flows of peace, bliss and cooling delight that can satiate our inner being, which are released into our minds and nervous systems through Yoga and meditation that are more exhilarating than any drug, sensation or media show, breed no dependency, have no side effects, rely on no equipment and have no price.

The true spiritual alchemy, the way of Yoga and meditation, is to learn to extract the inner Soma directly, apart from any external stimuli, through the light of awareness hidden in our own hearts. This involves discovering a deeper inner contentment, detachment, peace and bliss through spiritual and creative practices, through our own individual experience and direct perception of life that itself is a movement of cosmic joy.

Soma and Cultural Renewal

Our culture, particularly its artistic, philosophical and spiritual forms, represents our collective Soma. It is not enough to strive to develop our personal Soma; we also should strive to uplift the Soma of our culture. Our current culture is sunk in lower level commercial Somas that are making us more insensitive and less gentle or refined. Our primary Somas are of drugs, machines, fast foods and mass production. These do not provide a suitable vehicle for the soul in us, our eternal being to emerge.

To renew our culture and take us beyond our current global crisis, we need to develop a new cultural Soma. This is to develop a culture not only of beautiful art and music, sophisticated science and profound philosophy, which are certainly important; it also means to develop a culture of Yoga and meditation, a culture born of self-control, not of seeking to exploit the world around us. To develop our own individual Soma, we must also strive to connect with and develop the world cultural Soma. We should bring more Soma into our lives and into our environment, not for our own enjoyment, but for enhancing the world in which we live and helping nature to evolve and manifest the Divine light.

One of the first signs of our inner Soma beginning to awaken is a greater sense of beauty in nature, which can lead us into the artistic realm as well. Nature is full of Somas, rasas or nectars, not just in dramatic storms of sunsets but also in the subtle hues of the moss, lichen and rocks, in the very textures of the Earth. When we start to live in nature more than in the media, we can access a new level of Soma and delight. We can once more integrate our human world into the greater conscious universe. We can also integrate more of nature and spirituality into the media, which will then become more a means of our secondary expression than our primary activity that will shift to the inner worlds.

The Spiritual Search for Soma

The awakening of devotion to the Divine within our hearts is the main spiritual sign that our inner Soma is coming to the front of our being. This also means honoring the sacred nature of all life. On the level of emotions, it is love that allows our Soma to flow. The higher the love, the purer and more lasting will be the flow of Soma. This inner devotion is not a matter of mere emotionality, but a more refined sensitivity to the Divine ground of existence as an unbounded expansion of beneficence and grace.

As our inner Soma develops, we become conscious of ourselves as an immortal soul, seeking divinity through many lives, many births and deaths, connecting to our undying aspiration to the internal and the infinite. We seek our happiness in expanding our sense of divine love, awareness and higher perception, not only through formal yogic or mystical practices, but also through a change of our attitude and values in life. We enter into various yogic or mystical experiences, including the unity consciousness called samadhi, in which the inner currents of Soma-bliss flow throughout the channels of the nervous system and subtle body, improving our health, well-being, happiness and joy. The Shakti or electrical power of Soma brings a rain of higher knowledge into every corner of our minds.

Each one of us has a certain amount of inner Soma that we are born with, depending on our level of awareness from previous lives. This is our inherent capacity for peace, happiness, creativity, love and spirituality. Not all of us use our inner Soma wisely. Most of us deplete it in transient and trivial pursuits through the body and senses. The pursuit of the outer forms of Soma through sensory enjoyments depletes our internal Soma. Once our inner Soma is depleted, we easily fall into depression, anxiety or anger. Our innate happiness, curiosity and will to live get reduced. Therefore it behooves us to protect our inner Soma as the treasure of immortality it is for us, and to seek to develop it in a way that will not fail us. Soma leads us to the rejuvenation of body and mind, aligned with the awakening of the spirit. But if we do not first turn away from the outer Somas, we may not be able to access those that are within.

We need to create a new inner body of bliss or 'body of Soma', which is a receptacle of love, compassion and delight. We must move out of our physical body as our vehicle for happiness and move into our bliss body, which is ultimately a power of awareness, not any outer body or external vehicle at all. When we fully enter into our body of bliss, we have true immortality, whether we continue to use a physical body or not.

Longevity and Happiness

The main reason we pursue longevity is because we are happy to be alive and healthy and see aging and death as suffering. However, longevity itself does not provide happiness. We can live long physically infirm or psychologically distressed. Some people linger on for years in chronic diseases. Others can last long in a state of depression or decreased mental functioning.

The first thing we need to realize is that happiness is our very nature; bliss is the core of our being. Our inner happiness does not depend upon a good physical longevity. In fact, we can live happy and fulfilling lives that are not long in duration. Many great yogis and sages have lived lives that were ordinary in length or even short, like Shankara, the greatest philosopher of India, who only lived to the age of thirty two or Jesus who only lived to thirty three. We should not confuse longevity with happiness, or a short life with a failed life.

Our happiness does not depend upon living long but upon realizing the truth of our inner being and connecting to the bliss within. This may take decades or lifetimes to fully accomplish, but is a realization that ultimately takes us outside of time altogether. Our eternal being is not increased by a long life, nor decreased by a short life. In this regard, the search for our inner Soma is more important than the seeking of greater longevity. Without that inner Soma, longevity will not fulfill our soul. It may become something artificial or distorted, a continuation of selfish and sensate drives and passions beyond their normal or natural span.

Rejuvenation and Immortality through the Inner Soma

A healthy and harmonious physical rejuvenation depends upon developing and strengthening our physical and vital Somas. Rejuvenation of the mind depends upon developing and strengthening our mental and emotional Somas. Immortality of the spirit depends upon developing and strengthening our connection with the supreme Soma of universal love, joy and compassion. There are several aspects to these processes, which can work together.

- Soma-increasing foods (fruits, nuts, dairy, root vegetables, whole grains) to nourish a higher quality energy and tissue in the body.

- Soma-increasing herbs (tonic, nervine and rejuvenative agents) for strengthening the body and mind.

- Soma-increasing sensory impressions (sights and sounds born of nature and spiritual aspiration) to nourish and revitalize the mind and senses.

- Turning within and slowing down: rest, relaxation and deep sleep, stillness, silence and spacing, learning to hold and conserve our energy within.

- Soma-increasing emotions, devotion and associations born of the spiritual heart.

- Soma-increasing pranayama and pranic exercises, calming and deepening the breath and vital force.

- Soma-increasing mantras, visualizations, thoughts and affirmations to increase the Soma of the mind.

- Soma-promoting deep meditation and samadhi, to unfold the deepest Somas of the bliss of awareness.

Soma increasing diet and herbs are part of the Ayurvedic approach to Soma. They are covered under Ayurvedic rejuvenation or *rasayana* practice, which is an important aspect of Ayurvedic treatment starting with the ancient classics of *Charak* and *Sushrut Samhitas*. The section relative to the treatment of disease in *Charak Samhita* deals with rejuvenation first![34] For Ayurveda, the development of Soma is the key to good immunity, good longevity and optimal health, as well as to good progeny.

Inner factors for developing Soma come under Raja Yoga or Yoga in the broader sense of the combination of knowledge, devotion, service and energy practices. Classical Yoga can be defined as a means of developing our inner Soma, particularly through the state of samadhi, to uncover our inner immortality in our true Self. This Soma is sometimes referred to as nectar or as the Moon in yogic thought.[35]

Yet Soma is the essence of all healing and well-being and is present in whatever allays our suffering in any manner. This means that Soma-increasing approaches have great relevance for everyone, as we all want to avoid pain and gain happiness. Life itself is Soma or we would not want to live. The inner Soma takes us into the universal life, which is our true existence.

Becoming the Soma Ourselves

We must carefully prepare ourselves in order to be able to hold and carry the higher forms of Soma. You cannot store nectar in a dirty or broken vessel. This preparation requires purification and detoxification of body and mind, along with a willingness to give up our old personality and its memories to embrace our cosmic being, even if it means letting go of all that we thought we were or wanted to become. Should the old ego seek rejuvenation, it will only cause more sorrow and unhappiness, or at best a new form of self-indulgence to distract us.

Our real spiritual adventure begins when we shift our goals and begin to seek the inner Soma, which requires that we let go of our outer Somas. The inner Soma awakens our higher perception and lifts us out of the shadowy human world into the Divine realm of light. This inner Soma is the true Holy Grail that we must find in order to go beyond death and sorrow.

We ourselves must become that Soma or immortal nectar for the Gods to drink. Our lives must become an offering and a sacrifice to the higher powers. To accomplish this, we must refine our nature to its essence, like extracting gold from the crude ore that holds it. We must extract the deepest motivation of our souls out of our base desires and expectations. Our life movement must become an alchemy of Soma; not seeking a personal immortality but honoring the universal immortality that underlies all life as both its origin and end. We should be a source of Soma, healing or well-being not only for ourselves but also for others and the entire world.

When we consider how we can imbibe this nectar of immortality or Soma, we must therefore also ask the question: "Who can drink the Soma?" The Soma is a beverage of the Gods or a Divine drink. A mere mortal cannot simply drink the Soma and survive. The immortal transcends the mortal. What is immortal can be a poison for mortals. In the *Vedas*, it is only Indra, the king of the Gods, who can drink the Soma, which he must do so alone, even apart from all the other Gods.[36] Soma serves to give him power and allow his energy to expand. We need to awaken that Indra consciousness within us in order to be able to drink the immortal juice. Indra consciousness means Self-aware-ness, independence, fearlessness and deep powers of perception born of patient observation.

In later Yoga teachings, Shiva is the main deity who drinks the im-mortal nectar, but he must also be able to drink poison and survive. He takes the poison only to his throat, in which form he is called *Nilakan-tha* or 'Blue-throated'. It is only through a deep Yoga practice, which can face and overcome negativity, that one can truly access and imbibe the immortal nectar. All else is a support or preliminary.

Whatever promotes our inner Soma, promotes our longevity, with-out creating any further clinging to life. These inner Somas are real substances and energies that we can learn to perceive and work with, just as we can work with the different forms of water and food around us. It is not a matter of belief or faith but of understanding the secret energies of life, which is an endless stream of transformation.

Strive to learn this language of Soma both in yourselves and in the world around you. Strive to cultivate the highest form of Soma pos-sible for you. It is something that you can take with you beyond this world and will be a source of joy for you forever.

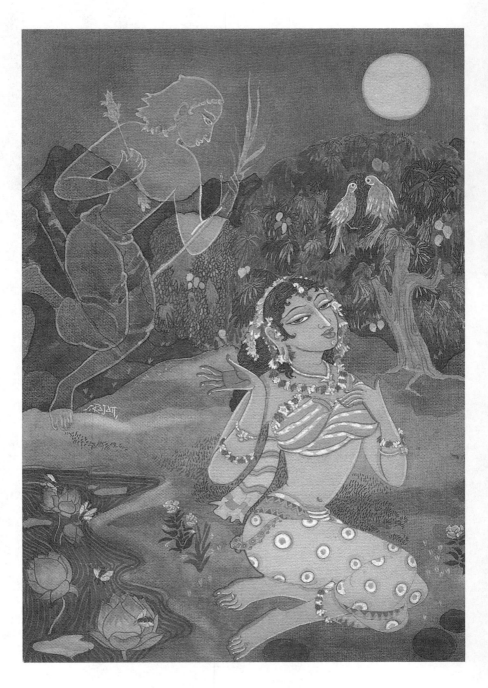

Soma as the Feminine Principle

AGNI AND SOMA:
THE ETERNAL FIRE
AND THE IMMORTAL NECTAR

From the sacred fire (Agni), the Soma nectar develops, by the Soma nectar the fire grows. Thus the offering is extended throughout this universe consisting of Agni and Soma.

Brihadjabala Upanishad II.4

The universe is a manifestation of dualistic forces and polarities, complimentary energies of various types, which serve also as the basis for our own physiology and psychology. Two forces and their interplay are necessary for the dynamism that keeps the entire cosmos vibrating. These two universal forces have been described in various ways in different spiritual traditions. Vedic thought speaks of this prime polarity of energy in the cosmos mainly in terms of *Agni* and *Soma*. *Agni* refers to spirit, fire and light on all levels, and *Soma* refers to nature, water and matter.[37]

Agni indicates to the power of heat and transformation. Soma means that which swells and overflows. The two are part of a cosmic symbolism much like yang and yin of Chinese thought and just as intricate. Below is a simple listing of their main dualistic reflections, though we should recognize that they intertwine on various levels, and that each is ultimately contained within the other.

AGNI AND SOMA: PRIME SYMBOLISMS

Agni	Soma
Fire	Water
Harsh	Soft
Electric	Magnetic
Sun	Moon
Day	Night
Ascending Force	Descending Force

Agni	Soma
Ascending Triangle	Descending Triangle
Aspiration	Grace
Mountain	Lake/ Valley
Speech - expression	Mind - reception
Male	Female
Martial or aggressive	Receptive or responsive
Seer	Seen
Subject	Object
Enjoyer	Enjoyment
Thought - Knowledge	Emotion - Feeling
Spirit	Nature/ Matter
Purification	Rejuvenation

Agni and Soma, as the prime cosmic duality, pervade all of nature. Agni is the Sun, which shines of its own accord, and Soma is the Moon, which has a reflected light. Agni is the ascending force that strives upward; Soma is the descending force that moves downward. Agni represents our Godward aspiration, while Soma is the descent of grace.

Agni is the power of movement, perception, energy, and effort. Soma refers to the powers of nutrition, enjoyment, rejuvenation and ecstasy. These actions occur on all levels of life and all planes of the universe. Generally Agni as fire is a masculine force and Soma as water is a feminine force, but there are masculine and feminine sides of both Agni and Soma. The feminine also has its special fire or Agni and the masculine has its coolness or Soma. There is an Agni within Soma and a Soma within Agni.

Agni as fire represents light (Jyoti) in the broadest sense, which includes the light of perception and the light of consciousness, not simply light as a material principle. Soma as water (Apas) is the medium on which light can be reflected, which is ultimately a quality of light itself. In this regard Soma is not only water, but also the mind and ultimately, the reflective power of consciousness itself.

Soma as a cosmic power, however, is not simply watery in its nature. It has an oily quality that can nourish and sustain fire. In this regard it has been compared to ghee (ghrita) in texture. All objects that we see are like fuel for the flame of our awareness. Soma also has a sweet quality and has been compared to honey (madhu). All that we see is like a flower, from which the honey of bliss can be extracted. These properties that sustain light and provide joy pervade all of space. Soma is the delight that is the counterpart of light. On the deepest level, Agni is the fire of consciousness that is reflected in the Soma or water of bliss. In this regard Agni and Soma are ultimately the same, two complementary aspects of Brahman.

However, rejuvenation and immortality depends upon accessing a higher power of Soma, either externally through plants, or internally through the plant of our own nervous system, the subtle body and its chakras, particularly the crown chakra, which is connected to Soma in yogic thought. Yet without some corresponding purification through Agni or fire – especially enkindling the fire of prana and awareness – the higher Somas cannot be accessed. This means that *whenever we consider Soma, we must remember Agni.* Deeper powers of fire and light are necessary for us to discover the immortal essence of Soma and to extract it, which requires some sort of cooking or ripening process. We need a powerful and clear Agni in order to prepare the most enduring Soma. This higher fire is not one of anger or aggression but of the inner light of seeing, born of sharp discernment between the outer and the inner, the transient and eternal aspects of our existence.

Biological Aspects of Agni and Soma

As the prime factors of natural existence, Agni and Soma have specific biological forms in the body and mind on which health and well-being depend. Agni exists primarily as the digestive power in the body as a whole, which is centered in the belly and small intestine. This is called 'the digestive fire' or *Jatharagni*, the fire in the belly, which is the main physical form of Agni. There are additional biological forms of Agni or digestive energies in the liver responsible for the digestion of the five elements,[38] in the seven tissues of the body,[39] in the five senses, particularly the eyes, in the prana and in the mind.[40] In fact, every cell in the body has its own Agni or digestive/metabolic power contained in the nucleus. Agni governs over metabolism in the body and perception in the mind and senses. It is our guiding light, sustaining fire and metabolic force.

As a complimentary force of a watery nature, Soma exists at a physical level as the bodily tissues that are built up by the action of Agni as the digestive fire. These tissues are seven in nature according to Ayurveda as 1) plasma, 2) blood, 3) muscle, 4) fat, 5) bone, 6) marrow and nerve, and 7) reproductive.[41] Our deeper tissues, the nerve and reproductive, have the greatest power of Soma among all the tissues and can afford us the greatest enjoyment in life accordingly.

Food itself is the main Soma or factor of enjoyment for the physical Agni as the digestive fire. There are additional Somas or food/enjoyment factors for each of the Agnis or fires of the five senses. Each of our sensory inputs is the Soma for the respective Agni, like sound as the Soma for the Agni of the ear. Soma governs form in the body and feeling in the mind and senses. It is our supporting ground and invigorating delight.

BIOLOGICAL FORMS OF AGNI AND SOMA

Digestive Capacity	Nutrients Taken In
Digestive Fire - Jatharagni	Food
Pranic Fire - Pranagni	Breath
Fire of the Senses (fires of hearing, touch, seeing, tasting and smelling)	Sensory impressions (sound, touch, sight, taste and smell)
Emotional or Volitional Fire	Emotions
Fire of Intelligence	Knowledge, truth
Fire of Consciousness	Bliss, love

Soma relates to the receptive side of our nature through our ability to take in food, breath, impressions and experiences. Agni relates to our ability to digest these intakes and to develop energy, action and expression out of them. Our sense organs overall, like the eyes and ears, are more receptive or Soma based, while our motor organs, like speech, hands and feet, are more active or Agni/fire based. The contemplative and emotional aspects of the mind are more Soma or lunar based, while the judgmental, discriminating and expressive sides of the mind are more Agni or fire based. But the two forces are intertwined on all levels, each offering itself to the other and each becoming the other.

Both Agni and Soma are connected to the mouth and tongue through the processes of eating and speaking. Soma governs the sense of taste in the mouth and the drinking of liquids, along with the water and sugar metabolism in general.[42] Agni governs our appetite and the eating of food, particularly our digestion of solids.[43] Soma represents the refined and creative aspect of speech, as in poetry and song. Agni represents the critical and perceptive aspect of speech, as in science, mathematics and philosophy.

Soma is called *rasa*, a juice. One imbibes the Soma rasa or drinks the Soma juice. Yet rasa is not just an external juice but also refers to taste and the essence extracted from whatever we experience in life. Our Soma reflects our sense of taste, both at a literal level of the food and drinks that we like and at a figurative level in how we have developed our overall sense of taste, whether in food, art, ideas or relationship. Our sense of taste reveals how we have developed our Soma. Similarly, our power of speech and expression, particularly its clarity, reflects our Agni.

Agni as the Digestive Fire and Power of Purification

The key to physical well-being resides in maintaining our power of digestion, regarded as a biological fire in Ayurvedic thought. The digestive fire or *Jatharagni* is responsible not only for the digestion of food but also for the prevention of impurities from entering into the body through the digestive tract. In this way Agni upholds the immune system and removes all toxins. *Agni is so central to the functioning of the body that the physical body itself is sometimes called Agni.*

Ayurvedic treatment emphasizes the management of Agni. Health depends upon the proper functioning of the digestive fire, which should be neither too high, nor to low in how it burns and functions, properly adjusted like the flame on a stove. If the Agni is too low, toxins will build up from the improperly digested food mass called *Ama* in Ayurveda, literally meaning something that is raw. Low Agni is like eating uncooked food that may contain toxins within it. Ama is the root of the disease process, just as Agni is the basis of health. Health and disease reflects the balance of Agni and Ama within us. Taking in wrong food substances and irregular eating habits, including an Agni out of balance, cause Ama to develop instead of healthy tissues.

As we age, Ama or this toxic mass increases in the body and accumulates in the tissues, fermenting within them and causing various forms of decay. For example, entering into the bone tissue, Ama causes arthritis and degeneration of the bones. Some of this Ama is simply the result of the inertia and entropy born of time, even if our life habits are good. Our Agni or metabolic power tends to decrease with age. With aging we usually gain weight, particularly after forty. This weight is usually held in the belly but often also in the hips and buttocks. It reflects this natural decline in the power of Agni

The pursuit of rejuvenation at a physical level begins with the normalization of the digestive fire and the removal of any Ama or toxic undigested food particles from the digestive tract and the tissues. This is the 'preliminary purification' behind rejuvenation, the 'development of Agni to support Soma'. It is the basis of Ayurvedic palliation or *shamana* therapy, which largely rests upon heating methods like spicy herbs and fasting to improve the digestive fire.

This balancing of Agni in turn leads to a radical purification or *shodhana*, particularly *Pancha Karma* in Ayurveda, which involves eliminating the disease causing toxins and doshas directly from the body through therapeutic use of emetics, purgatives and enemas. We will examine these practices in more detail later. They are important for making the body ready to handle the higher Soma essences, though in themselves are not rejuvenative.

Soma and the Mind

Soma has subtler forms and aspects beyond the bodily tissues that are its physical counterparts. The ultimate product of nutrition is not just the tissues of the body but the mind itself.[44] Soma relates to the mind in Vedic thought, and to the Moon, which is said to be the cosmic counterpart of the mind. The *Vedas* say that the moon is born from the mind of the Cosmic Being or Purusha.[45] The mind like the Moon has a reflective nature, and functions best when kept cool, calm and in state of composure. *As Agni rules the body through the digestive fire, Soma rules the mind through its reflective nature. We can even say that while Agni is the body, Soma is the mind.*

In this regard, it is curious to note that in ancient Greek thought Soma means the body, from which our term 'somatic' arises. Even in Vedic thought, Soma can refer to the body as our vehicle of physical enjoyment or the bodily structure or tissues that complement Agni as the digestive fire. In fact, Soma can refer the body that is a means of enjoyment for the spirit symbolized by fire. However, Soma has a deeper meaning as well, referring to the mind which through the senses is our inner instrument of enjoyment and experience. The mind is the essence of all that we take in, not only through the mouth but also through the senses.

Soma relates both to the mind as a non-physical principle and to the brain and nervous system as a physical principle. *We could also say from a physical level that Soma is the brain.* The brain is our Soma center from which we experience sensory impressions and all the enjoyment and fascination that goes with them.

Our cerebrospinal fluid is the Soma of our nervous system. Our nervous system is our body's Soma system and its transmissions and secretions constitute the flow of our biological Somas. We can include the endocrine system under this greater Soma system, as our endocrine secretions are the main Somas that drive our nervous system and through it all our other bodily functions.

The key to the well-being of the nervous system, mind and emotional nature is to develop and sustain the Soma within us. The essence of the food that we eat, which is digested by Agni, serves to build up the Soma of the mind. Yet not only solid food, but liquids, air, impressions, thoughts and emotions are part of our greater food or nutrition equation, with each having its own importance to our overall well-being.

When our organism is functioning normally, we are naturally healthy and happy and derive great enjoyment in life through the simple acts of living like eating, breathing, walking, or observing the natural world around us. This natural joy in our everyday functions is a sign that our inner Soma is intact, and along with it that our physical and psychological well-being is stable. We don't need anything special to be truly happy. Life itself is happiness in movement when we are connected to the core of our being.

However, just as *Ama* or poorly digested food particles causes physical disease and an impairment of Agni, Ama in the mind causes psychological diseases and an impairment of Soma. Ama in the mind, we could say, is unconverted Soma, life experiences that we have not been able to assimilate into peace and contentment. Undigested experiences and negative emotions ferment in our minds, creating a kind of emotional poison that depletes our Soma.

Taking in of wrong sensory impressions and harmful life-experiences cause this emotional Ama to build up within us and result in psychological disease, impairment and unhappiness. We should keep our Soma pure in order to remain happy and healthy. If we mix our Somas with impurities, disturbed or darkening forms of experiences, then our mind's nectar will become a poison. This means that we should always keep our minds pure, clear, relaxed, receptive and observant, with our senses sharp and attentive. We should not let negative thoughts and emotions accumulate within us, but should let them go every day.

Agni and Soma in Hatha Yoga

Classical Yoga, such as is discussed in the *Yoga Sutras*, can be defined as a pursuit of immortality at a practical level, teaching us how to use the body, prana, senses, mind and heart in order to reach and dwell in the eternal and undying essence of our being, the *Purusha* or 'higher Self' of yogic thought. Yoga is perhaps the most developed spiritual science available for achieving immortality, and all its millennial experience and wisdom take us in this direction.

Agni and Soma are key concepts not only in Ayurvedic medicine but also in Yoga, particularly in Tántric and Vedic forms of Yoga, notably in the system of Hatha Yoga itself. Hatha Yoga originally is defined as a 'Yoga of the Sun and the Moon', which is also the Yoga of Agni and Soma. 'Ha' refers to the Sun, which is Agni, and 'tha' to the Moon in yogic thought, which is Soma.[46] Hatha Yoga aims at developing and balancing Agni and Soma at a higher level, but with regard for their physical functions as a foundation. The asana component of Hatha Yoga reflects this higher pursuit of energy balancing, which is its real concern, orienting the asanas to balance and protect the Sun and the Moon.

In Hatha Yoga,[47] Agni and Soma relate to two important sites in the body:

- Agni: the digestive fire in the navel, including what is called the solar plexus in western thought.

- Soma: the soft palate of the mouth, which is said to be the region of the Moon or Soma in yogic thought.

The palate is where we take in the enjoyment from our food but also where we can experience the descent of a higher delight from the brain, enjoyment from the senses, mind and consciousness. The navel reflects the digestive fire on all levels from body to spirit, not just the digestive fire but also the fire of Prana manifests from this location.

The palate rules over the sense of taste and the tongue. That is why we speak of food as being "pleasing to the palate." The soft palate is the inner and lunar counterpart of the third eye, which has a fiery nature. Like the third eye, it is a place where all the five senses meet and can all be controlled along with the mind. As the third eye controls the perceptive aspect of mind and senses, the soft palate controls the nutritive and enjoyment aspect.

The soft palate is said to be the birthplace of Indra (Indra yoni), the supreme consciousness, the Purusha or the seer, in Vedic thought. The Divine consciousness that enters into the body through the point at the top of the head manifests from this location.[48]

Concentrating on the soft palate with deep focus can reveal all the secrets of bliss and immortality. That is why when Yogis meditation they place the tongue at the roof of the mouth, and in some approaches, gradually aim at bringing the tongue back to the soft palate itself. This helps them drink the inner Soma.[49]

According to Hatha Yoga, longevity depends upon protecting the Soma in the soft palate, which is the nectar of life, from being burned up by the heat of the fire of Agni in the belly below.[50] If our Soma is burned up both our longevity and happiness are impaired. The key to do protect the Soma is to prevent the Agni from rising adversely and to maintain a protective barrier between the Agni and the Soma. It requires keeping the mind cool and calm, the senses from being over stimulated, and our digestive fire balanced. It also depends upon proper hydration and oleation (lubrication) of the tissues, starting with the plasma itself, our prime nutrient pool. We must avoid drying out the nervous system. The intake of proper liquids is part of this, as are various Yoga practices (like Jalandhara bandha). We will discuss these procedures later in the book.

Soma and Tarpak Kapha: Controlling our own Brain Chemistry

Among the different forms of Soma in the body, probably most important is what is called *Tarpak Kapha* or the form of Kapha that gives contentment. This is one of five types or subdoshas of Kapha dosha, the biological water humor, which specifically provides lubrication and nourishment to the brain, senses and nervous system.

The other Kapha subdoshas are *Bodhak Kapha*, which governs the sense of taste and the tongue; *Avalambak Kapha*, which supports, cushions and lubricates the heart and chest; *Kledak Kapha*, which lubricates and protects the digestive tract; and *Sleshak Kapha*, which lubricates and cushions the joints of the body. Bodhak Kapha is closely connected to Soma and as our inner Soma increases its nature changes and it begins to secrete a kind of nectar, in which our own sense of taste is sublimated. Avalambak Kapha also has its place for keeping the heart calm. All five Kapha subdoshas can be regarded as types of bodily Somas, preserving which sustains health and longevity. All tend to be depleted by disease and by the aging process.[51]

Tarpak Kapha is the most crucial of these for overall well-being and can be regarded as the key to happiness and the absence of pain for body and mind. Endorphins that counter pain and promote well-being derive from Tarpak Kapha. The depletion of Tarpak Kapha or the 'Soma of the brain' causes psychological diseases and emotional unhappiness, including chronic pain, depression and anxiety. Managing Tarpak Kapha is the Ayurvedic key to overall well-being and countering pain and sorrow. It is the main Soma therapy approach of Ayurveda, one could say.

CONDITION OF TARPAK KAPHA

Sufficient Tarpak Kapha	Contentment, peace, happiness, calm, composure, forgiveness, compassion, devotion, independence
Deficient Tarpak Kapha	Unhappiness, depression, sorrow, insomnia, anger, fear, anxiety, attachment, dependency, addiction

Modern medicine has developed many new powerful designer drugs that can regulate our brain chemistry and make us feel better, that in Ayurvedic parlance can artificially manipulate our Tarpak Kapha. Chemical drugs, both medicinal and recreational, affect Tarpak Kapha, our brain's Soma in various ways, stimulating it or sedating it. Such drugs include antidepressants, analgesics, and sleeping pills, on the medicinal side, and narcotics, intoxicants and psychedelics on the recreational side, though there is some crossover of these types of drugs and their usage, with opiates being a good example.

Taking such medications, we come to rely upon the external drug for the secretions of our own Tarpak Kapha or inner Soma. The result is that our brain gradually stops secreting its own Tarpak Kapha and relies upon the drug instead. A similar process occurs with any form of addiction. Our own Tarpak Kapha shuts down in favor of an external essence, stimulant or sugar that serves to calm, sedate or entertain us instead. To gain control of our own lives and destiny, we need to develop our own Tarpak Kapha so that we can access contentment within and need no external drugs to do so. This is what Yoga and Ayurveda help us to do. Otherwise our lives will become a pattern of addiction leading to long-term depletion and despair, not only at a personal but also at a societal level.

The main reflex point for the Tarpak Kapha in the body is the soft palate of the mouth, the same place as the yogic Soma. It connects externally to two *marmas* or energy points, one on either side of the base of the cheek bone called *Shringataka*.[52] It is closely connected to the tongue in terms of the nerves.[53] The tongue is the sense organ that expresses and energizes Tarpak Kapha. The tongue also relates to the *Bodhak Kapha* or the Kapha governing taste and saliva, which develops from Tarpak Kapha.[54]

Longevity depends upon protecting our inner Soma through the right management of Tarpak Kapha, the lunar energy in the brain that manifests through the soft palate of the mouth. If we meditate or hold our awareness on the soft palate, we can create an enduring state of inner contentment and allow the nectar of immortality to flow within us.

Our ordinary activity, particularly when emotionally agitated, burns up or dries up this nectar. If our digestive fire is too high, it can also burn it up. If our digestive fire is too low, it can prevent this nectar from properly forming, causing its energy to become heavy and congested. Stress that stimulates our adrenal glands and fear and flight reactions easily depletes Tarpak Kapha as well. Diabetes is an example of a malady that arises when the Tarpak Kapha is impaired through the digestive system.

Yoga and Ayurveda provide various methods of developing, stimulating and transforming the Tarpak Kapha within us, turning it into a spiritual Soma. On that screen of the inner Soma one can experience the entire universe as a play of one's own consciousness. It is the ultimate media experience compromising time and the timeless, space and the sizeless. Yoga and Ayurveda teach us how to develop our own internal Soma so that we can access the nectar of immortality within our own minds and hearts and need no longer depend upon any external experience for our happiness in life.

Though Ayurvedic herbs and Yoga practices of pranayama, mantra and meditation we can gain mastery over our brain chemistry and make sure that we are developing a divine nectar in life, not a mortal or emotional poison! Unless we gain control over our own brain chemistry and cease to be under the control of external stimuli or drugs, we cannot access the wellsprings of immortality that lie within us. And we must eventually end up in boredom, depression or sorrow.

The true fountain of youth is the flow of Soma in the calm and quiet brain and mind, the flow of Soma and Tarpak Kapha. Only those who have complete stillness within can fully drink of it. Soma requires the right vessel in order to hold it. We must ourselves become a true Soma vessel, which means to make our minds and hearts receptive to the inner flow of grace that lies at the core of our being. Rejuvenation of the body is allied with rejuvenation of the nervous system, brain and mind through Tarpak Kapha. We will discuss methods for developing Agni and Soma, particularly Tarpak Kapha throughout the book.

However, longevity and rejuvenation is not just a matter of information or technique, it requires awakening an inner power, the 'Shakti of rejuvenation', and an inner intelligence, the consciousness of eternity. If that inner power is awakened, rejuvenative practices will be much more effective and guided from within. We cannot find real transformation mechanically. There is no fixed formula for life, creativity or awareness. It is not accessible to any sort of manipulation or self-assertion. Ultimately, a flow of grace is required, which rests upon our ability to honor all life as sacred and to embrace the whole of nature within ourselves.

Spiritual Aspects of Agni and Soma:
Appreciating the Universal Culture

Agni is the striving of the soul upward towards the divine, while Soma represents the descending grace of God. Agni represents our will or aspiration to the truth, while Soma represents what inspires us and also the goal that we seek. That is why Agni or fire is represented by an upward facing triangle, while water or Soma is represented by a triangle that faces downward.

In this regard, Agni represents *Jnana Yoga* or the Yoga of Knowledge, which proceeds through the heat and friction of introspection and self-inquiry. This is the main upward movement of the soul. Similarly, Soma represents *Bhakti Yoga* or the Yoga of Devotion, which proceeds through the flow of surrender. This is the main descending movement of grace.

For both individual and social harmony, we need to honor the sacred presence of Agni and Soma within and around us. These two factors are the basis of the cosmic order that is an offering of the Self to the Self, the Divine to the Divine. In ourselves we need to honor the digestive fire, the fire of Prana, the fire of perception, the fire of the mind and the fire of consciousness itself, not simply as factors of personal well-being but as sacred forces within us. Similarly, we need to honor the corresponding Somas of our foods, air, impressions, ideas and experiences, not simply as means of personal enjoyment but as aspects of the cosmic play of delight.

We should learn to appreciate not only the gross Somas of food and pleasure but also the subtle Somas of art, devotion, perception and meditation. In the outer world, we need to honor the sacred fire in nature, in the rocks, the plants, the day, the Sun and lightning. We need to similarly honor the sacred Soma in the waters, the clouds, the night, the Moon and the stars. The inherent beauty of the universe as a play of consciousness far outweighs our personal sorrows and offers much more satisfaction to our inner being than the achievement of any amount of external wealth or recognition.

Having this reverence for the cosmic powers and the inner Somas is to be truly cultured in the spiritual sense of the term. Our current culture, pursuing sensory and media Somas on the outside, has become vulgar, if not crude. This breeds a certain rudeness that some find fascinating, like movie images of violence and seduction, but does not create finer sensitivities within our hearts or in our nervous systems, much less in our relationships. To be aware of Soma everywhere is to appreciate the culture of the universe, which is a culture of awareness, light, subtlety and mystery.

These two cosmic powers are also the basis of science in all of its forms. We must learn to recognize the subtle Agnis and Somas at a biological level within ourselves and other creatures, which are the basis of our physiological functioning. We must strive to discern these two forces in the realm of physics from the subtle Agnis and Somas at a subatomic level, to those operative at a supragalactic level. The entire universe is the expansion of a primordial explosion of a cosmic fire ball from a point of Soma or pure delight by the power of Agni. To gain our full immortality, we must honor the Soma of the universe and its eternal play of delight. We must learn to consume and digest the entire universe with the fire of knowledge, finding within all things the Soma of endless bliss.

Soma Ayurveda and Soma Yoga

Soma Ayurveda is a name that can be given to this Ayurveda of rejuvenation or rasayana allied with Yoga. It aims at longevity for the body, rejuvenation for the mind, and awakening our inner consciousness allied with the immortality of the soul. It emphasizes Soma increasing practices, therapies, diet and herbs.

Soma Yoga is the name for the corresponding Yoga that aims at developing our inner Soma, particularly through pranayama, mantra and meditation, and unfolding the Soma of the chakras and the spiritual heart.

These two approaches aim not simply at rejuvenation but well-being and harmony of all aspects of our nature and their interface with the corresponding cosmic powers.

Individual Constitution and Rejuvenation: The Role of the Three Doshas

Ayurvedic medicine is the traditional natural healing system of India and the greater Yoga tradition. It provides a complete system of medicine and right living for body and mind rooted in yogic principles and philosophy, including the pursuit of longevity and immortality. The term *Ayur* itself means longevity and *Veda* means knowledge or science. Ayurveda's aim is not simply treating disease but improving both the length and the quality of our lives. Rejuvenation is therefore the ultimate, if not primary concern of all Ayurvedic treatment. Ayurvedic self-care and personal well-being ends up in Ayurvedic Self-care or care of the Divine Self and essence within us.

Ayurveda bases its view of health and disease upon an understanding of the three *doshas* or 'biological humors' of *Vata* (air and energy), *Pitta* (fire and light) and *Kapha* (water and form) and their interactions within us. These doshas themselves are manifestations of the life-force or prana working through the five elements. According to Ayurvedic medicine, the three doshas are responsible for health, disease, longevity and the potential for higher consciousness. They are the key to the movement and evolution of life, reflected through all the forces of nature.

The three doshas are the basis of our biological functioning and govern the different tissues, organs and systems of the body. Most importantly, the doshas provide the foundation for our individual typology, our unique constitution or energetic formation. Each person is usually dominated by one or two of the three doshas as his or her characteristic nature (Prakriti). Understanding the doshas is essential for everyone for health and well-being, just as we should all know what to eat or how to breathe properly. The three doshas are also the foundation for understanding the disease process in a person (Vikriti), which usually involves one of the three doshas becoming excessive.[55] Diseases are nothing but manifestations of doshas out of balance.

Nature of Vata Dosha

Vata, the biological air humor, is the first and foremost of the three doshas as it reflects the Prana or life-force itself. Vata, on the positive side promotes energy, vitality, movement, growth and change. On the negative side, excess Vata causes disequilibrium, degeneration, disease, and the aging process.

Vata's main manifestation is through the nervous system for which it is the activating electrical force, but it provides the motivation and energy for all the systems and organs of the body and their functions. Vata like wind causes dryness, coldness, lightness and mobility in the body. It is stimulating and energizing but can be disturbing and destabilizing.

Psychologically, Vata gives sensitivity, creativity, adaptability, and wide comprehension on the positive side. On the negative side, excess Vata promotes agitation, fear, anxiety and emotional swings.

Vata is the biological manifestation of Prana, the cosmic life-force. It guides and directs the other two doshas that are considered to be lame or incapable of movement without it. Vata is our portion of the cosmic energy. Yet it tends to return to its origin in air and space and is not easily held within the confines of the body.

Vata is the main factor behind both physical and psychological disease. Old age is the Vata time of life, which increases over time. Old age increases Vata qualities of dryness, lightness and instability. Vata causes most of the chronic and debilitating conditions of old age and hastens the aging process. Unless we first understand and learn how to control Vata, it is difficult for any rejuvenation practices to really work.

Nature of Pitta Dosha

Pitta, the biological fire humor, on the positive side promotes digestion, metabolism, light, warmth and luster in the body. On the negative side, it causes heat, inflammation, toxicity, fever and bleeding. Pitta's main manifestation is through the digestive system, of which it is the active force. Pitta causes heat, dampness, lightness and color in the body. It grants motivation and determination but can be harsh and disruptive.

Psychologically, Pitta grants courage, strong will, good intelligence, perception and leadership skills. On the negative side, excess Pitta causes anger, envy, jealousy and aggression, with an overly critical mind.

Pitta is the biological manifestation of Agni, not simply as the digestive fire, but as the cosmic fire and light energy pervading body and mind. Through it we can access the forces of light both within and around us, including fire and the Sun.

Pitta dosha is aligned with the process of cooking, ripening or maturation, which requires heat and light. It governs the mature or adult phase of life from around the age of twenty to that of sixty. Pitta gives us warmth and light but too much Pitta overheats and burns us up. Pitta helps purify us for rejuvenation practices.

Nature of Kapha Dosha

Kapha, the biological water humor, on the positive side promotes proper development of all bodily tissues and fluids, giving lubrication, stability, fertility, and endurance. On the negative side, Kapha causes overweight, accumulation of water, mucus and fat, inhibiting movement and circulation, and blocking perception.

Kapha's main manifestation is through the tissues of the body, particularly the liquids, plasma, fat and reproductive system. Kapha causes dampness, coldness, heaviness, slowness and compactness in the body. It is protective, soothing and nurturing but can become congesting, blocking and inhibiting.

Psychologically, Kapha gives patience, devotion, steadiness and calm on the positive side. On the negative side, excess Kapha results in desire, greed, attachment and clinging to the past.

Kapha is the main manifestation of Soma, or the watery enjoyment factor, in the physical body. It grants us access to the many forms of Soma and water on both lower and higher levels, from food and drinks to love and devotion.

Kapha is the main factor of positive health and longevity and must be sufficient to sustain any process of rejuvenation. Childhood is the Kapha stage of life, in which tissue and mucus production is high. Kapha provides us with endurance, strength and support, but too much Kapha slows and weighs us down and prevents positive change and development.

Your Doshic Type

Determining your doshic type is essential for a deeper examination of Ayurveda. Below is a simple chart for helping you to figure this out. You can consult an Ayurvedic practitioner if you are in doubt as to the outcome.

AYURVEDIC CONSTITUTION CHART[56]

	VATA (Air)	PITTA (Fire)	KAPHA (Water)
Height	tall or very short	medium, average	usually short can be tall and large
Frame	thin, bony	moderate, good muscles	large, well developed
Weight	low, hard to hold weight	moderate	heavy, hard to lose weight
Skin Luster	dull or dusky	ruddy, lustrous	white or pale
Skin Texture	dry, rough, thin	warm, oily	cold, damp, thick
Eyes	small, nervous	piercing, easily	large, inflamed
Hair	dry, thin	thin, oily	thick, oily, wavy, lustrous
Teeth	crooked, poorly formed	moderate, bleeding gums	large, well formed
Nails	rough, brittle	soft, pink	soft, white
Joints	stiff, crack easily	loose	firm, large
Circulation	poor, variable	good	moderate
Appetite	variable, nervous	high, excessive	moderate but constant
Thirst	low, scanty	high	moderate

	VATA (Air)	PITTA (Fire)	KAPHA (Water)
Sweating	scanty	profuse but not enduring	low to start but profuse
Stool	hard or dry	soft, loose	normal
Urination	scanty	profuse, yellow	moderate, clear
Sensitivities	cold, dryness, wind	heat, sunlight, fire	cold, dampness
Immune Function	low, variable	moderate, sensitive to heat	high, slow
Disease Tendency	pain	fever	congestion, inflammation edema
Disease Type	nervous	blood, liver	mucous, lungs
Activity	high, restless	moderate	low, moves slowly
Endurance	poor, easily exhausted	moderate but focused	high, steady
Sleep	poor, disturbed	variable	excess
Dreams	frequent	moderate, disturbed	infrequent, colorful, romantic
Memory	quick but absent-minded	sharp, clear	slow but steady
Speech	fast, frequent	sharp, cutting	slow, melodious
Temperament	nervous, changeable	motivated	content, conservative
Positive Emotions	adaptability	courage	love
Negative Emotions	fear	anger	attachment
Faith	variable, erratic	strong, determined	steady, slow to change
TOTAL	**Vata**	**Pitta**	**Kapha**

Note the total number of items you have checked from the total of thirty. The dosha with the highest number will likely be your main doshic type. If you have two doshas in relative balance, you are likely a dual or two dosha types. It does rarely occur that a person has all three doshas in relatively equal proportion. In these cases, we usually aim at treating the dosha that is most out of balance within us or most active seasonally.[57]

Rejuvenation, Longevity and the Balance of the Three Doshas

Longevity depends upon the proper balance and function of all three doshas, but has specific doshic ramifications as well.

- Kapha dosha individuals normally have the best longevity of the doshic types as Kapha provides a good bodily structure, well-developed tissues and endurance to resist the damaging influences of time and the disease process.

- Vata dosha types normally have the shortest longevity as Vata causes dryness and depletion of bodily tissues that reduces resistance to disease factors and weakens overall immunity.

- Pitta dosha people have medium longevity, with a good digestive power to sustain positive health but suffer from tissue damage, inflammation, and infection through excess heat and aggression.

Dual doshic types have their special longevity considerations as well. Pitta-Kapha types usually have a good longevity, combining the endurance of Kapha with the warmth of Pitta. Vata-Kapha types have challenges owing to their tendency to suffer from cold-natured diseases and a lack motivation. Vata-Pitta types, though usually highly intelligent, are limited by their lack of Kapha, which allows them to easily burn themselves out. Yet we usually treat dual types according to the dosha that is most out of balance within them at any particular time or season.

This means that rejuvenation therapies are primarily anti-Vata in nature and promote the development Kapha dosha, yet secondarily aiming at reducing Pitta as well. They include a nutritive diet, cool, moist and nutritive herbs, adequate rest and relaxation, stillness, reduction of activity, letting go of stress and reduced stimulation.

Rejuvenation is most connected with Kapha dosha, which as the biological water humor, provides for nourishment, growth, calm and contentment of body and mind. Kapha reflects the cool watery energy of the Moon that is the force of Soma. Proper Kapha is necessary for rejuvenation, which means not only avoiding an excess of the other two doshas, but keeping healthy Kapha in balance as well. This requires control of weight and avoiding the accumulation of mucus in the body, which means maintaining good exercise and activity patterns.

Rejuvenation therapies work to build a subtler, lighter, cleaner and more sattvic (pure) form of Kapha, using sattvic, natural and light substances in diet and herbs. Heavier forms of Kapha including heavy foods, sedentary life-style and self-indulgence are not helpful. In addition, rejuvenation therapies work to sustain and regulate the Agni or the digestive fire for overall metabolic balance. In this regard, the doshic ability to apply rejuvenation therapies must be considered.

- Kapha dosha people are usually the poorest at implementing positive health therapies because they are slow to change, tend towards lethargy and find it hard to let go of bad habits. However, once they adopt a positive therapy they are also best at continuing it, as they are steady, patient and enduring in what they do.

- Vata constitution people are initially good at adapting positive health therapies, as they are creative and open to new ways and methods, liking change and experimentation. However, they lack consistency in maintaining therapies over a long period of time as they tend to be impatient, expect quick results and get easily distracted by new options.

- Pitta type people can be good at implementing positive health therapies and determined to pursue them as they have a strong motivation, focus and concentration in what they decide to do. Their main limitation is that they can be fanatics or use too much personal effort and strain. They do not always choose the right therapies to follow. Their success depends upon the right balance of effort and grace.

While Vata people have the lowest physical longevity potential in terms of the strength of their bodily tissues, they also have the greatest capacity of change and so can adjust their life-styles as needed, giving them the best ability to implement rejuvenation therapies.

While Kapha people have the greatest physical longevity potential in terms of their bodily tissues, they are the slowest to correct wrong habits and adapt better life-styles, meaning that they can lack the will to apply their rejuvenation potential for its best results.

While Pitta people have a medium physical longevity potential in terms of their bodily tissues, they are the most intelligent and determined in applying positive health therapies once they learn them in the right manner, giving them a good capacity for rejuvenation as well. In short, doshic potentials must be judged relative to both body and mind and each doshic type has its strengths and weaknesses relative to longevity.

- *Kapha people have the best longevity potential but only if they control their weight.* Overall, excess body weight is worse than deficient body weight for longevity, a fact that Kapha people should not forget. This does not mean that they should aim to be skinny and anorexic but that they have to avoid obesity.

- Vata people have a good longevity potential if they develop the proper nutrition to support their activities, but they must do so in a consistent and regular manner.

- Pitta people have a good longevity potential if they follow the right therapy and don't go to any extremes, not overheating their systems.

If we look at the world of nature, we find that among the oldest plants in the world are Bristlecone pines. These live in high mountains in the Southwest United States, in near tree line conditions of low moisture and high wind; what is essentially a strongly Vata dosha climate. These trees are also Vata in nature, growing in irregular and gnarled forms, with little sap flowing in their bark. Yet because they have adapted to the Vata energy of their environment they can survive for long periods of time.

The coastal redwoods in California, on the other hand, which also live very long, show an opposite type adaptation. These are Kapha in form, being large in size and girth and able to hold much water in their tissues. They grow in very Kapha climates of heavy rainfall and nearly constant damp fog along the Pacific coast.

Both types of trees show how longevity can be gained by adapting to the environment. We must not forget these examples from the natural world in looking at human health. Each doshic type has its strengths and weaknesses that we can learn to benefit from.

Doshic Caused Factors of Aging

Each of the three doshas in excess promotes the aging process according to its inherent qualities. Make sure to avoid increasing these in your own life-style.

- Vata-Caused Factors of Disease and Aging

- Coldness and dryness, lack of nutrition, excess movement, depletion of the tissues, lack of sleep and rest, exposure to wind and temperature changes, worry, fear, anxiety, and insomnia, lack of emotional support and peace of mind, irregular life-style habits.

- Kapha-Caused Factors of Disease and Aging

- Coldness and dampness, overweight, clogging of the channels, accumulation of mucus, water retention and edema, excess eating, lack of exercise, too much sleep (particularly during the day), greed, attachment, lack of motivation, discipline and effort, lax life style habits.

- Pitta-Caused Factors of Disease and Aging

- Exposure to excess heat, fire and light, too high appetite, toxic blood, infections, inflammation, fevers, anger, aggression, overly critical mind, overheated emotions, compulsive need to control and dominate, inability to relax or let go, overly assertive life-style habits.

Doshic Caused Factors of Longevity

Each dosha in its proper and balanced condition promotes longevity and positive health. Make sure to seek to increase these in your own life-style.

Vata-Caused Factors of Longevity and Rejuvenation

Ability to connect with Prana or creative energy, adaptability, flexibility, willingness to change, enthusiasm, creativity, ability to forget and detach.

Pitta-Caused Factors of Longevity and Rejuvenation

Ability to connect with the Cosmic Agni or power of light, strong digestion, warmth, light, perception, friendliness, clarity, discrimination.

Kapha-Caused Factors of Longevity and Rejuvenation

Ability to connect with the Cosmic Soma or forces of cohesion, strong bodily tissues, endurance, patience, consistency, faith, devotion, contentment.

The Three Doshas in the Aging Process

Your particular doshic type is an important consideration for any therapies you may choose to undergo, which must be adjusted accordingly. Any rejuvenation procedure should consider one's doshic type and work on balancing it as part of the overall treatment.

Vatas are the main doshic types that most benefit from tonification and rejuvenation practices. They need deeper nourishment rather than detoxification. Yet everyone needs some degree of rejuvenation which increases the older that we get. Vata dosha accumulates with the aging process as our bodily tissues and fluids become depleted. Yet the negative aspect of all the doshas tends to increase with age as our immune system declines and our digestive power weakens, particularly the dosha of our constitutional type. Note the following factors of doshic based aging and how they may impact your constitution.

DOSHIC ASPECTS IN THE AGING PROCESS

Vata	Pitta	Kapha
Low body weight, irregular weight gain	Average body weight, moderate weight gain	Excess body weight, obesity
Variable or nervous digestion	Excess appetite	Steady appetite
High metabolism	Medium metabolism	Slow metabolism
Dry or cracked skin	Red or inflamed skin, skin rashes	Thick skin, skin growths
Weak bones and joints	Toxic blood	Excess fat and water
Constipation, bloating	Acidity	Congestion
Weakness of the nervous system	Weakness of the liver and gall bladder	Weakness of the lungs and lymphatic system
Loss of hearing	Loss of sight	Loss of sense of taste, excess salivation
Excess bodily movement	Medium bodily movement	Lack of bodily movement
Instability, tremors	Red discolorations, inflammations, intolerance of light	Inertia, lethargy
Lack of sleep, insomnia	Disturbed sleep	Excess sleep, lethargy
Arthritis	Hypertension	Heart disease
Loss of memory	Crankiness	Dullness and non-responsiveness
Nervous sensitivity	Mental reactiveness	Emotional torpor
Fear, anxiety	Anger, irritability	Attachment, greed
Erratic behavior	Obsessions and compulsions	Lack of motivation
Debility conditions	Chronic infections and inflammation	Mucus congestion and water retention

Vata	Pitta	Kapha
Sensitivity to cold and wind	Sensitivity to heat, fire and light	Sensitivity to coldness and dampness
Wind based diseases	Fire based diseases	Mucus based diseases

Doshic Sites of Accumulation and the Disease Process

The three doshas have their respective sites of accumulation in the body where they breed disease and from which they spread to the rest of the body, damaging its various tissues and organs. Ayurveda works to prevent the doshas from accumulating at these three locations, and also to remove them from the body from these three sites as well.

• Kapha and the Stomach

Kapha's main site of accumulation is in the stomach, from which as mucus it overflows into the plasma, lymphatic system, lungs, chest, heart, head, and body as a whole, causing various Kapha diseases. Such conditions include nausea, frequent or chronic colds and flu, allergies, edema, asthma, diabetes and heart disease. Preventing Kapha from accumulating in the stomach inhibits the disease process and reduces premature aging.

• Pitta Dosha and the Small Intestine

Pitta's main site of accumulation is the small intestine, from which as toxic heat or toxic blood it overflows into the blood, liver, heart, sweat glands and body as a whole, causing various Pitta diseases. Such conditions include hyperacidity, fever, bleeding disorders, skin diseases, liver diseases and hypertension. Preventing Pitta from accumulating in the small intestine inhibits the disease process and reduces premature aging.

• Vata Dosha and the Large Intestine

Vata's main site of accumulation is in the large intestine, particularly the colon, from which as dryness and toxic gas, it overflows into the bones, joints, nervous system, bladder and body as a whole, causing various Vata diseases. Such conditions are bloating, constipation, insomnia, arthritis, tremors, and nervous debility. Preventing Vata from accumulating in the large intestine inhibits the disease process and reduces premature aging.

Of these three factors of doshic accumulation, the accumulation of Vata dosha in the large intestine and its overflow into the deeper tissues is most detrimental toward health and longevity. It is most allied with the forces of gravity, entropy and decay. It is a common occurrence during old age, the Vata stage of life.

Broader Usage of Ayurvedic Rejuvenation Therapies

Ayurvedic rejuvenation therapies are not only of great value for the middle-aged or the elderly. They have a broad relevance for treating a wide variety of diseases of all ages, particularly severe, chronic and debilitating diseases of both body and mind. They are essential to the recovery phase of disease in general and so form the last phase of many Ayurvedic treatments. All of us of whatever age or condition can benefit from some degree of rejuvenation and restoration of our energies.

- Rejuvenative therapies can be very helpful for childhood diseases, such as a rejuvenative diet and herbs for children suffering from malnutrition or poor growth and development, particularly of the muscles, reproductive and nervous systems.

- Rejuvenation therapies cross over with therapies to treat patients in convalescence or recovery from serious diseases, including febrile diseases that burn up the body fluids or damage the lungs, or diseases and injuries that result in blood loss.

- Rejuvenative therapies are important for reproductive system disorders associated with sexual debility, infertility and impotence.

- Rejuvenation therapy can be a helpful support in the treatment of chronic and degenerative diseases of all types like heart disease, diabetes, epilepsy, asthma, arthritis, cancer and Aids.

• Rejuvenative therapies are excellent for treating all low energy conditions, whether caused by short-term overwork or long-term depletion. This includes all diseases of the immune system, nervous debility and chronic fatigue. Psychologically, it extends to depression and loss of attention that lower our mental and emotional energy levels.

Rejuvenation therapy is gaining particular importance as our population suffers from more and more diseases of depletion of energy caused by our stressful and high tech life-styles and environments. In addition, rejuvenative therapies promote positive health, strengthen immunity and improve performance in sports for those seeking to improve their energy levels. Rejuvenative therapies provide a good basis for any deeper Yoga practice and development of the subtle energies of the psyche. *In short, rejuvenation therapy (rasayana) is the essence of all wellness therapies and all therapies that aim at improving our nutrition, vitality and level of awareness.*

PRANA, TEJAS AND OJAS: THE MASTER OR SOMA FORMS OF THE DOSHAS

The three doshas of Vata, Pitta and Kapha are portrayed in a negative light in Ayurveda relative to their disease causing-consequences. This is because when the doshas become excessive they set in motion the disease process. However, the three doshas do have positive implications and in their proper function serve to sustain positive health and well-being. This beneficial role of the doshas is best revealed by the factors of *Ojas*, *Tejas* and *Prana*, the subtle counterparts of Kapha, Pitta and Vata doshas.

Ojas, Tejas and Prana are the master forms of the doshas that sustain overall organic harmony immunity and longevity. They uphold the body from within, just as food, water and air uphold the body from the outside.

- Ojas, which means strength, is our inmost vital fluid essence, the subtle form of Kapha dosha, the biological water humor. Eight drops of Ojas in the heart are said to sustain us at an inner level, though its influence pervades the entire body. Ojas is closely connected to brain activities and our mental and emotional balance, calm and vigor.

- Tejas, which means radiance, is our inmost vital fire, the subtle form of Pitta dosha, the biological fire humor, particularly as the fire of the prana, emotions, senses and mind. It provides light, warmth, color, motivation and determination to all our efforts and actions.

- Prana, which indicates the primary life-force, is our inmost vital energy, the subtle form of Vata dosha, the biological air humor. It is the master form of life energy or

Prana behind our physical, vital, mental and emotional functions, affording them impetus, movement, adaptability and balance.

Ojas is more specifically connected to Soma and Kapha dosha, as these three powers are interrelated subtle essences; however, we can also speak of Prana, Tejas and Ojas as aspects of Soma and as the 'Soma essences of the three doshas' of Vata, Pitta and Kapha.[58]

Prana, Ojas, Tejas and Prana can be added to the seven dhatus or tissues (plasma, blood, muscle, fat, bone, nerve and reproductive) as the main factors that make up and support our bodily existence.[59] They can be looked upon as the three factors of our subtle or energy body behind the physical.

1. **Plasma** – nourishes and hydrates all the tissues.

2. **Blood** – warms, oxygenates and brings Prana to all the tissues.

3. **Muscle** – gives strength and stability to the body.

4. **Fat** – cushions and protects the body.

5. **Bone** – provides structure and support.

6. **Nerve and Marrow** – guiding intelligence and enervation.

7. **Reproductive** – capacity for procreation, enjoyment and rejuvenation

8. **Ojas** – sustains immunity, endurance and contentment.

9. **Tejas** – gives vitality, warmth and luster.

10. **Prana** – gives healing, adaptability and creativity.

Ojas is said to be the essence of the seven tissues of the body, like an eighth tissue element, specifically the essence of the seventh or subtlest tissue, the reproductive tissue, with which its functions are closely associated. Tejas and Prana are regarded as the ninth and tenth such supportive factors, though unlike Ojas, which has a fluidic nature, do not have material forms.

Tejas and Ojas reflect the cosmic forms of fire and water that exist in the world of nature and can be found in our deeper psyche. Prana is a result of their union and balance.

- Ojas reflects the Cosmic Soma or universal power of cohesion, attraction and nourishment in the cosmic waters and in all gravitational and magnetic energies.

- Tejas reflects the Cosmic Agni or universal power of fire and light shining everywhere along with its heating, ripening, coloring and illuminating powers.

- Prana reflects the Cosmic Vayu or universal energy, the subtle electrical currents at work everywhere in the universe, causing the stars and planets to revolve in their orbits, and stimulating life at a biological level.

Prana, Tejas and Ojas are aligned with the *subdoshas*, or subtypes of Vata, Pitta and Kapha, which reflect the health sustaining functions of the doshas, particularly the subdoshas active in the brain.

- Prana connects to the subdosha of *Prana Vayu* that is the form of Vata dosha governing the head, brain and nervous system and the intake of nutrients and energy through the mind, senses, breath and mouth.

- Tejas connects to the subdosha of *Sadhak Pitta*, which is the form of Pitta governing the brain, nervous system, perception, reason, logic, discrimination and judgment.

- Ojas connects to the subdoshas of *Tarpak Kapha*, which is the form of Kapha governing the brain and nervous system and their secretions, lubrication, stability, harmony and contentment.

Ojas, Tejas and Prana are closely aligned with sexual vitality. Prana and Tejas, like Ojas, are rooted in the reproductive system, its tissue, secretions and functions. That is why sexual debility or exhaustion can weaken our health overall. Ojas reflects our basic reproductive vital energy reserve. Tejas is the warmth, drive, passion and aggression that arises from Ojas. Prana reflects its creative energy and vitalizing effect.

Ojas, Tejas and Prana are ultimately rooted in the heart that is our primary source of vitality and our connection with the soul or immortal consciousness within us. Prana provides energy and functional power to the heart. Tejas provides it warmth and radiance, including its heat giving functions through the blood. Ojas reflects the hearts underlying energy reserve, strength capacity and endurance.

Ojas, Tejas and Prana are the basis of our immune system. Ojas is our basic power of immunity, our ability to ward off disease.[60] Tejas is our ability to activate the immune force, which largely occurs through the body's fever response. Prana is our capacity for deep healing after recovering from acute diseases.

Tejas and Ojas are opposite as fire and water, male and female energies. Ojas is sometimes said to provide power in the hips and legs and Tejas in the arms and hands. They also connect to the solar and lunar currents, the Pingala and Ida of yogic thought. Prana is the background force behind Tejas and Ojas, at once their result and their origin.

Ojas, Tejas and Prana are the higher energies that we seek to develop in Yoga practice. They not only improve health and well-being but set in motion our higher consciousness and deeper feeling nature. They provide us the strength to handle the currents of spiritual energy that Yoga connects us to.

Prana	Tejas	Ojas
Positive side of Vata dosha	Positive side of Pitta dosha	Positive side of Kapha dosha
Prana Vayu	Sadhak Pitta	Tarpak Kapha
Vayu – Cosmic energy	Agni – Cosmic light	Soma – Cosmic harmony
Vital Energy	Vital Warmth and Radiance	Vital Endurance

Prana	Tejas	Ojas
Power of the breath	Power of perception	Power of consistency
Lightness and ease of movement	Light and illumination	Strength and steadiness
Expansiveness	Clarity	Stability and composure
Adaptability, creativity	Fearlessness, courage	Patience, fortitude
Ability to heal from chronic diseases	Ability to fight acute diseases	Strength of the immune system
Tolerance, ability to understand a number of points of view	Good perception and discrimination	Loyalty, faith and devotion
Rejuvenating Prana	Rejuvenating heat and light	Rejuvenating fluids

Ojas, Tejas and Prana, Yoga and Rejuvenation

Rejuvenation depends upon developing more of Ojas, Tejas and Prana as positive energies while reducing the doshas of Kapha, Pitta and Vata as factors of disease, decay and the aging process. *We could say that Prana, Tejas and Ojas are the rejuvenative forms of Vata, Pitta and Kapha dosha, which in turn are the disease-causing aspects of Prana, Tejas and Ojas.*

Rejuvenation depends upon developing more Ojas, Tejas and Prana but in an integral and balanced manner. This requires first developing the proper Ojas. Ojas is the key to Tejas and Prana as well. Soma develops primarily out of Ojas and Ojas develops out of Soma. Both are aspects of the same nutritive lunar energy. Plants and foods that increase Ojas, such as we will discuss in the next chapters, also can increase our inner Soma.

Prana, Tejas and Ojas are closely interrelated and depend upon one another. Ojas provides the fuel for the fire of Tejas and the sustenance for the energy of Prana. Prana and Tejas arise out of Ojas and rely upon it for their proper development. This means *of these three factors, Ojas is the most important, as Tejas and Prana require the support of Ojas to keep them at a positive level of functioning.*

The aging process depletes the seven tissues, starting with drying up of the plasma and its nutrient essences. It also weakens Ojas. However, Tejas and Prana can increase in a positive way if one lives a spiritual life, but they become more difficult to ground in the body. Only if Ojas is sufficient will Prana and Tejas stay in the physical body. For rejuvenation and for opening up deeper spiritual energies, we must learn to create more Ojas, Tejas and Prana.

Developing Prana, Tejas and Ojas[61]

- To develop Ojas requires emotional calm and balance in life, a strong psychological immunity as it were, which does not react to the fluctuations of pleasure and pain, success and failure in life but remains steady and composed within. Ojas is aided by steadiness of mind, consistency of motivation, and the ability to master our impulses in life. It requires that we do not drain away our energy through the senses or motor organs. Ojas develops through self-control and also through the power of devotion and calm meditation. A yogic lifestyle and dharmic values provide a field in which Ojas can grow and develop.

- Ojas is supported by good nutrition (a yogic and Ayurvedic diet), rejuvenating tonic herbs (like ashwagandha, shatavari and bala), adequate rest and deep sleep. It is fostered by attitudes of love, faith, devotion, compassion, forgiveness, peace and silence, particularly the Yoga of Devotion or Bhakti Yoga. One can also draw in Ojas from the Earth, waters, mountains and rocks.

- Tejas can be developed through yogic practices like mantra, concentration, especially fixing the gaze, and by inquiry, the Yoga of Knowledge or Jnana Yoga. Certain fiery or spicy herbs and nervines like calamus, sage and tulsi can increase it. One can draw in Tejas from the Sun, fire or other natural light sources. Certain heating forms of pranayama are helpful like right nostril breathing. Practice of tapas, self-discipline, and occasional fasting are good as well.

Prana can be developed through the practice of pranayama overall, particularly types of pranayama that are slow, deep, calming and nourishing and help develop the unitary prana within us. It can be increased through accessing the cosmic Prana through the plants, water, Earth, wind, stars and sky. One can draw Prana in from the lightning and the electrical energy flowing everywhere in nature, and through meditation on space or the void. Certain herbs that contain air and ether like brahmi and manduka parni are helpful.

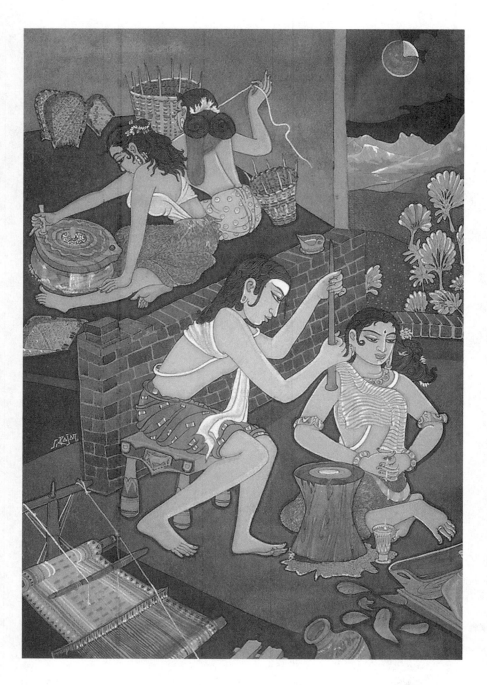

Preparing the Soma

PART II

Soma Ayurveda:

Physical Rejuvenation and Longevity through Ayurveda

The Gods starting with Brahma, the Creator, created at first the Soma nectar for the elimination of old age and death.

Sushrut Samhita Chikitsasthana XXIX.2

From rejuvenation (rasayana) arises longevity, good memory, wisdom, health, youth, lustrous complexion, excellence of voice, strength of the body and senses of the highest order, power of speech, respect and beauty.

Charak Samhita Chikitsasthana I. 7-8

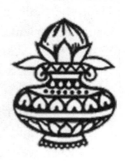

The Soma of Food:
Diet for Yoga and Longevity

Appropriate diet means moist and sweet vegetarian food, leaving one-quarter of the stomach free, and taken as an offering to the Lord as Shiva.

Hatha Yoga Pradipika I.58

Physical well-being depends upon the proper food. One cannot change the nature and function of the body without a corresponding change in diet. Exercise and herbs can be of great help but without a proper diet to back them up will lack the foundation to have a transformative effect. Unless we address our diet first of all, it is difficult to benefit from other health-promoting practices. Even the mind is greatly impacted by our eating habits and cannot be successfully treated without dietary changes. Yet while right diet is the foundation for rejuvenation of the body and mind, without the proper herbs, pranayama and deeper yogic practices to go along with it, it is also not complete.

The right food sustains our life but the wrong food weakens our vitality, promotes disease and can eventually kill us. Disease is as much a product of wrong diet as health is of right diet. The effects of wrong diet, however, may not manifest for some years or even decades, so that it is often difficult to know the consequences of the types of food that we have taken in. Yet right diet is not just a matter of the particular food items we happen to ingest. It implies right eating habits and attitudes, not overeating or undereating, and gaining the right taste or rasa from what we imbibe. Only when we touch the sacred essence in food, in which eating becomes a ritual, sacrament or communion with the cosmos, will the real Soma of food be felt by us.

Food is our main Soma or source of enjoyment for the physical body. Eating is our favorite physical pastime, starting from infancy to old age, an attitude that we share with the entire animal kingdom. We all have our favorite foods or physical Somas, particularly as desserts or sweets to finish off and highlight the meal. However, many of our prime enjoyment foods do not possess good nutritional qualities. We could describe them as 'low quality Somas' that weaken and deplete us in the long run. We also have gourmet food items, such as found in great restaurants, which like the beauty of great art, have a higher aesthetic or Soma value. Yet even these can prove unhealthy, like a surfeit of fine wines and cheeses! However, there are many high quality natural foods that increase the Somas or vital juices of the body and help promote well-being rejuvenation in a lasting manner. Such 'food Somas' form the basis for 'herbal Somas', which are highly nutritive and tonic herbs that constitute a deeper form of food or nutrition.

Different individuals may find that different diets work better for them. These may reflect their constitution, life-style or habituation patterns. It also depends upon the kind of Somas that we are seeking in life. In this regard, we should seek the type of food that sustains the highest Soma or elevation of mind and heart possible for us. This implies food that promotes a greater acuity of the senses, depth of feeling and power of perception.

Light but Nutritive Diet

Longevity depends upon only being present lightly in the body, not weighed down by body consciousness and its inertia but allowing the spirit to freely move within us. This requires a nourishing diet but one that is not too heavy. The diet should also be supplemented with good herbs, pranayama and meditation for deeper levels of energy.

Excess eating is probably the first dietary habit that promotes the aging process, particularly if the foods involved are heavy, oily, very sweet or hard to digest. Light eating, particularly of natural food items, promotes longevity unless one is not eating adequate amounts. Excess eating produces excess weight that clogs and congests the body and slows down our movement, metabolism and perception. This weakens immunity, longevity and enthusiasm in life. It promotes many degenerative diseases like heart disease, diabetes, asthma, arthritis and cancer.

Often we combine excess eating along with the taking in of low quality food items. The use of too much sugar, salt, oily and fried foods, refined flour, and processed food items –what increase *Ama*, or internal toxins in Ayurvedic thought – all contribute to the aging process and to disease in general. This includes fast food and junk food, and the general tendency of the modern diet in which few people cook and most of the diet consists of processed food items.

The rampant overweight and obesity in modern society is a sign that the overall longevity is likely to decrease, or at least the quality of our energy in life is bound to be reduced. It is a reflection of our sedentary and spectator way of life in which we seek to find our Soma outside ourselves and apart from our own creative activity. To develop a higher quality of bodily tissue, which rejuvenation implies, requires that we do not accumulate unhealthy or unnecessary weight. An overweight body hides nutritional deficiencies and weakness of the muscles, organs and tissues. It is the ideal place for disease to develop.

Yet an overly thin or anorexic body will not promote longevity either. It causes ungroundedness, dryness and debility, disturbing the mind and the nervous system. The goal is not to lose weight for appearance purposes but to have a good quality of tissue in the body, energy in the prana and attention in the mind. One must have the proper weight relative to one's body type, which is a little stocky for Kapha, average for Pitta, and a little thin for Vata, but not too extreme for any type. As we age, we naturally tend to hold more weight, which is not entirely bad. Such extra padding of maturity, however, should not be allowed to develop into real obesity.

The type of food we enjoy reflects the type of Soma we are seeking in life. Some individuals, like certain artists, intellectuals or yogis, have little regard for food-based Somas because they are seeking Somas at a subtler level. Other people seek the Soma of food to compensate for a lack of love (Soma) in relationship or success in life. Yet to maximize whatever we wish to accomplish, a proper diet is helpful, particularly one that is allied with long-term rejuvenative effects.

Yogic Sattvic Diet and Ayurvedic Rejuvenative Diet

A yogic diet is described in many Yoga texts including the *Hatha Yoga Pradipika*.[62] It consists of good quality vegetarian food, including dairy products, whole grains, beans, vegetables, fruit and nuts. This is called a 'sattvic diet' as it increases *sattva* or the quality of purity and clarity in the mind. The rejuvenative diet, such as found in Ayurveda is similar to the sattvic yogic diet, but usually emphasizes the nutritive side of the vegetarian diet, with special care to reduce Vata dosha.

Vegetarian food holds the power of prana, the cosmic life-force, in which immortality resides. Meat items, derived from killing a creature, carry an energy of death and communicate this to the cells of our body, promoting degenerative processes within us. In eating killed and dead food, we are also teaching our body to die. In eating vegetarian food we uphold the energy of life.

However, both Yogic and Ayurvedic diets, particularly on the rejuvenative side, do give importance to dairy products. Dairy products are used in the preparation of Ayurvedic rejuvenative herbs as well. Milk in particular can help increase the Ojas or primary vital force that rejuvenation rests upon. Yet only natural and organic dairy products have this value, meaning those that are produced along with a proper care of the cow. Dairy products produced by modern factory farming and its cruel methods can prove harmful. They can promote the energy of death by holding the negative emotions of the mistreated animals, not to mention the chemicals and pollutants that their tissues hold.

While a rejuvenative diet is vegetarian, not all vegetarian food is necessarily rejuvenative for everyone, though it may have other health providing effects. Vegetarian items that are light, drying, reducing or diuretic are not usually rejuvenative, which includes certain beans, cabbage family plants and many greens. The main vegetarian items that are aid in rejuvenation are fruits, seeds and nuts, whole grains and heavier root vegetables.

Ayurveda holds that the fresh juice of plants has the greatest capacity for rejuvenation. This is particularly true of fruit juices. Vegetable juices have strong healing powers, no doubt, and can be rejuvenating in small amounts, but in large amounts are usually more detoxifying. They can help remove Ama or the disease causing toxins from the body, so that rejuvenation can be more effective.

Vegetable juices, particularly of the green variety, have their main healing effects on Kapha and Pitta doshas, for whom detoxification is usually more important than rejuvenation. However, they are not usually effective for Vata dosha types, who need heavier grounding foods and are the main doshic type needing rejuvenation. Vegetable juices and raw vegetables, particularly greens, serve mainly a supplementary role in rejuvenation and are more properly for detoxification, and if taken in excess can be depleting or disturbing to Vata dosha.

Raw vegetables and greens do carry large amounts of Prana, but for this to be truly rejuvenating we need Ojas increasing foods like dairy, nuts, grains and root vegetables to ground and hold that prana. This means that the Ayurvedic rejuvenation diet is not simply a raw food diet, much less a raw juice or green juice diet. Most raw vegetables and green juices predominate in astringent and bitter tastes, which are reducing to our weight and our bodily fluids. They are often diuretic in effect and have a drying effect upon the tissues. While this can be beneficial for reducing toxins and cleansing the blood and lymphatic systems, it is not helpful in building up the tissues and bodily fluids that have become depleted.

We may think that raw food approaches are rejuvenating because in removing toxins they make us feel better. This is why raw food diets can be helpful for diseases like cancer, in which there is an excess of tissue formation of a toxic nature. As most people today tend to be overweight, such reducing diets may give them more energy and make them feel better and may be quite necessary, but for those of low body weight or high Vata dosha, living in cold climates or the winter season, or those who are elderly and weak, these diets can be debilitating.

However a predominately raw food diet for a short period can be helpful as a preliminary purification diet to prepare the body for rejuvenation. A certain amount of raw food in the diet, around ten to twenty percent, is also necessary for health maintenance and providing the minerals that we need, more so in the late spring and summer when such food items are fresh. Sprouts are also good for raw food supplementation. As part of a larger rejuvenative diet such raw food items have their place but in a secondary way.

Besides raw food diets there are vegan approaches, which avoid dairy as well as animal products, but that use cooked food in the diet, particularly soy and brown rice. Vegan diets can be useful for health and longevity, particularly for people who do not have the ethnic background to benefit from dairy products, especially if they are Kapha types. But for those who can benefit from dairy products, like most Vata and Pitta types, Ayurveda does not consider that vegan diets are the best way to go.

I have observed that a number of Yoga centers and alternative health centers in the West emphasize a raw food or vegan diet, and consider it to be good for long-term health maintenance, if not rejuvenation. They may dismiss dairy products in any form as unhealthy. They tend to reduce or avoid salt, sugar, spices, wheat and other foods commonly involved in food allergies. They are likely to promote soy products or a macrobiotic approach. They seldom examine the traditional yogic and Ayurvedic wisdom about food.

We do note that some Yogis, particularly in the Himalayas, can live on prana alone and do not need much by way of solid food. Others can live on Prana along with a diet of wild plants, leaves, herbs, roots and berries. This is because their Agni or digestive fire has become very powerful through their yogic disciplines, particularly pranayama. Yet such Yogis are quite exceptional and may not be a good model to emulate, particularly those who have a weak digestion, poor immunity or low body weight, notably Vata type individuals, especially when they may need to do physical work or face the stress of the modern work field.

More commonly in India, Yogis live on whole grains, mung and other dals (beans), milk, ghee and dairy products, particularly in the winter, which is a safer grounding and nutritive diet. Many traditional Yoga centers in India have their own cows and their own fruit, herb and vegetable gardens to assure a high quality of food items.

GUIDELINES FOR AN AYURVEDIC REJUVENATIVE DIET

Below are some Ayurvedic dietary guidelines for rejuvenation, but remember that these rules must be applied on an individual basis. They are suggestions, rather than rigid prescriptions. They need to be adjusted relative to climate, season and geographical setting, emphasizing freshly produced and freshly cooked items.

In addition, these diets rest upon prior purification of the body and are best taken up if we have already done internal cleansing and developed a good Agni or digestive fire. For this reason, a rejuvenative diet usually includes mild spices for promoting Agni. If one is overweight or has a body filled with toxins, one may not be ready for a rejuvenation diet, and should begin with a reducing approach, in which raw foods, fasting and stronger exercise can be helpful.

Generally speaking, the ordinary Ayurvedic diet prescribed according to one's doshic type has long-term rejuvenative effects, though mild in nature. Rejuvenative food items can be added to one's ordinary diet as nutritional and energy supplements. Special strict rejuvenative diets are followed for shorter periods of time, usually one to three months. For longer rejuvenation practices, it is a matter of the predomination of the foods that we take in, so more latitude in the diet is allowed.

Use of the Six Tastes

Ayurveda recognizes the existence of six primary food tastes – sweet, salty, sour, pungent, bitter and astringent – with their corresponding qualities and effects. We all need all six tastes in our diet for balanced nutrition. However, three tastes tend to increase and three tastes tend to decrease each of the doshas. We should take comparatively more of the tastes that reduce our doshic type and less of those increase it.

Taste	Elements	Potency	Doshic Action	Effect on Rejuvenation
Sweet	Earth and Water	Cooling	Decreases Pitta and Vata, Increases Kapha	Promotes rejuvenation in a primary way in right quantity and quality, but in excess promotes disease and aging
Salty	Water and Fire	Heating	Decreases Vata, Increases Pitta and Kapha	Promotes rejuvenation only in a supplementary manner, particularly using special mineral salts
Sour	Earth and Fire	Heating	Decreases Vata, Increases Pitta and Kapha	Does not promote rejuvenation, with a few exceptions like amalaki, but does aid in digestion

Taste	Elements	Potency	Doshic Action	Effect on Rejuvenation
Pungent/ Spicy	Fire and Air	Heating	Decreases Kapha, Increases Pitta and Vata	Promotes rejuvenation in a support role, as stimulating digestion by itself is not rejuvenating
Bitter	Air and Ether	Cooling	Increases Vata, Decreases Pitta and Kapha	Does not support rejuvenation except special herbs for the mind like brahmi
Astringent	Earth and Air	Cooling	Increases Vata, Decreases Pitta and Kapha	Does not promote rejuvenation, with a few exceptions like haritaki

Sweet, salty, and sour tastes, which increase Kapha dosha, are more common in tonification rejuvenation therapies, along with predominantly cool natured substances.[63] Bitter, astringent and pungent tastes, on the other hand, that reduce Kapha tend to be depleting and detoxifying. A typical rejuvenative diet therefore combines anti-Vata and anti-Pitta items and aims at increasing Kapha in its higher essence of Soma. In the case of Pitta or heat caused depletion conditions, the herbs and foods should be cold natured. For Vata, some warming substances can be used as well, particularly mild spices to aid in the digestion of rejuvenative foods and herbs.

This means that a *rejuvenation diet is not an anti-sugar or anti-sweet diet, but one that rests upon high quality natural sugars.* Such rejuvenation promoting natural sugars include honey, cane sugar, fruit sugars, milk sugars and special fruit jellies like Chyavan Prash. One needs special sugars as a central part of a rejuvenation diet because its concern is rebuilding a higher quality of tissues, not simply detoxification, which requires less of any sugar types.

Yet using natural sugars does imply taking low quality sweets such as refined sugar and high fructose corn syrup, or taking large amounts of sugar in a body that is already clogged with toxins. Excess of any type of sugar tends to block the channels and breed Ama (toxic undigested food residues), becoming acidic and damaging the blood. A rejuvenative diet does not give us a license to indulge in the sweet taste without discrimination. Sugar is the basic Soma or enjoyable substance that we find in foods, which we naturally seek and easily become addicted to. The problem is that we have moved from high quality natural sugars towards heavier low quality sweets and oils, such as abound in junk foods. For rejuvenation, *Ayurveda recommends the sweet taste, but only in more refined and sattvic items.*

An important aid to make our intake of sugars more rejuvenative is to balance them with the right spices. Best for this are sweet and aromatic spices like ginger and cardamom. Such spices help counter the heaviness inherent in the sweet taste and make it lighter and easier to absorb. They also bring an additional flavor to the sweets they are combined with.

Because of our cultural indulgence in low quality sugars, many modern health food diets may reject sugar or at least cane sugar as something bad. They may accept honey and maple syrup instead. The fact is that we do need sugar as part of our nutritional requirements. Yet sugar can be both the worst and the best thing for us, depending upon its type, nature and quantity. Low quality sugars build up Ama (undigested food particles) and toxins in the body and promote many diseases such as diabetes, arthritis, asthma, heart disease and obesity itself. Yet high quality sugars can be the best thing to provide us with energy and to allow our body to produce the best quality of fluids and tissues.

Sour taste is usually not rejuvenative but there are some important exceptions like amalaki or yogurt (particularly yogurt that is a bit sweet and not too sour). Ayurveda has special herbal wines that are good for convalescence and for the early stages of rejuvenation therapy, as they are easier to digest, but are not used in stricter rejuvenative procedures. Some sour items can aid in the rejuvenation of the blood.

Salty taste is also usually not rejuvenative as it can accumulate in the body and clog the channels, but a certain amount of salt is necessary in order maintain proper hydration of the tissues and to regulate elimination through the colon. In this regard salt in moderation can aid in the rejuvenation of the rasa dhatu (plasma) and the skin. Mineral salts also aid the skin externally.

Some rejuvenative items for Kapha dosha can have a spicy or pungent taste, like pippali (long pepper) or garlic, though spicy articles by themselves are not rejuvenative. In addition, some exceptional rejuvenative items for the mind can be of a bitter or astringent taste. This is because the mind relates to the air and ether elements that abound in such tastes. Rejuvenation of the mind can be aided by the lighter tastes of bitter, astringent and pungent.

Spices

A rejuvenative diet, being heavy and nutritive, benefits by good spices to aid in digestion. Good spices are strongly revitalizing to our body, mind, prana and senses. A number of spices have if not rejuvenative powers, at least a strong capacity to sustain positive health and well-being. Spices are an integral part of a rejuvenative diet and of rejuvenative herbal formulas for the body and mind.

Sweet and mild aromatic spice like ginger, turmeric and cardamom are best for a rejuvenative diet, improving digestion and circulation in a powerful but gentle manner. Hot spices like chilies and mustards can be too strong, overheating the digestive fire or drying up the body fluids and tissues, though this is not so much the case for those habituated to hot spices from childhood. However, under certain strict rejuvenative diets, particularly for rebuilding the bodily fluids, few or no spices may be used temporarily owing to their drying nature. This is particularly true for individuals suffering from high Vata dosha, debility and fatigue.

The best spices for longevity and rejuvenation include ginger, turmeric, cinnamon, cardamom, fennel, cumin, coriander, basil, fenugreek, mint, saffron, bay, and rosemary. Those to be used with caution owing to their hot and drying nature include black pepper, mustard, horseradish, cayenne, red and green chilies.

A few spices have special rejuvenative qualities: garlic is an important rejuvenative to the heart, long pepper (pippali) is rejuvenative to lungs, basil aids in rejuvenation of the mind, and asafoetida (hing) is helpful for the rejuvenation of the colon. Garlic and asafoetida are often avoided for rejuvenation of the mind owing to their strong fragrance, so their usefulness in rejuvenation is more for the body. Fresh ginger root and fresh turmeric root are great to use in the cooking or as foods and help improve health overall.

Preparation of Food

The best food items for rejuvenation are those local, naturally grown, freshly picked, organic and home cooked, better yet if home grown. Food cooked with love by a person close to you has an emotionally rejuvenative quality as well as greater physical value. It is not just the technical issues of food types or chemistry that we must consider but the awareness, prana and emotion that goes along with its growth and preparation.

Food that is overcooked or recooked should be avoided. All dead food in general should be avoided. This includes most canned food, processed food and "junk" food of all types. Food that has chemical additives, has been canned or frozen too long, or food items that combine too many different ingredients in their packaging should also be avoided. It is best to begin with whole grains, fruit and vegetables. Fried food should be avoided, along with any food that is very greasy or oily. Only a good quality natural cooking oil should be used (ghee, coconut, olive). Food that is microwaved should be avoided as well. It is best if you have a relationship with the food yourself, being involved in its growing, cutting or cooking.

Timing of meals is very important for proper assimilation. The main meal should occur around noon, when the digestive fire is strongest. Eating after sunset, particularly of heavy foods, should be avoided; as such food does not digest easily and easily clogs the system. One should also avoid heavy, sweet and mucus forming foods for breakfast. Best is to start the day with a mild spice tea like ginger, cinnamon or basil to clear any residual Kapha or Ama held over from sleep. Then one can take heavier foods in another hour or two, if one needs to work.

A lighter and more detoxifying diet is best in the late spring and summer. Heavier, more nutritive and rejuvenative diet is better in autumn and winter. However, a rejuvenative diet can be very good in the late spring or summer after a preliminary phase of detoxification.

Good Food Items for Rejuvenation

Below we will outline food items that are in harmony with a long-term mild rejuvenation therapy. *Note that these recommendations are general indications and should be modified on an individual basis, according to your body type and the foods you are accustomed to or grow in your environment. What is important is the overall diet and the main staple foods that one eats regularly. You need not be a food fanatic. Other rejuvenative practices like herbs, exercise, pranayama and meditation are important as well.*

Fruit

Most fruits are excellent foods for rejuvenation, particularly freshly picked fruit, as well as freshly made fruit juices. Note that we are not necessarily recommending that we juice all the fruits that we take. There is a kind of prana that is lost when we juice a fruit as opposed to eating it that is most noticeable with more substantial fruits like apples or bananas, than with fruits that have high juice contents like oranges. Tropical fruits are perhaps the strongest rejuvenating fruits. Yet fruit may not be sufficiently nourishing by itself and will need to be combined with dairy products, whole grains, seeds and nuts for a complete rejuvenative diet.

Good fruit items for longevity and rejuvenation include dates, mango, papaya, bananas, grapes (raisins), pomegranate, mulberry, guava, pears, apples, peaches, cherries, plums, prunes and berries of all types. Sour fruit is of less value but can aid in a secondary as a digestive stimulant, particularly limes. Some special rejuvenative fruit include amalaki and bilva or bael fruit of India.

Vegetables

Mainly sweet vegetables, freshly picked, are best for rejuvenation, emphasizing heavier root vegetables, particularly as taken with whole grains and appropriate spices and oils. Most such vegetables need to be cooked. However, it is important to have a small amount of raw vegetables and sprouts in the diet as well, particularly cucumbers, sprouts and mixed greens, for their special nutrient effects. This can include some raw vegetable juices, particularly seasonally, though not a strong raw juice diet, which will become more detoxifying.

Good vegetables for rejuvenation include asparagus, sweet potatoes, yams, squash (particularly winter squash), green beans, green peas, carrots, beets, and celery. Cabbage family plants should not be heavily used (broccoli, cauliflower, brussel sprouts), nor certain lighter root vegetables like radishes, parsnips and turnips. Mushrooms can be helpful only if the digestion is good.

Greens (spinach, lettuce, chard, arugula, kale, mustard greens) are good for helping to rejuvenate the blood but can be depleting to the other tissues, if taken too much. They are helpful in a rejuvenative diet in small amounts. Potatoes, tomatoes, peppers, eggplant and nightshade family plants in general require some discretion in their usage owing to their alkaloids that can cause diseases like arthritis in some people and should be well cooked and spiced. Cooked potatoes are the safest among the nightshades. Onions and leeks can be helpful but are sometimes irritants in their effects upon the nervous system.

Whole Grains

Whole grains are central to a long-term rejuvenation diet for most people. Only a few yogis with a great pranic power can get by without them. Generally cooked whole grains are better than breads. Yet non-yeasted breads are better than the yeasted breads, like the Indian chapattis and nans. Breads are also better taken freshly baked.

There is a tendency of modern health food diets to reject wheat and gluten along with white flour. According to Ayurveda, while white flour should usually be avoided owing to its heavy and sticky nature, wheat is an excellent grain. Wheat aids in building the muscles and gives strength. It is a good food for those living in northern climates or doing a lot of physical labor, better than rice, which has less protein in it. It is particularly good for Vata dosha.

Best for rejuvenation are grains that are sweet and demulcent, particularly rice and wheat. Rice is excellent for all long-term health issues, particularly basmati. Brown rice can be taken but does not mix as well with vegetables. Oats are also calmative. Grains that are light and drying like corn or barley are not as helpful. Corn, millet, barley, buckwheat, rye and amaranth can be good for Kapha types but care must be taken relative to their drying properties.

Beans

Most beans should be taken with discretion during strict rejuvenation practices with the exception of mung, as beans have a tendency to disturb Vata dosha. Yet for general dietary and milder rejuvenation practices, beans along with whole grains form the basis of a healthy diet. Generally soy is not a good rejuvenative food, though tofu is much better than the whole bean itself.

Some beans from India like urad or kulattha have special good nourishing and rejuvenative properties. Other beans like lentils, kidney beans, lima beans, aduki beans, black beans and tur dal should be properly cooked to reduce their irritant properties and not overly used during strict rejuvenation practices.

Kicharee, consisting of equal part of split yellow mung and basmati rice, is the foundation of Ayurvedic diets and helps restore weakened digestive function. It is taken along with ghee, a little salt and simple mild spices like ginger or turmeric. Kicharee also forms a good food base on which to add other vegetables, particularly the heavier root vegetables like yams, sweet potatoes, potatoes and Jerusalem artichokes. There are many Ayurvedic kicharee recipes that can be part of a rejuvenative or restorative diet.

Nuts and Seeds

Nuts and seeds carry a strong rejuvenative energy and the power to create new life. They are excellent for rejuvenation but should be taken in moderate amounts, as they can be heavy or hard to digest. They should not be old, rancid, overly roasted or salted.

Sesame seeds, almonds, coconut, cashews, pecans, walnuts, pine nuts, Brazil nuts, macadamia nuts, hazel nuts and pistachios are particularly good. Almonds are best soaked overnight in water with their skins removed, in which case they are very helpful. Cashews can be taken raw or used in cooking. Sunflower seeds are light and more reducing in their properties, while peanuts (which are a legume) can be irritants to some people.

Cooking Oils

Oils are important nutritive and rejuvenative agents for the deeper tissues, particularly the nerves. In fact, rejuvenation therapy is essentially an 'oleation' or *snehana* therapy, requiring increased internal and external usage of oils. All oils should be as fresh as possible and of good natural quality.

Ghee or clarified butter is probably the best of all rejuvenative oils, particularly for the nervous system, and for Vata and Pitta doshas. Coconut is also very good, particularly for the skin and plasma. Olive is probably the best vegetable oil. Safflower and sunflower are weaker but can be good for Pitta. Drying and reducing oils like mustard, corn, canola and soy are of limited value and are not appropriate for strict rejuvenation therapies. They are better for detoxification and weight reduction approaches. One should avoid all animal fats and margarines as these easily clog the channels.

Dairy Products

Dairy products are excellent for rejuvenation and form the basis of many traditional Yoga and Ayurveda rejuvenation diets. But it is best if all dairy products are raw (unpasteurized, unhomogenized), organic and taken from animals that are treated well, which requires a special effort in these days of factory farming.

During a strict traditional Ayurvedic Rasayana therapy fresh cow's milk is usually the first thing to be taken, derived from a cow that has been well treated. The milk is the Soma of the cow; even better yet the cream. Cows' milk is the easiest thing to digest and does not interfere with the working of rejuvenative herbs, functioning like an infusion of pure plasma or nutrient fluids. Yet milk should be taken warm, preferably with mild spices like ginger, cinnamon and cardamom, not cold. Ayurvedic rejuvenative herbs like ashwagandha, shatavari, or bala may be taken along with the milk as well, with the powder of the herbs cooked in milk, with some natural sugar added and taken warm. Milk sugars also can be very nourishing and form the basis of many traditional Indian and European sweets. Goat's milk is of a weaker quality for rejuvenation and mainly for Kapha types.

Ghee (clarified butter) also very good and can be taken along with milk. Butter is good as well. Whey is an excellent good dairy source of protein and is good for rejuvenation, particularly strengthening to the digestive system. A good quality fresh yogurt is helpful but better if a little sweet and not too sour. Indian buttermilk or *takra* is very good for a weak stomach and poor digestion. Many cheeses can be too heavy and salty for strict rejuvenation diets, though light cheeses can be good like paneer, cottage cheese and cream cheese. Sour cream can be too acidic.

One simple rejuvenation method is to live in a pleasant natural surrounding while subsisting primarily on fresh cow's milk for three months. For this purpose it is best to have one's own cow, which is cared for properly. Pranayama and meditation should be practiced along with the recitation of mantras, control of the senses and control of the sexual energy.

Sweeteners/ Confections

Good natural sugars include raw sugar, sugar cane juice, molasses, maple syrup, fruit sugar, and fruit jellies. Raw honey, less than six months old, is a powerful rasayana, particularly if taken from the wild. Ayurvedic jaggery or gur, made from natural sugarcane, is one of the best natural sugars and used along with many herbs and beverages.

There are many Ayurvedic 'rasayana confections' that combine fruits, natural sugars, milk sugars, seeds, nuts, spices, whole grains and oils like ghee. These often constitute the 'prasad' or sweets given out at Hindu temples after rituals are performed. These form a higher quality 'Soma sweet', one could say. In this category one may include some of the better quality whole grain and protein bars of the western health food business.

Salt

Too much of salt, particularly mixed with fried food, clogs the arteries and promotes aging of the heart, circulatory and nervous systems. But good quality natural salts in moderation helps sustain the plasma and strengthen digestion. Indian rock salt is best; a small amount of black salt (kala namak) is good. Sea salt in moderation, some kelp or seaweed can be helpful. Excess salt in the diet is harmful and reduces the longevity, but some salt is needed to keep Vata dosha from accumulating as salt is very helpful for reducing Vata.[64]

Vitamins and Minerals

Vitamins and minerals can also be regarded as Somas or subtle essences of a kind. Vitamins can act as powerful rejuvenative agents, particularly the B and E vitamins. But they are best derived from food. One cannot simply take a lot of vitamin pills and get the same results. However, one can take a good multiple vitamin to counter any vitamin deficiencies that may occur in one's food.

Minerals are similarly best derived from food, particularly green vegetables taken raw or lightly cooked, like lettuce, mustard greens, fenugreek leaves, arugula, spinach, and kale, or by kelp and seaweed.[65] Yet mineral supplements can be of some value when special deficiencies are there or when good quality fresh food is hard to get.

OUR SOMA DRINKS:
REJUVENATING WATERS AND BEVERAGES

Soma spoke to me that in the waters are all medicines and Agni that gives well-being to all, and the waters are medicines for all.

Rigveda I.23.20

Just as Agni is connected with the digestion of solid food and the earth element, Soma relates to the water element and the beverages that we take in. In general, liquids nourish prana and mind, which are light in nature, as solids nourish the body, which is heavy. Soma as the nectar of immortality was always something that was drunk, a beverage. Yet Soma is not only water but also anything that has a liquid, moistening, softening and nourishing effect. Soma in the *Vedas* is an essence, extract, ferment, juice and nectar – a liquid pressed out of plant fibers. Soma is an elixir that revitalizes the core of body and mind. True Soma is a liquid that is deeply refreshing, which cools and fortifies the mind and heart, helping us let go of all fever, friction, stress and agitation.

Our favorite beverages, one could say, are our personal Somas, be they herbal teas, coffee and black tea, fruit juice or wine. The beverages we drink feed our Soma or sense of taste, however we have oriented that Soma to be. The water or liquid that we take in serves to hydrate the body and its tissues, particularly the brain, affording us a sense of well-being. Our beverages influence the brain and mind, refreshing, nourishing, stimulating or calming them. Look at your own habits and see what your favorite beverages or Somas are and what they say about you and your interests in life.

Beverages that are overly stimulating, too sweet or habit forming can deplete our inner Soma. Soft drinks in particular are a kind of false liquid Soma, like the Coca Cola cult that ties our metabolism to strong sweeteners that are addictive in nature. These stimulant Somas inhibit our inner sweetness and weaken the natural resilience of the nervous system, pumping us up with a quickly moving energy that depletes our deeper vitality. The use of soft drinks is one of the worst things for our health and well-being, particularly when taken during a meal and along with ice that suppresses the digestive fire.

Our daily stimulant beverages like coffee also are kinds of Soma beverages for us, but can be depleting as well. Coffee has stimulant and addictive qualities and should be taken with some discretion, particularly the commercial and instant types. Fresh natural brews are better. Yet coffee should be avoided during strict rejuvenative approaches. Tea is usually better than coffee, but too strong or in excess has a lot of tannins that can be depleting to the body. Green tea is milder than black tea. Black tea if taken with milk and spices like cinnamon or ginger can be alright, but again not for strict rejuvenation approaches. Chocolate as a drink is similar to coffee but milder in properties and does better taken with milk. It can be a kind of Soma for the heart. Combined with large amounts of sugar, however, it becomes more addictive. We should not allow such beverages to substitute for our own inner Soma. We should remember that the type of beverages we take in nourish the type of Soma we are developing in life. Good quality beverages are essential for physical and psychological well-being.

Soma and Alcohol

Vedic texts usually discriminate between Soma, which heightens our inner perception, and *Sura* or alcohol, which dulls the senses. Somas are herbs that promote a heightened awareness, greater clarity and right judgment. Suras are drugs that cause addiction, including not just alcoholic beverages but narcotics, in which our awareness and judgment are usually impaired or inhibited.

Alcohol, particularly wine, is part of many poetic metaphors throughout the world. Mystic poets have often compared spiritual ecstasy to the state of drunkenness, including Chinese poets, Sufis and Sanskrit poets. Often this drunkenness is experienced at night by the light of the Moon. Such a metaphor is really about the inner Soma, in which the alcohol is but a symbol. Alcohol also occurs as part of negative metaphors, the drunkenness of ignorance and lack of consciousness. The Maya or illusion of the world is said to make us drunk.

Alcoholic beverages, particularly wine in small amounts, can have mild health benefits such as improving digestion and circulation or easing menstruation, but that is another matter. Ayurvedic medicine has an entire range of medicinal herbal wines, like *Ashwagandharishta* or Ashwagandha herbal wine, which has restorative powers, particularly for those with a weak digestive power, but these are more medicines than beverages.

Tantric Yoga employs alcohol and intoxicants as part of its left-handed path (Vamachara), which includes sacred sex practices. Intoxicants like wine or cannabis are taken in a sacred way in limited amounts in order to evoke higher mystical states. These methods, however, are largely eschewed on the right-handed path of Tantra (Dakshinachara), and contradicted in traditional Raja Yoga with its yamas and niyamas, its strict rules of ethical conduct.

Soma Beverages

Below are a few important Soma beverages in traditional Ayurveda.

Water

It is important, first of all, that we have good quality water for rejuvenation purposes. This is water has that power to quench not only our outer thirst but also our inner thirst. There are many natural and sacred waters that are great for this purpose, like water from mountain rivers, springs and lakes. Yet any good natural water is fine for this purpose.

For our long-term well-being, we should also make sure to drink water that is full of prana. We can aerate our water for this purpose (exposing it to the sunlight and pouring it back and forth in the air a bit). Best is to keep water overnight in a copper vessel with a little mint or basil (tulsi) in it and chant some healing mantras over it. The herbs will provide additional prana to the water. The mantra will bring a higher consciousness into the waters. One of the reasons that we like carbonated water and carbonated beverages is because of the air in them, but it is not true prana that they have.

Ganga Water

In India, the main such mountain water used is that of Ganga water, water from the Ganges river in its Himalayan course above Rishikesh. But many other Himalayan rivers can be used for the same purpose. Ganga water carries the rejuvenative energies of the Himalayas, along with their glacier and snow melts, and rain falls. Ganga water is also sacred and carries the meditative energy and mantras of the many yogis and sages who have lived along its course over thousands of years. Ganga is not simply regarded as a river but as a Goddess and form of Shakti. Her water carries the grace, blessings and power of the Divine Mother.

One can sprinkle Ganga water to purify ones meditation seat, meditation room or clinic. One can drink Ganga water by itself as a rasayana or place certain herbs in it like Tulsi (holy basil). Or one can add a few drops of Ganga water to one's herbal teas or fruit juices. Ganga water is now commercially available in India and in the West.

Amalaki Juice

The fresh juice of amla or amalaki fruit is an excellent rejuvenative. It is ready available in India and now exported to the West. What we drink with amla juice tends to become a rasayana itself. Best is to mix a couple of tablespoons of amla juice with some pomegranate juice or, if that is not available, apple juice. It can also be added to water.

Coconut Juice

Coconut juice has such vitalizing properties that it was used for blood transfusions in World War II when the blood banks ran out of blood for wounded soldiers. Coconut juice hydrates all the tissues, with its influence extending to the nerve tissue and the brain, bringing in not only natural sugars but also oil. Coconut juice is readily available, including in various mixtures with other juices. Coconut is an important Soma plant overall and indicates the mind and crown chakra.

Sugar Cane Juice

Fresh sugarcane juice is a rasayana or rejuvenative medicine in Ayurveda. It builds up the plasma and body fluids and serves to counter fever, thirst, dryness and fatigue. It is not easy to get in North America but is common in tropical countries and may be added to other fruit drinks or beverages.

Aloe Juice

Aloe juice can be a helpful rejuvenative drink, particularly for women, or for Pitta types, though it can also be mixed with other fruit juices. It is better taken in small amounts before meals or as diluted with other juices. One must be careful in that it tends to have a laxative effect.

Fruit Juices

Sweet fruit juices in general are natural Soma beverages, though sour fruit juices are not as useful. A few important fruit juices are pomegranate, mulberry, guava, mango, blueberry, grape and acai. Pomegranate juice is especially good for women. Taking natural fruit juices during the day helps keep our Soma flowing, but fruit juices should be avoided during meals as they can interfere with the digestive process, or they should be diluted in water.

Herbal Teas

Many herbal teas are natural Soma beverages, particularly nervine herbs as Soma beverages for the brain and mind. We will discuss these more relative to herbs for the mind. Typical in this regard are holy basil (tulsi), brahmi, licorice, hibiscus, rose, lemon grass and many mints and sages. Mild sweet spices like ginger, cinnamon, cardamom, fennel, nutmeg and cloves can be helpful as well. Green tea is good and has many varieties. Black tea can be taken light and mixed with spices as in Indian chai or masala tea.

Milk as a Beverage

We have discussed milk as a food but it is also an important rejuvenative beverage, either by itself or with certain herbs and spices cooked in it. Milk is an important carrier for other herbs or foods and augment their properties. It can serve as a vehicle for rejuvenative herbs and spices, particularly if taken with a little natural sugar, honey or ghee. Yet as a beverage, milk is better taken warm and not consumed during the meals as it does not combine well with a number of food items.

Saffron milk, milk taken with a little saffron cooked in it, is very good for rejuvenation of the blood and the female reproductive system. Milk with turmeric powder is good combination for the liver. Milk with ginger powder is good for the lungs and stomach. Milk with nutmeg helps calm the mind and promote deep sleep.

REJUVENATIVE HERBS AND SOMA PLANTS

Filled with vigor, filled with Soma, filled with energy that increases Ojas,
I have found all the herbs for our well-being.

Rigveda X.97.7

Herbs are our natural medicine, the healing gift of Mother Earth along with her wonderful life-energy or prana that permeates the ground, air and waters around us.

Herbs can be found that promote all our biological processes: diaphoretics that induce sweating, diuretics that cause urination, digestive and circulatory stimulants, alteratives or blood purifiers, and nervine sedatives. Herbs also exist that promote immunity, longevity, well-being and higher consciousness, and a special class of rejuvenative agents.

Rejuvenative herbs are called *rasayanas* in Sanskrit meaning what enters (ayana), the rasa, the plasma or essence of our tissues, and can revitalize us from within.

Many rejuvenative herbs form a special class of 'nutritive tonics' (*brimhana* or weight-increasing in Sanskrit), providing a deeper level of nutrition than food, for not only building up the tissues but for strengthening Ojas or our deeper vitality. Other rejuvenative herbs are powerful function-promoting agents, improving our natural activity on various levels, particularly stimulating awareness, perception, immunity and adaptability, as well as developing Tejas and Prana. There are rejuvenatives that can work on the different tissues of the body and for the mind as well. Such rejuvenative herbs are a key factor in physical longevity and help keep the mind youthful. They are probably the most important herbal medicines and one that we should all know about and learn to benefit from.

Soma is a Vedic name for rejuvenative plants and plant preparations in general, a point that we will explore at several places in the book. Therefore, we can speak of many different types of 'herbal Somas' and 'herbal Soma preparations'. *Soma or rejuvenation effects are an important type of herbal properties. This means that there are always Soma plants available for us, though some plants will possess more Soma than others. Plants abounding in Soma qualities are rare, but some can be found in every geographical region.* A few important and accessible of these Ayurvedic rejuvenative or Soma plants will be introduced in this chapter.

Rejuvenative Properties and Plant Parts

Rejuvenative properties are prominent more in certain plant parts than in others. Flowers, fruits, seeds, nuts and roots all can carry rejuvenative properties. Only a few leaves have rejuvenative properties, mainly owing to aromatic oils that they may carry. Important in this regard is tulsi or holy basil and other mints and parsley family relatives.

Roots work more on the physical body and connect us with Earth energy, strengthening the root chakra that governs the earth element and the muscles overall. Rejuvenative roots include ashwagandha, shatavari, bala and ginseng. They include various bulbs and rhizomes that have moistening and nourishing qualities, including members of the lily and orchid families.

Seeds and nuts work more on the nervous and reproductive systems, providing high quality nutritive oils. Most common in this regard are sesame seeds and almonds. They help calm the Vata dosha behind the aging process. Fruit works more on the brain and mind, yet in a mild way mainly through the plasma or bodily fluids. Amalaki is the best of such rejuvenative fruits, which include various Soma beverages.

Flowers work more on the mind and emotions but in a more subtle way than fruits. Some flowers function as good herbal teas and elixirs. These include saffron, rose, hibiscus, and Himalayan rhododendron. Many provide fragrant oils that can be used as aromas or incense. These include rose, jasmine, saffron, iris, lily, gardenia, honeysuckle, and champak. Flowers reflect an astral essence and bring the creative astral light into our world. They affect our feeling nature and finer sensitivities.

Tree resins can be helpful in rejuvenation or in an associated purification process, as they promote healing of the bones, muscles and blood. Guggul, myrrh, frankincense, benzoin and shallaki are good examples. Some milky tree saps like those of the tropical fig trees have Soma holding powers as well.

Plants that contain strong juices are often good for rejuvenation. These are most common in fruits but other like sugar cane or moist roots like shatavari can contain a fair amount of juice as well. The fresh juice of plants is a good way to take in their rejuvenative properties, including for herbs like brahmi (gotu kola relative) that do not contain large amounts of juice. Rejuvenative herbal roots can be taken in milk decoctions or cooked with certain grains to increase their strengthening properties.

In addition, rejuvenative properties may require picking the plant at a proper time of the day or season of the year. Soma relates to the Moon, so the right alliance of the plant with the movements and phases of the Moon has its importance. Other time and place considerations, including those of astrology and *vastu* (directional) influence can be important.

Along with considerations of location is the nature of the soil and water depending upon which the Soma plants grow. Generally wild plants will have greater Soma qualities than cultivated items, though there are ways of making sure that we preserve the Soma in the plants that we cultivate. Wild plants cannot provide enough herbs and can be easily picked to extinction, as seems to have been the case with a number of ancient Soma plants in Vedic times.

Preparing Somas and Rejuvenative plants

Vedic Soma is usually referred to as something that is extracted.[66] It is described as purified through a filter or sieve,[67] suggesting some kind of distillation process. Heat or Agni was often used in its extraction. Soma was prepared in other natural ingredients, particularly milk, ghee and grains like barley to bring out and increase its properties. Soma is compared to ghee or honey in its constituency.[68] If we look at these factors, one is drawn to the following conclusion: *Soma is not just a type of plants but a way of extracting plant essences, an entire herbal alchemy.*

The existence of Soma herbal preparations and an entire Soma pharmaceutical science is reflected in the Vedic Soma. Getting the essence or the active ingredients from a plant is a concern for all herbalists. We can identify several types of plant essences or extracts.

The juice of the plant can be extracted through simple grinding procedures. Heavy oils in plants like sesame oil in the sesame seeds, can be extracted in a similar manner but because of their greasy nature are more difficult to get out and harder to clean. Extracting aromatic oils like those from mints or various flowers requires yet a more refined distillation process because of the subtle nature of such oils. Sugars and starches in plants can often be brought out and removed through cooking. Some herbal properties can be extracted directly in a sugar or juice base, like glycerin extracts. Other herbal essences are better extracted in alcohol or in vinegar.

Besides these different means of extraction, there is the issue of preservation of the plant essences. The two are related as many mediums of extraction can serve as mediums of preservation as well. One simple way to preserve herbs is through sugar, which is an excellent natural preservative, particularly for any nutritive type of herb. Here we find various Ayurvedic sugars, jellies and confections, like the famous Chyavan prash. Herbal honeys or herbs preserved in a honey base also have their place as important Soma preparations and a large variety of these can be prepared.

Another natural preservative for herbs is oil, which we find in Ayurveda in abundance through using herbs cooked in oils like ghee, sesame and coconut. While many of these oils are used externally, a number, particularly the medicated ghees, can be used internally.

Alcohol is another good preservative as in the case of herbal tinctures. In Ayurveda, herbal wines (asavas and arishtas) are more common as they better organically develop the herbal essences. Yet another way is to preserving herbs by cooking them in special plant resins.

In Ayurveda, guggul, a relative of frankincense and myrrh, is used as a base to hold and carry various herbs. A number of other methods could be mentioned. The main point here is that *we need to learn not only to properly identify Soma plants but also how to extract and preserve their Soma qualities.* Plant Somas may not be useful for us unless they are produced and prepared in the right manner. Here we can connect the Vedic idea of Soma with the alchemical preparation of herbs and minerals and the preparations of various herbal 'elixirs'. Ayurveda has developed such herbal extraction methods as well.

This means that we can identify a number of Vedic Soma preparations still found in modern Ayurveda. These include the use of the fresh or cooked juice of the herb, preparing special herbal ghees, oils and resins, herbal honeys and sweets, preparing herbs in milk, cream, or yogurt, preparing herbs in whole grains, the use of herbal wines and herbal plus mineral preparations. The medium of extraction or preparation can enhance the properties of the herbs used, giving them more food value or taking them more specifically into different tissues and organs of the body.

However, we must remember that getting the Soma essence of a plant is not merely a matter of outer methods. It also requires that we approach the plant in a sacred manner with prayer, ritual, mantra, pranayama and meditation, with yogic methods of bringing the Cosmic Prana and Cosmic Soma into the plant, and with communion with the plant spirits or Devas that grant access to the powers of the plant.

Types of Rejuvenative Herbs

The main class of rejuvenative herbs is that of rejuvenative tonics, which work to improve the quality and quantity of our bodily tissues. They nourish us at a deeper level of Kapha, Ojas and Soma, our subtle vital fluids, secretions and hormones or deeper lunar and watery forces. These powerful tonic herbs are the main herbal Somas and can be like nectar to our deeper tissues. Most are sweet in taste and cool in their energetic effect.

Many rejuvenative herbs are aligned with aphrodisiacs or reproductive system tonics (*vajikaranas* in Sanskrit or 'what gives the power of a horse'), as what strengthens the reproductive system can aid in rejuvenation of the body overall. Yet not all rasayana herbs are aphrodisiacs as some target other tissues, systems or functions than the re-

130

productive. Nor are all aphrodisiacs are rasayanas either, as some may not support the conservation and internalization of energy that rejuvenation requires. Rejuvenative herbs are also commonly described as *jivaniya* or 'protecting the life', and *vayasthapana* or 'upholding vitality'. Some additionally are *hridya* or 'good for the heart', which is the source of vitality, or *medhya*, 'rejuvenative for the mind' and nervous system.

Besides the main group of 'tonic rasayanas', which have a nutritive nature and increase Ojas, are 'functional rasayanas' or rejuvenative agents for various bodily functions and actions. These functional rasayanas include stimulants for reviving consciousness, improving circulation and digestion, or herbs that keep the blood pure and the immune system strong, protecting us from fevers and infections.

Rejuvenative herbs, particularly the nutritive type, can be taken in small dosages as 'energy supplements' to an ordinary Ayurvedic diet, and so can be helpful for everyone. In higher dosages, they function as part of rejuvenative therapies. Rejuvenative herbs also vary in their strength. Some rasayana herbs have strong rejuvenative properties like shilajit or ashwagandha. Others are mild like lotus seeds or licorice. However, rasayana herbs only give their best results if taken along with a rejuvenative diet and life-style and should be viewed as part of a larger overall rejuvenative therapy.

Types of Rasayanas by Herbal Effects

- Cooling, sweet and nutritive rasayanas that increase Kapha dosha, the bodily tissues and Ojas and largely reflect a lunar energy. Examples: shatavari, bala, safed or white musali, pueraria (vidari kand), lotus seeds, water lily seeds (makhanna), and the ashtavarga or group of eight herbs in Ayurvedic medicine. Amalaki, though sour in taste, comes in this category as well. These often have a calmative effect upon the mind and nourish the nervous system.

- Stimulants for reviving energy and promoting awareness (many are more properly speaking rasayanas for the mind). Examples are camphor, calamus, sanjivani, ephedra, and basil. These often have a stimulating effect upon the mind and its higher perceptions.

- Spicy, bitter herbs and resins for purification of the blood, countering fever and protecting immunity. Examples are saffron, myrrh, guggul, guduchi, shallaki, saussurea, aloe, and sandalwood.

Rasayanas by Dosha

Rasayanas can be classified according to the three doshic types or biological humors of Ayurveda.

Vata	Most rasayanas work well on Vata, which is the main dosha behind the aging process, particularly combining nourishing, warming and calmative herbs	Ashwagandha, bala, shatavari, vidari kand, shilajit, calamus, shankha pushpi, haritaki, amalaki, guggul, garlic, sesame seeds, ashtavarga herbs
Pitta	Pitta does best with cool, sweet and moistening rasayanas as well as those that purify the blood	Shatavari, bala, white musali, vidari kand, licorice, lotus seeds, amalaki, brahmi, saussurea, sandalwood, ashtavarga herbs
Kapha	Kapha does best with pungent, warming and stimulating rasayanas	Shilajit, pippali (long pepper), bibhitaki, haritaki, calamus, garlic, guggul, ashwagandha

Primary Ayurvedic Rejuvenative Herbs

Below are listed a number of important Ayurvedic rejuvenative herbs that are accessible. There are many other herbs of this type, more which are listed in the appendix. We are introducing these herbs here, not providing a full delineation of their constituents, energetics or usages.[69]

Shilajit

Shilajit is a special mineral and plant residue or pitch, exuded by various rocks in the Himalayas and few other mountain ranges in the world (like the Altai or Caucasus mountains). Such residues are millions of years old and carry the healing powers of the ages.

Just as the Ganga carries the sacred water of the Himalayas, Shilajit carries the sacred essence of the rocks and plants. Shilajit holds the concentrated essence (rasa) of the Himalayan earth element as the Ganga River carries its water element. Shilajit grants one the strength and power of the mountain, the support of the Earth. Some regard it as the best of all rasayanas and the very 'Soma of the earth'. It has a powerful Shiva energy, revitalizing and rejuvenating us from within. Shilajit reflects the Somas of the mineral kingdom and the powers of different minerals, which is another important study in its own right.[70] There are several varieties according to the mountain ranges where it is taken, with much of the best Shilajit coming from Nepal.

Shilajit is a great mineral supplement and improves both digestion and elimination. It is astringent and bitter in taste, pungent in post-digestive effect and warm in energy but not too hot in its effects. It can be good for all three doshas of Vata, Pitta and Kapha. Though pungent in post-digestive effect, it does promote the building of bodily tissues.

Shilajit is probably the simplest and most powerful rasayana to take, as well as one of the most balanced in its properties. One can take Shilajit pills or capsules or get the fresh resin and take it mixed warm water and honey. Shilajit can be combined with ashwagandha or other rasayanas. One should drink more milk when taking Shilajit, which aids in its absorption.

Shilajit is good for a variety of diseases including asthma, arthritis, kidney diseases, sexual debility and general debility. Rare for a rejuvenative herb it is also good for weight reduction (in Kapha types) and for removing gall stones and kidney stones. Yet it does promote energy development and energy consumption in body and mind, and is not for those who need to function on reduced activity.

Amla or Amalaki – Emblica officinalis

Traditional Ayurvedic rejuvenation therapy emphasizes three herbs, which are related tropical fruits. These are amalaki (Emblica officinalis), haritaki (Terminalia chebula) and bibhitaki (Terminalia baelerica). All are fruits of tropical trees called 'myrobalan plums'. They have no relationship with regular plums, we might add, but do vaguely look like them.

Amalaki (Emblica officinalis) is the most commonly used of the three and the most important rejuvenative plant used in Ayurvedic medicine, both by itself and as a part of larger formulas. Amalaki is an unusual fruit. It contains five tastes, though predominantly sour, and is cooling and nourishing in nature. It builds up all the tissues, particularly the plasma and blood, extending to the reproductive system. It is good for all doshas but more specifically anti-Vata and anti-Pitta, as well as antacid, laxative and blood purifier. If a person had only one rasayana herb to rely upon, Amalaki, particularly the fresh juice, would probably be the best.

Amalaki fruit can be made into a jelly that becomes the basis of various rasayana preparations, notable the many different types of Chyavan prash, for which it is the main ingredient. Amalaki juice can be used as a base to carry other rasayana herbs. Amalaki is also available in powder or pill form. Dried and lightly sugared and salted Amalaki fruit is available as a kind of candy. Good quality amalaki can be found throughout India. The best quality comes from the Himalayas, and should be collected in the proper season. The best quality rejuvenative medicines are prepared with fresh amalaki fruit.

Haritaki – Terminalia chebula

Haritaki is the herb that the medicine Buddha carries. It is one of the most important of all Ayurvedic herbs. Haritaki has the five tastes - astringent, sweet, sour, pungent and bitter. The only taste it does not have is salty. It is warming in energy and auspicious in its effects. It gradually removes all excess doshas and is light in properties. It promotes both digestion of food and burning up of toxins. It improves longevity, nourishment and well-being. It is often said to be the best substance to take for preventing aging. It helps alleviate all diseases. It gives intelligence and power of the senses.

Haritaki works quickly to help counter skin diseases, tumors, abdominal distention, consumption, anemia, hangover, hemorrhoids, malabsorption, chronic and intermittent fevers, heart disease, diseases of the head, nose and throat, diarrhea, poor appetite, cough, diabetes, constipation, enlargement of the spleen, laryngitis, poor complexion, jaundice, parasites, edema, asthma, vomiting, impotence, debility, blockage of the channels, congestion in the chest and heart, poor memory and bad judgment. Those suffering from chronic weak digestion, who have eaten too much dry food, indulged in excessive sexual activity, taken alcohol or drugs, or those afflicted by hunger, thirst or heat, should not use haritaki, however, as it can be drying.

Haritaki is taken in pills and powders and in formulas with other herbs, particularly the other Triphala herbs. Amalaki softens its effects.

Bibhitaki – Terminalia baelerica

Bibhitaki is the third of the myrobalan fruits of the Triphala combination. Though helpful for all three doshas, it is specific for Kapha and the lungs, for chronic cough and asthma, and for the throat and sinuses, but has a wide usage for many health complaints extending the circulatory, urinary and digestive systems. It can be taken in pill and powder form, or as mixed with honey.

Ashwagandha – Withania somnifera

Ashwagandha is perhaps the prime Ayurvedic rejuvenative agent. It is similar to ginseng in its properties, though unrelated botanically and more calmative in its effects on the nerves. Ashwagandha is an excellent tonic for the reproductive system, the nervous system, the bones and the muscles, adding a higher quality weight, bulk and energy to the body. It calms the mind and aids in concentration, meditation and deep sleep. It is good for the lungs, heart, and kidneys. Unlike most rejuvenative tonics, Ashwagandha is warming and so can be used by Kapha types who would find the cooling rasayanas to be unhelpful. Its actual taste is a bitter and usually some natural sugars are added to it to make it easier to take.

Ashwagandha powder or pills are available in western herb stores. The powder is good cooked in milk or mixed with honey (taken one-half teaspoon morning and evening, as a mild dosage).

Bala and Related Plants

Bala means strength in Sanskrit and this is an herb that provides it. There are several varieties of bala, a kind of wild mallow, used as tonic and rejuvenative medicines in Ayurveda. Such herbs are cooling and nutritive in nature, but give energy and help build up the reproductive system. Other mallow roots may be examined for the same purpose, including wild mallow or marshmallow in the West. Bala is similar to vidari kand and shatavari and like them with its powdered roots taken in milk. Apart from bala are atibala and nagbala as related plants. Atibala is usually taken with water and nagbala with honey.

Vidari kand – Pueraria tuberosa

Vidari kand is an excellent nutritive tonic with rejuvenative powers for the plasma, blood and reproductive system and is cooling and strengthening to the body overall. It is good for both the young and the old, helping create strength in children. It can be taken with ghee, sugar and milk or even with wheat. Vidari and bala are often taken along with ashwagandha to promote strength, particularly as powders cooked in milk and sugar.

Shatavari – Asparagus racemosus

Shatavari is a kind of wild asparagus. Its root has powerful tonic, rejuvenative and aphrodisiac properties, particularly for the plasma and for the female reproductive system, for which it is probably the best tonic herb. Shatavari is great for improving the skin and complexion as well as for recovery from febrile diseases and diseases born of dryness and dehydration. It restores our bodily fluids and soothes the entire body.

Shatavari is readily available in pill and powder form. It can be taken cooked in milk, which is often the preferred form. Mild dosage is one half teaspoon of the powder or one gram of the pills, morning and evening. Shatavari ghee is available and is very soothing to the heart and nerves. Shatavari mixed with raw cane sugar is good for building the plasma and improving the skin.

Black or Kali Musali – Curculigo orchioides

One of the more powerful rejuvenative members of the orchid family, good for convalescence, debility and longevity and strengthens the reproductive system. Often combined with shatavari.

White or Safed Musali – Asparagus adscendens

Another asparagus species plant with qualities similar to shatavari and often used along with it. Very good for the reproductive system, debility and convalescence from fever, strengthens bodily fluids.

Lotus – Nelumbo nucifera

The lotus flower, seed, root and stem have important herbal powers, extending into rejuvenation effects for the reproductive and nervous systems. The flower is best known for its aroma. The seeds and root have more nutritive power. Lotus is sacred to Lakshmi, the Goddess of Devotion, and is a symbol of spiritual unfoldment.

Lotus seeds can be taken as an herb or as a food, mixed with sugar, milk, rice or ghee and used for rejuvenation purposes. Either the fresh, dry or powdered seed can be employed. The root can similarly be used.

Water Lily (Makhanna) – Eurayle ferox

Water lily (kumuda in Sanskrit) is much like lotus in its effects. The puffed water lily seeds, called *makhanna* in Hindi, are often included along with foods and items for Prasad or sacred offerings in Hindu rituals. The seeds can be used like lotus seeds or taken along with them. They strengthen the reproductive and nervous systems, promote moisture and dispel heat, fever and inflammation.

Bilva (Bael) – Aegle marmelos

Bilva is sacred to Lord Shiva as it has three lobes on its leaves like Shiva's trident. Bilva fruit is good for longevity and rejuvenation. In the unripe state the fruit has astringent properties for strengthening absorption in the colon and intestines, particularly good for a weak or collapsed colon and hemorrhoids, including conditions of chronic diarrhea and dysentery. In the ripe state it has good nutritional properties. In this regard Bael is made into a type of candy, which is sold in Ayurvedic stores. Other parts of the plant can also be used. Powdered bilva roots, mixed with honey and ghee and taken every morning is an old Ayurvedic rejuvenative mixture.

Licorice – Glycyrrhiza glabra

Licorice is one of the most common rasayana herbs, aiding in rejuvenation of both body and mind. It is mainly a secondary or adjunct rasayana. Licorice is cool and sweet, counters pain, stops cough, moistens the mucus membranes, soothes the nerves and harmonizes the stomach. A simple Ayurvedic rejuvenation formula is powdered licorice one part, lotus seeds and water lily seeds one part each, taken in a milk decoction. The dosage varies from one gram on the low end to five grams on the high end morning and evening.

Garlic – Allium sativa

Garlic, at first hand, seems like the antithesis of the sweet Soma roots, but it is one of the most important rejuvenative agents among our common foods and herbs. It is an important rejuvenative for the heart and for Kapha dosha, excellent for coronary heart disease. It also aids in lung diseases, arthritis and nervous indigestion. It helps deal with obesity, lethargy, edema and lymphatic congestion.

It is best to take the garlic cloves whole with honey, three cloves morning and evening. Alternatively, one can press the cloves and take the garlic juice with honey. This mixture also aids in weight reduction and removal of excess mucus from the body.

Aloe vera - Kumari

Aloe vera is a mild but commonly available rejuvenative agent. One can use the fresh gel, but it is easier to take it diluted into a juice. The dried power is more of a laxative and does not have the same value.

Aloe is excellent for revitalizing the plasma, blood, liver, gall bladder and female reproductive system. It is particularly good for Pitta and Kapha types. It balances rejuvenative and detoxification properties and can cleanse the blood and lymphatic systems and aid in weight reduction when necessary. Its Sanskrit name as *kumari* or a young girl, indicates its power to make a woman youthful.

We can enhance Aloe's power by adding various spices to it. For example, aloe juice with a touch of saffron is good for the female reproductive system. Aloe juice with turmeric is great for the blood, liver and gall bladder. Aloe juice with ginger is good for digestion.

Guduchi – Tinosporia cordifolia

Our longevity is weakened by fever, infections and a decline in our immune system. Exposure to various forms of radiation also weakens the blood. Guduchi is an important herb for countering the effects of such conditions. It can increase the white blood cell count in the body.

Guduchi extract (sattva), a starch taken from the plant, is a very important rejuvenative agent for Pitta, the blood, and for chronic febrile diseases. It strengthens the heart, liver and kidneys. It can be taken with milk or with other rejuvenative tonics. It is particularly important for a compromised immune system, including conditions like cancer and Aids. Guduchi is also called *amrit* in Sanskrit, which means nectar, indicating its properties.

Bakuchi – Psoralea corylifolia

Discoloration of the skin and the consequent inability to absorb sunlight are a common problem in the aging process. These usually reflect malabsorption in the intestines and other metabolic imbalances. Bakuchi (Psoralea) is a helpful rasayana for the skin, countering leucoderma, vitiligo and other dermatoses, as well as for improving overall skin luster and complexion. It is also a good rejuvenative for the mind along with amalaki. Bakuchi seeds are reduced to a fine powder, to which jaggery is added. Bakuchi seeds can also found in Chinese herb stores.

Bhringaraj – Eclipta alba

Bhringaraj is a prime Ayurvedic restorative herb for the hair and is also good for the eyes. It combines well with amalaki for these purposes. It can be found in many Ayurvedic hair oils and is overall very good for the head and the scalp. The fresh juice of the leaves is excellent for promoting longevity. Or the powder can be taken along with ghee, honey and sugar.

Pippali or Long Pepper – Piper longum

Pippali is Indian long pepper that is similar to common black pepper, which it is closely related to, but is more rejuvenating in action. It is used in the Ayurvedic digestive aid *Trikatu*, consisting of black pepper, long pepper and dry ginger, which is excellent for reviving the Agni or digestive fire.

By itself pippali is an important rejuvenative agent for Kapha and the lungs. It also is a stimulant to the brain and has nervine properties. Cooked in milk, five pods per cup of milk, it can help rebuild the lung tissue and restore lung function. It is particularly good for countering the effects of chronic asthma.

Guggul – Commiphora mukul

Guggul is a tree resin similar to myrrh and frankincense. It is used as a base for preparing many Ayurvedic herbal formulas called 'gugguls'. Guggul is known for its ability to treat high cholesterol, heart disease, diabetes, asthma, arthritis and other degenerative diseases of the aging process. It has strengthening properties that are useful for rejuvenation, that improve mental function and aid in weight reduction.

Certain guggul formulas are very useful restorative agents. Some of these like *Triphala guggul*, *Yogaraj guggul* and *Mahayogaraj guggul* have powerful healing effects upon the tissues.

Rejuvenation Preparations and Formulas

There are many different rasayana herbal preparations used in Ayurveda. Some are complex and hard to make, others are simple to prepare, and a few consist of a single herb only. Some of these herbs are becoming common in the West, like ashwagandha, amalaki or shatavari. While Ayurvedic rasayana preparations are not as commonly available in stores in the West, except for the Ayurvedic jelly Chyavan Prash; many of them can be purchased through the Internet or through mail order companies.[71]

Often the best rejuvenative effects derive from the fresh juice of the herbs, particularly those herbs growing in mountain regions or wild crafted like brahmi juice. Some rasayanas are eaten and most are prepared with foods. Many rasayana herbs are taken with sugar, particularly raw sugar cane juice, as this is also a rasayana. Fresh honey (less than six months old) is another rasayana that can be used and another ancient form of Soma. There are many rasayana honeys depending upon the plants the bees gain their pollen from. Nectar from flowers or dew collected from them are other special types of Soma.[72]

Milk decoctions of rasayana herbs are very effective as milk itself is a rasayana. Yet for real rejuvenative purposes raw cow's milk should be used from an animal that has been raised with love and care. Milk decoctions are also good mixed with ghee, raw sugar or honey.

Ghee (clarified butter) is another substance that can increase the rejuvenative effects of many herbs, particularly for the nervous system. So is sesame oil, which is a natural rejuvenative for the skin, hair, bones, teeth and nails. Many rasayanas are made as herbal jellies combining the herbs with ghee, honey, sugar and other substances.

Tinctures and herbal wines are not usually considered to be rasayanas. Alcohol itself is counter to the process of rejuvenation. Yet some herbs prepared in alcohol or as herbal wines may be taken in small amounts when the digestion is weak (like Ashwagandharishta or Ashwagandha herbal wine) or as herbs for the mind.

Various food items strengthen the rejuvenative properties of herbs including milk, ghee, sesame seeds, almonds, cashews, pistachios, raw sugar, fresh honey, and coconut juice or grains like rice and wheat. Different fruits can be used like amalaki, pomegranate, dates or raisins. Various rejuvenative jellies, ghees, beverages, gruels or confections are made with such ingredients.

Most Ayurvedic rejuvenative formulas feature primary rasayana herbs like ashwagandha, shatavari and bala. Some may use these herbs along with nutritive agents like lotus seeds, water lily seeds, almonds, sesame, sugar, honey, milk and ghee. They are usually balanced by spices like ginger, cardamom, cinnamon, cloves. A good herbalist can make such formulas and preparations.

Different Ayurvedic companies have their own proprietary medicines that are often based upon traditional formulas, including many new modern rasayana products. Sometimes formulas may be named after their chief ingredient. Other times they are given modern names that require an examination of their constituents to know what their effects may be. These rejuvenative medicines can be very valuable but care must be taken to understand their usage and their potency. Below are listed a few common traditional rasayana preparations.

Chyavan Prash

Amalaki is often said to the best rasayana as it helps rejuvenate all seven tissues. Chyavan prash, a kind of jelly made with amalaki and many other herbs, is the best preparation based on Amalaki. Chyavan Prash is named after Chyavan Rishi who received the special knowledge of Soma and immortality from the Ashwins, the twin horseman deities who symbolize the transformative power of balanced prana and apana. It is an ancient Vedic formula.

Chyavan prash uses amla as the base to which it adds raw sugar, honey and ghee to give it more substance, and certain spices to aid in its digestion. It adds special rejuvenative herbs like ashwagandha, shatavari or the ashtavarga (group of eight formula), as well as other powerful herbs of various kinds for body and mind. Sometimes gold and silver are added. The amla fruit serves as a base to hold, carry and improve the potency of these rejuvenative herbs added to it.

Available forms of Chyavan prash differ in their secondary herbal ingredients, as well is in the proportional amounts of amalaki, sugar, honey, sesame oil and other primary ingredients. Many modern and proprietary medicines are types of Chyavan prash or variations on it, though they may have different names.

Triphala

These three herbs together form the famous Ayurvedic compound Triphala. Triphala is an important rasayana for the colon and aids in the proper absorption of prana in the large intestine. It is a good healing astringent for the mucus membranes. It is also helpful for the bones and for the nervous system. It is often an adjunct in larger rejuvenative formulas. Prepared as a ghee, Triphala is very good for the eyes.

Brahma Rasayana

This is an important rasayana preparation made originally primarily with haritaki and amalaki. Many nervines like brahmi (gotu kola), calamus, and shankha pushpi are also used in its preparation. It combines many of the rejuvenative properties of Chyavan prash for the body along with additional rejuvenative powers for the mind and nervous system.

Chandraprabha

Chandraprabha means the light of the Moon and can strengthen the Soma within us, while reducing any excess Kapha. It contains numerous herbs notably camphor, shilajit, guggul and many anti-Kapha agents. It is a tonic and rejuvenative for the urinary system and reproductive system, counters arthritis, reduces obesity and improves overall strength and immunity. It is a good example of more complex Ayurvedic restorative formulas of which there are many both in classical and modern Ayurveda.

Ashtavarga Plants

Ashtavarga is a famous traditional group of Ayurvedic rejuvenative herbs, often used in combination and added to Chyavan prash. They work to increase Kapha, Ojas, bodily fluids and bodily tissues, including reducing fever and heat. There is some doubt as to their original species and many substitutes are now used. They have been discussed in the appendix of the book.

Rejuvenative Herbs in Other Traditions

There are important rejuvenative and nervine herbs in herbal traditions from all over the world. Chinese medicine in particular has its entire set of tonic and rejuvenative herbs, most notably the different types of ginseng and ginseng substitutes, and its various chi, blood, yin and yang tonics that are quite powerful in their effects. The yang tonics like aconite overall relate to Agni and Tejas, the yin tonics like rehmannia or asparagus for Ojas, the chi tonics like ginseng, astragalus and codonopsis to Prana and perhaps Ojas as well, and the blood tonics like dang gui can be very revitalizing as well. Lycium berries, a powerful yin tonic, make a particularly good rejuvenative juice that can now be found in many natural food stores mixed with other fruit juices.

Powerful rejuvenative properties are common in the plants of the tropical rain forests, like the Amazon, where many orchid, lily and aquatic plants prevail as well as special tropical fruits like acai, papaya or jabutikaba as well as nuts like Brazil nuts and cashews. The rain forests of Kerala in South India and Assam in the northeast are similar ecosystems, with similar types of plants. Much research needs to be done in this area.

IMPORTANT AYURVEDIC REJUVENATIVE AND RESTORATIVE SOMA PLANTS

Common Name	Latin Name	Properties and Actions
Aloe/ Kumari	Aloe vera	Rejuvenative for the liver and female reproductive tissue, for Pitta and Kapha; carries Shakti energy as house plant
Amalaki	Emblica officinalis	Rejuvenative for all tissues, particularly plasma and blood, for Pitta and Vata
Arjuna	Terminalia arjuna	Restorative for the heart, promotes healing of soft tissue
Ashtavarga	Group of eight plants	Soma and Ojas promoting properties, cool and moistening; traditional component of Chyavan prash
Ashwattha peepal, bodhi tree	Ficus religosa	Astringent and tonic to the reproductive system, carries spiritual Shiva energy as a house plant, sacred to Agni
Ashwagandha	Withania somnifera	Rejuvenative for Vata and for muscles, bones, nerves and reproductive system, good for Kapha
Bakuchi	Psoralea corylifolia	Rejuvenative for the skin, normalizes skin color; possible ancient Soma
Bala	Sida cordifolia	Rejuvenative for Vata and Pitta, promotes Ojas, gives strength

Common Name	Latin Name	Properties and Actions
Bhallatak	Semecarpus anacardium	Rejuvenative for the lungs, skin, nervous system, for Vata and Kapha doshas; increases immunity
Bhringaraj	Eclipta alba	Restorative for the hair, skin, blood
Bibhitaki	Terminalia baelerica	Rejuvenative for Kapha and the lungs
Bilva (Bael)	Aegle marmelos	Rejuvenative for colon, astringent
Black or kali musali	Curculigo orchioides	Rejuvenative for the liver, lungs, kidneys and reproductive system, mainly for Vata and Kapha
Chyavan prash	Amalaki based rejuvenative formula	Rejuvenative for all the tissues, main classical Soma formula
Deodar cedar	Cedrus deodaru	Protects the lungs and immune system; carries Shiva energy
Durva, darbha, kusha	Cynodon dactylon	Strengthens reproductive system and nervous system, improves the skin, counters Pitta and Vata doshas; sacred Soma grass
Garlic	Allium sativa	Rejuvenative for heart, lungs, reproductive system, Kapha and Vata
Gokshura	Tribulis terrestris	Rejuvenative for kidneys and good for the heart, lungs and reproductive system.
Guduchi	Tinospora cordifolia	Rejuvenative for liver and blood, removes chronic fevers and infections, special for Pitta
Guggul	Commiphora mukul	Rejuvenative for heart, bones, Kapha and Vata
Haritaki	Terminalia chebula	Rejuvenative for colon, throat speech and Vata dosha
Kapikacchu	Mucuna pruriens	Ayurvedic tonic and rejuvenative for reproductive system and nerves, good for Vata dosha

Common Name	Latin Name	Properties and Actions
Licorice	Glycyrrhiza glabra	Rejuvenative for nervous system and lungs, analgesic, calmative, anti-spasmodic
Lotus	Nymphaea nucifera	Rejuvenative for reproductive system and nervous system; ancient Soma plant
Pippali/ long pepper	Piper longum	Rejuvenative for lungs, brain and Kapha systems
Punarnava	Boerhavia diffusa	Rejuvenative for kidneys and blood
Saffron	Crocus sativa	Stimulant and rejuvenative for blood and female reproductive system
Shalmali/ Silk cotton tree	Bombax malabaricum	Rejuvenative for the blood and reproductive system, reduces Vata; sacred to Agni
Shankha pushpi	Convolvulus microphyllus	Rejuvenative for mind and brain, revives perceptive and sensory powers, as well as memory; for Pitta and Vata
Shatavari	Asparagus racemosus	Rejuvenative for plasma, skin, and reproductive system, particularly for women; mainly for Pitta and Vata
Shilajit	Shilajita	Rejuvenative for the kidneys, lungs and nerves, good for Vata and Kapha types, a good mineral supplement
Trikatu	Three spices of dry ginger, black pepper and long pepper	Adjunct for reviving the digestive fire and aiding in the absorption of heavier herbs; mainly for Kapha and Vata
Triphala	Combination of Haritaki, Bibhitaki and Amalaki	Rejuvenative for colon, nerves and bones; widely used for all doshic types, particularly Vata
Turmeric	Curcuma longa	Balances digestion, promotes healing of soft tissue injuries, guards against cancer

Common Name	Latin Name	Properties and Actions
Udumbar/ Cluster Fig	Ficus racemosa	Rejuvenative, especially for Pitta, particularly when taken with milk; sacred tree like Ashwattha
Vamsa rochana	Bambusa arundinacea	Rejuvenative for lungs, cooling and soothing; mainly for Pitta and Vata
Vidari kand/ Indian Kudzu	Pueraria tuberosa	Rejuvenative, reproductive system tonic, refrigerant; good for Pitta and Vata
Water lily or makhanna	Euryale ferox	Rejuvenative for reproductive system, refrigerant; reduces Vata and Pitta
White or safed musali	Asparagus adscendans	Rejuvenative for reproductive system, plasma and lungs; mainly for Pitta and Vata

HERBS TO REJUVENATE THE MIND

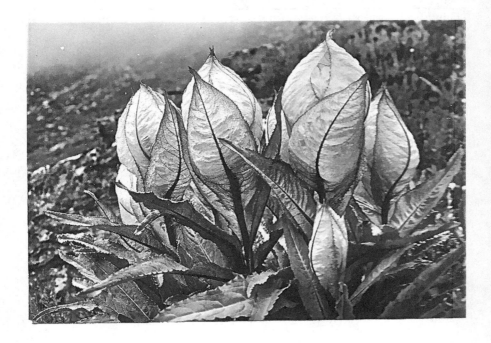

Brahma Kamal, Saussurea obvallata

In this chapter, we will examine the role of herbs, which play a powerful but support role to yogic methods like meditation that we will go into in detail in the next section of the book.

We live in an age of a widespread use of medicinal drugs not only for the body but also for the nervous, system, brain, and mind. Drugs for depression and attention problems are being given out in massive numbers almost like a new panacea. We are taught that we can change our brain chemistry and balance our emotions through the right drugs alone. We often do this without first considering any natural alternatives or trying to make changes in our own life-styles. In the process we are also losing control of our own brain chemistry. We are becoming dependent upon, if not addicted to, drugs for our sense of well-being and for our psychological balance in life. The older we get, the more our well-being and freedom from pain is likely to depend upon taking not one, but numerous such drugs, as well as trying to balance their side effects.

However, nature has not left us without any medicines for the mind, any more than it has for the body. There are special herbs that work to improve the functions of the mind, senses, brain and nerves. An important class of these nervine herbs consists of special rejuvenative agents.

Rejuvenative Herbs for the Mind – Medhya Rasayanas

Ayurveda calls its rejuvenative herbs for the minds *Medhya Rasayanas*, 'rejuvenatives of wisdom'. These are of great benefit in smaller dosages for improving brain function and in higher dosages for rejuvenation of the mind. They have a new importance in the modern age in which we spend long hours behind computers or television screens, whose rays can deplete the nervous system and disturb the mind.

Rejuvenative herbs for the mind are linked with our Soma beverages, as the drinks that we take serve to hydrate the brain and nervous system. They are often taken with honey and ghee as well.

Each of the three doshas can disturb the mind. High Kapha blocks the channels, causing congestion, heaviness and lack of perception. High Pitta causes excess heat and agitation in the mind, including turbulent and conflicting emotions, fever and inflammation. High Vata causes the mind to move too quickly, to be stressed and ungrounded, leading to mental and emotional instability, including nervous exhaustion. Many rejuvenative herbs for the mind can work on all three doshas, depending upon their combinations. However, different herbs for the mind do work more on different doshas, so doshic variations still need to be considered.

Brahmi - Centella asiatica

Brahmi is probably the most important and commonly used of the Medhya Rasayanas. Brahmi cools and calms the mind, creating space and clarity for deeper mental and spiritual activities, and is also good for the heart. It helps cleanse the blood, liver and urinary system and remove heavy metals, drugs and toxins from the body. It is particularly good for Pitta, but can be used for Kapha and Vata in the right combinations.

Brahmi is commonly used as a ghee, or prepared in coconut oil (Brahmi oil) as a massage oil for the face and hair. It helps maintain hair color or darkness and aids in protecting all the sensory openings in the head. It is very good for the eyelids and for the ears.

Brahmi makes a good tea if taken with Tulsi and a little honey to balance out its bitter taste. The fresh juice is said to be a powerful rejuvenative for the brain. Various types of brahmi or pennywort drinks can be bought from South Asia, particularly from Thailand, where it is a common beverage. However, these sometimes have various chemical additives and preservatives.

Relatives of brahmi and gotu kola, which is closely related to it, grow commonly in tropical regions growing among grasses or in watery areas. I have seen them commonly in India, Hawaii and Brazil. However, their chemical contents do vary and not all are as effective as rejuvenative agents, so some caution must be taken in using them.

Manduka Parni - Bacopa monnieri

Manduka parni is another common tropical plant resembling brahmi in appearance and usage, though botanically unrelated, often growing in moist areas or where water is flowing. It is similar in properties to brahmi, and sometimes regarded as better, being more demulcent and holding more nutritive powers. It is often used as a substitute for brahmi, when that is not available, or taken along with it. The fresh juice is very good if one can get it or it can be taken as a tea.

Shankha Pushpi – Convovulus microphyllus

Shankha pushpi is another important Ayurvedic Medhya rasayana and nervine tonic, much like brahmi and manduka parni, with which it is often combined. Sometimes it is even considered to be better than brahmi. It is commonly made into a syrup for improving memory and concentration, or by simply combining the powdered herb with honey. It cools down the nerves and mind and counters heat, hypertension, sunstroke and headache. It has a strong lunar nature.

Calamus – Acorus calamus

Calamus is an important stimulant for the brain, nerves and senses. It aids in the recovery of the power of speech and perception after strokes. It is pungent and heating in nature and increases Tejas and Sadhak Pitta. Calamus clears Kapha and Ama from the subtle channels of the mind, brain and nervous system, allowing for the clearer transmission of impulses, helping with such Kapha nervous system problems as epilepsy. It is also very good for Vata.

One of the best ways to use calamus is in nasya therapy, prepared in a sesame oil base. One puts several drops of calamus nasya oil into the nose. This helps rejuvenate the mind and prana. One can also sniff the power of calamus, particularly for clearing congestion from the head.

Calamus and brahmi in equal amounts make an excellent rejuvenative agent for the mind that is very balanced in its properties. Together they make an excellent herbal tea that can improve the powers of speech and memory and are good for working with mantras.

Jyotishmati – Celastrus paniculata

Jyotishmati means what is full of light. It brings light and energy into the mind, much like calamus in its usage, improving perception and promoting insight, intelligence and Sadhak Pitta. The plant is the source of a good oil that has a powerful stimulating effect.

Tulsi or Holy Basil - Ocimum sanctum

Tulsi or holy basil is another important herb that has special properties that can aid in right function and rejuvenation of the mind and senses. It improves perception and brings clarity to the mind, along with good judgment, carrying the grace of Lord Vishnu. In some respects tulsi resembles calamus in its powers but is milder in nature, also improving Tejas and Sadhak Pitta and is best for Kapha and Vata. It aids in meditation and devotion. In addition it is good for colds, fevers, flu and lung disorders. It is an excellent tea and combined with herbs like brahmi will improve their flavor and balance their function.

Jatamamsi – Nardostachys jatamamsi

Jatamamsi is a special calmative agent for the mind and antispasmodic for the nerves, like it relative valerian, but cooler, gentler and more restorative in its effects. It is the main mild sedative and analgesic agent used in Ayurvedic medicine. It is an important ingredient in most formulas for strengthening the brain and mind and settling the nerves. It can be good for all the doshas. It is more commonly taken as a pill or powder.

Other Helpful Herbs for the Mind

Many nervine plants can be useful for rejuvenation of the mind in some way, aiding in reviving it, calming it or balancing its functions. These include ephedra, camphor, nutmeg, and asafoetida. Many mints and sages have similar properties and can be used as aids to clearing the mind. This includes sage, skullcap, peppermint, spearmint, pennyroyal and motherwort. Much depends upon combination and proportion in herbal formulas.

Many types of incense bearing herbs are good for the mind like sandalwood, lotus, rose and jasmine, including resins like guggul, frankincense and myrrh. Aromatic plants in general often have strong powers to affect the mind, as we will examine in the next chapter. Many rejuvenative herbs for the body can also be of benefit for the nervous system, brain and mind, including ashwagandha, shatavari, bala, licorice and lotus.[73]

Note the following two tables. The first consists of primary Ayurvedic rejuvenative, restorative and stimulant herbs for the mind. The second consists of various Ayurvedic rejuvenative herbs for the body, which also have a strong effect upon the mind.

AYURVEDIC REJUVENATIVE AND RESTORATIVE HERBS FOR THE MIND

Brahma kamal	Saussurea obvallata	Rejuvenative for the mind and nervous system, counters paralysis, revives the senses; ancient high altitude Soma plant
Brahmi	Centella asiatica	Rejuvenative for the brain, nervous system, liver, promotes awareness and meditation

Calamus	Acorus calamus	Rejuvenative for brain, eyes and speech, opens the sinuses; promotes Tejas, mainly for Vata and Kapha
Camphor	Cinnamom camphora	Nervine stimulant, revives mind and senses, clears head and sinuses, promotes perception, stimulates mind and senses, but must be used in proper small doses
Ephedra/ Somalata	Ephedra vulgaris	Stimulant for mind, brain, nerves and heart, mainly for Kapha; Persian Soma plant
Jatamamsi	Nardostachys jatamamsi	Rejuvenative and calmative for the mind and nervous system, calms Vata and Pitta
Jyotishmati	Celastrus paniculata	Nervine rejuvenative and stimulant, mainly for reducing Kapha and Vata
Manduka parni	Bacopa monnieri	Rejuvenative, calmative and clearing for brain and nervous system, like Brahmi
Sandalwood	Santalum alba	Calmative and anti-fever agent, reduces Pitta and Vata in body and mind
Saussurea/ Kushta	Saussurea lappa	Clears the mind and emotions, improves cerebral circulation, promotes intelligence, perception, and immunity; good also for skin diseases
Shankha pushpi	Convovulus microphyllus	Nervine tonic, nutritive, calmative and restorative; particularly good for Pitta and Vata
Tulsi	Ocimum sanctum/ tenuiflorum	Stimulant for mind, senses, nervous system and lungs, promotes devotion and meditation; regarded as a form of the Goddess

AYURVEDIC REJUVENATIVE TONICS
WITH ADDITIONAL ACTION ON THE MIND

Amalaki	Mild nervine tonic, nurtures the cerebrospinal fluid
Ashwagandha	Nervine tonic, sedative, improves memory and concentration for Vata and Kapha
Bakuchi	Nervine tonic, improves complexion and vision
Bala	Nervine tonic, calmative, strengthens physical and psychological immunity for Pitta and Kapha
Bhringaraj	Nervine tonic, cleanses the blood, promotes growth and color of hair
Garlic	Nervine sedative, anti-Vata for hysteria, anti-Kapha, but not sattvic
Guduchi	Cools and concentrates the mind, improves circulation, reduces anger and fever, good anti-Pitta
Guggul	Clears the channels, regulates endocrine system, balances metabolism
Haritaki	Balances mental functions, improves speech and voice, anti-Vata
Licorice	Nervine tonic, analgesic, harmonizing agent
Lotus seeds	Nervine tonic, nutritive, calmative, fortifies the heart; allays Pitta
Pippali	Stimulates perception, clears the channels, counters Kapha
Saffron	Mild nervine stimulant, improves cerebral circulation, fortifies heart
Shatavari	Nervine tonic, nutritive, calmative for Pitta and Vata
Shilajit	Nervine tonic, mineral supplement for the brain
Water lily seeds	Nervine tonic, nutritive, astringent, particularly for Pitta

Somas, Alchemy and Rejuvenation

In ancient Vedic times various plant Somas were lauded for their rejuvenative and mind-opening powers. Modern Ayurvedic rejuvenative plants have developed from this Vedic tradition, though the identity of certain Soma plants was lost over time. Yet there are suggestions that minerals, particularly gold and perhaps lapis lazuli, were used in the preparation of Soma in Vedic times as well. Soma was commonly called golden (hari) and connected with gold.

In post-Vedic times in India, from the early centuries BCE, various alchemical formulations came to be popular, particularly for rejuvenation purposes. Most important were special rasas or oxide ashes, including purified forms of numerous metals, minerals and gems, generally called *bhasmas* or oxides, owing to their preparation into fine powders. This alchemical use of minerals developed from the sacred Vedic fire ritual, out of which various ashes from plants, woods, resins, ghee and oils were prepared and had a healing as well as a spiritual usage. These ashes or bhasmas were also called rasas, referring to their nature as the refined or purified essence of material substances.

The metal mercury is regarded as having Soma like properties and to be Shiva in nature. Sulfur is said to be Shakti. Minerals like gold, silver and mica have also been used in this manner and are still added to Ayurvedic rejuvenative formulas like Chyavan prash in India today. Such minerals are prepared through special firing processes over a long period of time to 'humanize' them and make them safe for internal consumption. Special alchemical preparations continue to be used in Ayurvedic medicine in modern Ayurveda, particularly for their ability to work on the brain and promote rejuvenation. This includes the ashes of various gems like ruby and diamond.

A related alchemical tradition existed from China to Europe in the Middle Ages, though India probably had the most extensive development and the most sophisticated procedures for preparing metals for internal consumption. However, if one wishes to use modern Ayurvedic alchemical medicines, one must be very careful to get well made products from reliable sources as poorly made they can contain toxic heavy metals. In Tantric texts as in European alchemy, metals and minerals are also symbolic of inner spiritual practices and subtle energies.[74]

Probably the best and safest of these mineral preparations in Ayurveda are preparations of pearl (moti or mukta bhasma or pishti). Pearl, which corresponds to the Moon astrologically, has a special ability to heal the lunar or reflective essence of the mind, including cooling and calming the mind and reducing emotional stress and turbulence. Pearl ash can be taken by itself and is commonly added to other Ayurvedic formulas, particularly rejuvenative agents for the mind or for the female reproductive system.

An excellent Ayurvedic rejuvenative formula composed of various alchemically prepared minerals is *Vasant Kusumakar*, which is rejuvenative to the mind, heart, nervous system, and reproductive system and particularly good for diabetes as well as for sexual and general debility.

Soma, Psychedelics and Intoxicants

We all seek bliss, ecstasy or intoxication in life, which is the state in which our mind merges into a greater sense of unity, calm, contentment or happiness. We can gain that in a crude manner through alcohol and drugs, in a refined way through art, music and dance, or spiritually through mantras and chanting, pranayama and meditation. Yet, we should remember that all forms of intoxication or ecstasy gained by external circumstances, methods and substances are limited and must come to an end. They also easily breed addiction and cause dependency and depression. The *Yoga Sutras* indicates that herbs and drugs are one of several means of gaining siddhis or higher powers and mystic insights. Yet it ascribes them to Asuric or undivine practices that can be part of unspiritual motives and practices.[75]

Marijuana is regarded as one of the Soma like plants in the *Atharva Veda*.[76] Cannabis is a common component in Ayurvedic formulas as a decongestant, for pain relief or as an aphrodisiac, though generally used in small amounts along with other herbs. A number of yogis and sadhus in India, like many Naga Babas, commonly use marijuana, not just for its mind altering effects but to help them deal with the cold and physical hardship of living in the wilderness and mountains, which are usually their preferred habitats. However, great yogis usually do not recommend taking marijuana, especially over long periods of time. Even in terms of Ayurvedic medicine, cannabis is regarded as more dangerous than tobacco and can damage the lungs and the liver, as well as cause addiction, if taken in significant amounts or for long time periods. But there is no ban on its usage and a recognition of its considerable health benefits when used correctly. Marijuana along with such narcotic plants as dhatura are often regarded as sacred to Shiva, but meaning also that only Shiva can handle them!

Psychedelic herbs are another potential type of herbal Soma, such as found in peyote or various mushrooms, though we do not find much history of their usage in India. Soma is thought by some western scholars to be a narcotic mushroom (Amanita muscari), though this is not the Vedic Soma, which is described like plants of the reed, orchid and lily species, with nothing like mushroom characteristics.[77] Yet the Soma value of psychedelics, though stronger than alcohol and perhaps of some initiatory value, is limited and such plants can disturb or damage our nervous systems, particularly upsetting Vata dosha, sometimes in a significant manner.

Various shamanistic traditions from throughout the world have special sacred plants that can rightly be called types of Somas, taken either by themselves or in special combinations and preparations. These include such herbs as tobacco, cannabis, amanita muscari mushroom and ayahuasca. Yet here we must consider not only the type of plant but also how it is used. Such sacred usage of the plants, as in traditional cultures, is very different than modern recreational usage. Used recreationally, such plants are more likely to deplete our Soma. In traditional rituals, one strives to connect with the plant spirit, not simply regarding the plant as a drug, and one seeks a vision, message or higher awareness in order to improve one's life.

Modern medicine with its analgesic and anti-depressant drugs is creating its new forms of Soma that include various mood-elevating medicines like anti-depressants. These are powerful chemical Somas but not of a higher nature. Such chemical drugs do not serve to develop or increase our inner Soma but rather work to deplete it. They also accumulate in the tissues and can cause various health problems.

To counter the dangers of drug based Somas, we must develop a new set of Soma herbal preparations to bring true well-being to the mind, as well as the spiritual and yogic forms of Soma to help them really work. We should seek the highest Soma, the greatest refined essence, which requires an inner spiritual practice, not simply taking an intoxicant.

We cannot drink our problems away unless we are imbibing the bliss or Ananda of the Divine. This is the true Vedic Soma.[78]

Soma Herbs and Aromatherapy

We have discussed Soma as a type of herbal extract rather than simply as a particular plant. The most powerful extraction from plants is clearly their aromatic oils. The use of aromatic oils is an important type of plant Somas that deserves its separate examination. Such aromatic Somas or 'Soma aromas' are helpful for the rejuvenation of the body, but are more important for the prana, senses, mind and heart.

- Aromatherapy is another important rejuvenation therapy. Through the sense of smell it stimulates all the senses and brings Prana into the body and mind. Aromatherapy is probably the most powerful immediate therapy for revitalizing our energy. As aroma connects to the Earth element, it is the best means for nurturing the inner mind and senses. Aromatherapy strengthens our inner Earth, as it were, connecting us with all the healing powers of nature. The right fragrances or aromas stimulate the mind and senses, aiding in their rejuvenation, helping counter conditions of dullness and depression. Other aromas calm and nurture the emotions and the nerves, countering anxiety, anger and other negative emotions.

- Aroma and fragrance holds deep emotions. It is connected to both to human love and to religious devotion. Our memory, particularly at a deep subconscious level, is connected to various fragrances. Special aromas can be used to clear the mind and heart of negative memories, traumas and sorrow.

Aromatic Herbs

Aromatic herbs can be used like other herbs in teas in powders, as spices used with foods, or their aromatic oil can be extracted and used in its own right. They can be added to massage oils and other ways. Aromatic oils increase our Soma or sense of beauty and delight, as well as peace and contentment both in ourselves and in our interaction with our natural environment. Like rejuvenative herbs, aromas also can function as aphrodisiacs or vajikaranas for strengthening the reproductive system.

- The use of incense is another important part of rejuvenation and revitalization therapies as well as aromatherapy. The smoke of the incense can easily be transported and pervade the air. It can spiritualize the environment and atmosphere around us, as well as stimulating the mind and senses when inhaled.

The three types of Soma plants we have mentioned previously have their correspondences as aromas as well.

- Cooling, sweet and nutritive rasayanas that increase Kapha dosha, the bodily tissues and Ojas. This main type of Soma increasing rejuvenative tonics has its counterpart in aromatherapy mainly in sweet flower essences like lotus and rose, and in some barks like sandalwood.

- Stimulants for reviving energy and promoting awareness. These are mainly spicy aromatic herbs to begin with like camphor, calamus and tulsi that can be easily used as aromatic oils.

- Spicy, bitter herbs and resins for purification of the blood, promoting healing, countering fever and protecting immunity. These include plant resins that also have aromatic value like frankincense, myrrh and guggul.

Aromas like rejuvenative herbs are closely connected with aphrodisiacs. Sweet flower fragrances are particularly good for rejuvenation of the female reproductive system. They also help calm Pitta and reduce fever and agitation. Below is a more specific listing of several important aromas, though a few cross over and have properties in more than one of these three areas.

Types of Rejuvenative and Restorative Aromas

Nutritive sweet and generally cool fragrances	Lotus, rose, gardenia, jasmine, frangipani, lily, iris, champak, lavender, sandalwood, vertivert (khus)
Stimulating spicy/ pungent fragrances	Camphor, tulsi, calamus, cloves, cardamom, ginger, cinnamon, eucalyptus, basil, sage, thyme, mint, sagebrush, cedar, wintergreen, ajwan, heena, aloeswood (agaru)
Resins and blood purifiers	Myrrh, frankincense, guggul, loban (benzoin), shallaki, saussurea, saffron, turmeric

In other words, many of the same rejuvenative plants discussed from an herbal basis can be looked upon in terms of aromatherapy. However, we must remember that many tonic herbs are used for their food value, for which the use of their aromas, if they have these, cannot be a substitute. Some important rejuvenative tonics like ashwagandha have no corresponding aromatic oil. Aromatherapy is an addition to the herbal therapy, not a substitute for it. More importantly, aromatherapy is important for rejuvenation of the mind.

Soma as an Aromatic Plant

The question arises as to the identity of Soma as an aromatic plant. Clearly there is a diversity of aromatic plant Somas as of other types of Soma. Among these most obvious is the lotus itself, though there are many non-aromatic Somas as well.

In Vedic thought the head or crown chakra is called the realm of the thousand-petal lotus. It is also called the place of Soma or the Moon. The lotus symbolizes these aromatic or flowery Somas both in nature and in our own psyche. The lotus as a plant contains both nutritive and aromatic Somas.

Aromas and Bhasmas

In Vedic thought, Agni and Soma are always related. Fire produces fragrances as it burns and many plants, particularly woods with resins, yield good types of fragrance and incense when burned. Aromatic plants are another type of plant Soma offered into the sacred fire of Agni.

The ashes or *bhasma* from the Vedic sacred fire form another type of rasa, essence or Soma, though dry in nature. Such ashes also called *vibhuti* in Sanskrit are generally white in color and have an aroma of camphor, which is one of the main resins used in their preparation. These aromatic plant ashes are both another form of Soma and another type of aromatherapy. Many gurus give out the special bhasmas that their ashrams have made as a meditation tool, a means of attuning to the guru, which may be smeared on the forehead or the heart in order to connect with them. Incense is another important type of Soma aromatherapy, particularly for the rejuvenation of the mind. The entire universe is said to be the bhasma or sacred ashes created by the Divine fire.

Special Soma Aromas

Below are a few special aromas connected to Soma and the Moon, and often burnt as incense.

• Night-Blooming Jasmine

The intoxicating fragrance of jasmine is well known. It stimulates not only our outer emotions but also our inner devotion, carrying the emotional essence of the Moon. Other night blooming flowers carry such a Soma essence in their fragrances. In fact, many flower essences are stronger at night.

• Camphor, the Aroma of the Moonlight

Camphor is often compared to the rays of the Moon. It improves the mind, stimulates awareness, increases perception, relieves congestion and opens the subtle channels of the nervous system. Yet though it stimulates and revives, it does not damage the lunar essence as it not hot in nature. Though lunar in nature it reduces Kapha.

- Sandalwood, the Calm of the Moon

Sandalwood is the best calmative aroma. It has a special affinity with Soma as a power of peace and contentment, calm and equanimity. If there is one aroma to have to promote our inner Soma, sandalwood is probably the best. It is particularly good for reducing Pitta, fever and heat in the mind, but also reduces Vata, anxiety and fear.

- Benzoin or Loban - Styrax benzoin

Benzoin, called *loban* in India, is a sweet resin incense, with wonderful calmative and restorative properties for the mind and nervous system as well as for the bones, lungs and heart. It is the sweetest of the resins and makes a good incense. It is particularly good for the problems of Vata dosha.

Rejuvenation and the Skin: Ayurvedic Spa Therapies

There has been an amazing growth in spa therapies all over the world in recent decades. Sometimes it seems that spa is almost the new religion. Major hotels, particularly in big cities now feature spa therapies, not to mention special retreat, rejuvenation and vacation centers outside major urban areas. People travel not just for the scenery but for special spas, mineral baths, hot springs, mountain lakes or tropical waters all over the world. It has become an important component of eco-tourism as well as medical tourism.

Yoga is also now part of the spa scene worldwide, with asanas, pranayama and meditation. Yoga centers and retreats commonly offer or feature spa treatments or massage. Ayurvedic medicine has also gained an important place in the new spa therapy. It has become part of health tourism in India, where various Ayurvedic massage and spa centers can be found from Kerala now to the Himalayas, catering to clients from Europe and America.

In fact, as we age we naturally gravitate towards and find value in spa treatments of all kinds. Massage, oil therapies, aromatherapies, saunas, good food, good herbs and good exercise are part of healthy living and of rejuvenation. Many of the therapies discussed in this book work well in a spa environment, particularly if in a beautiful natural setting. Ayurvedic spa treatment is an important adjunct for any Yoga and Ayurveda rejuvenation therapy.

The Skin and Rejuvenation

Rejuvenation or rasayana begins with the skin, which is the outer face of the plasma or 'rasa' dhatu in Sanskrit, the first of the tissues of the body. The skin as our outer membrane connects to the mucus membranes of the body that form our internal lining or inner skin. This associates the skin with the plasma, the first of the seven tissues in Ayurveda, which reflects the entire process of digestion and the state of Kapha dosha within us. As connected to the plasma, the skin relates to the lymphatic system which sustains it.

The skin is connected to Vata dosha (the air humor) as our point of initial contact with the air, the atmosphere and the wind. Like Vata dosha, it is therefore involved in the aging process, which causes it to become dry and depleted, particularly for those who work outdoors or in the sun. The skin shows how the outer weather and climate affect us. Our wrinkles are chronicles of our years.

The skin is the largest organ in the body. It is the second most important tract in the body after the digestive tract. Its condition reflects that of our digestion as a whole, but its condition also has implications for the emotions, mind and nervous system as well. The skin is an important organ of absorption. After the lungs, the skin is the most important organ for absorbing prana and sunlight. Other nutrients can be absorbed through the skin as well, particularly as carried by various oils. The skin holds a certain luster or Tejas, reflecting the glow of our vital energy. We can tell a lot about a person through the condition of their skin.

Moreover, the skin forms our first line of contact with the external world and makes up an important component of our immune system, functioning like its initial protective wall. The health and vitality of the skin, and the power of circulation through it, reflects the strength of the immune system. We contact the forces of the environment through our skin and its sensitivity to weather changes. The skin can make us susceptible to the forces of heat, cold, dampness, dryness and wind. It can allow these forces to enter into our body and energy field and to set in motion the disease process.

Keeping our skin healthy is an essential part of any real wellness program, as well as any rejuvenation therapy. Applying herbs, aromas and oils to the skin can be helpful for everyone, including those on the spiritual path as it helps calm the mind and clear the emotions. We can bring rejuvenative medicines into the body directly through the skin, particularly by way of oil massage but also through the use of aromatic oils. Herbal powders and pastes can be applied to the skin, as can healing clay and mud. Special mineral baths are important as well. Saunas, and steam therapies work primarily through the skin and can

165

aid in its circulation, hydration or detoxification. Yet any rejuvenation therapy for the skin should be combined with other therapies for body and mind, particularly Soma increasing beverages to properly hydrate the skin, and herbs that nourish the skin like amalaki and shatavari.

Artificial Care of the Skin

Proper care of the skin, not simply for beauty but for the health of the body as a whole, is not just a cosmetic matter. It cannot be accomplished merely by using expensive cosmetics. Many cosmetics contain chemicals that deplete or damage the skin. Natural oils are much better, particularly sesame oil, which is extremely nourishing to the skin, though cosmetically speaking is greasy and messy to use. In addition to anything we put on the skin to make it look or feel better, we must improve our digestion and our intake of beverages, as well as develop better circulation through proper exercise and pranayama.

Today people are now changing their looks through chemicals and plastic surgery. Botox, a kind of poison, is the main such chemical used, which paralyzes the muscles beneath the skin, making the skin tight and removing wrinkles. Yet it is expensive and must be reapplied regularly and does not actually improve the skin itself. In fact, it weakens the muscles of the face and damages the skin over time.

Plastic surgery aims at tightening the skin of the face. Yet there are also surgeries to make larger, tighter, or smaller our other bodily parts. Here too we are not actually changing the energy or nutrition of the body but merely making it look good from the outside. Such procedures can make us more artificial and weaken our deeper creativity and spirituality. They are for the benefit of other people and our social image, not for how we ourselves feel. Natural methods can also be used to reduce our age and improve the quality of the skin and the muscles, but we cannot use them merely to escape the aging process. We must learn to age gracefully.

Oil Massage and Ayurvedic Oils

Oil application to the body, called *Snehana* in Sanskrit, is an important rejuvenation method as well part of ordinary health maintenance. It also serves as one of the preliminary practices of Pancha karma,

Ayurveda's radical detoxification procedure. Snehana consists of both the external and internal use of oils, with oil massage externally and taking of healing oils internally, particularly ghee or clarified butter in food, herbs or by itself.

Massage is one of the simplest and most powerful health-promoting and rejuvenation practices, particularly gentler methods that use a fair amount of oil in the process. The best massage oil for rejuvenation is sesame oil, which is warm, heavy, lubricating and nourishing in its properties. Sesame has the ability to penetrate deep into the bones and joints, carrying strong nutritive and calmative properties. It is specific for countering Vata dosha, which is the main factor behind aging and strengthens Ojas.

Other good massage oils for rejuvenation include almond, coconut, and ghee. Almond like sesame is strong to reduce Vata dosha, but not quite as heavy and so easier for short-term usage. Coconut is cooling and nutritive and most important for reducing Pitta dosha. It is great for inflammatory skin conditions and its cooling nature is good for the head, which we want to keep cool. Ghee is also good for Pitta and for inflammatory skin conditions. Stored in a copper vessel, it gains yet better properties for healing the skin, particularly for chronic and inflammatory skin conditions. There are special Ayurvedic sesame oil preparations that have rejuvenative powers as well. These include Narayana tail, Mahbhringaraj tail, Bhringamalaki tail, Dhanvantari tail and Kshirabala tail, among a variety of commercial preparations.

Regular oil massage is important for strengthening the skin, the plasma or rasa dhatu, particularly in dry climates, dry seasons (autumn and non-rainy seasons), and for those suffering from dryness in the body (like Vata types). Dryness of the skin can promote the aging process and the drying up of the other tissues as well. Oil massage is an important method for reducing Vata dosha, the main factor behind the aging process. Oil massage helps remove Vata dosha from its place of accumulation in the bones and joints and allows the healing prana to flow within us. Even as a general longevity practice, oil massage is important, and should be part of everyone's regular health regimen.

Full body oil massage is important. In Ayurveda, after a short massage that uses very little oil and aims more at the use of pressure, large amounts of warm sesame oil are poured upon the body along with a light massage. Traditionally, two massage technicians apply the oil in a simultaneous massage motion. Such extensive oil massage nourishes the skin as well as the nervous system. Special aromas are often used with massage oils and can add another healing dimension to massage.

Shirodhara and Oil Application to the Head

Shirodhara, or the slow pouring of warm sesame oil on the forehead while the patient is lying on a massage table, is another important massage and oil therapy, particularly good for improving Tarpak Kapha and also Sadhak Pitta. It can prove a little hot for Pitta types, however, who may need a more cooling oil application. It is helpful for rejuvenation of the mind, as it calms and nourishes the brain and nervous system. It relieves stress and anxiety and helps promote relaxation and deep sleep. It increases the sense of calm and contentment in the nervous system.

Saunas, Steam and Sweating Therapies

Sweating therapies, called *Svedana* in Sanskrit, are another powerful means of improving the health of the skin and circulatory system. The sweat not only purifies the skin but also removes toxins and stimulates blood and energy flow. However, one must keep adequately hydrated while undergoing any steam or sauna therapy or they can become depleting. That is why in Ayurveda, these usually come after oil therapy.

The use of spicy diaphoretic herbal teas like ginger and cinnamon will further promote sweating at an internal level, or the use of pungent herb like eucalyptus in the steam. Yogic pranayama can be used to develop a natural sweating even without herbs or heat, cleansing the Prana and the subtle body.

Sweating by itself is a reducing therapy, fiery in nature, and so is not normally part of rejuvenation therapy. The combination of oil massage and sweating therapies (snehana and svedana) is particularly important in Ayurveda. These conjoined therapies help drain the toxins from the deeper tissues so they can exit through the blood and plasma into the digestive tract for their elimination from the body in Pancha

Karma therapy.

Salt and mineral baths, which are largely heating in nature, can also be part of sweating therapies and can have their own special rejuvenative effects, particularly for the skin and the lungs. The hydrating effect of the mineral water is almost a kind of oleation and aids in the moistening of the skin. Salts are particularly good for reducing Vata dosha. Yet again care must be taken as any hot therapy will tend to be more reducing and must be applied with care when there is any significant weakness in the patient.

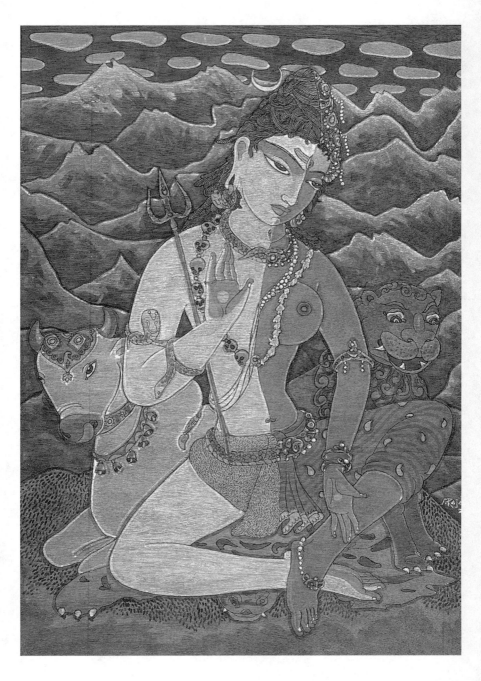

Ardhanareshvara: Shiva and Shakti in the same body

Sexuality and Rejuvenation:
Balancing Shiva and Shakti

Only when Shiva is united with Shakti does he have the power to act; otherwise he is not able even to quiver.

Shankaracharya, Saundarya Lahiri 1

Sex is perhaps our most powerful form of Soma, enjoyment or intoxication that we ordinarily experience in life. Sexual activity engages all the senses, as well as the mind and emotions. It has a power to allure, captivate, entice and absorb. How we use our sexuality is an important index of how we develop our Soma. Yet human sexuality reflects the polarity of energies through which the entire universe of duality operates and on which its dynamism depends. Sexuality is the most important biological force that we have and the basis of our mental energy as well. It has an essential role to play in rejuvenation and in the development of higher consciousness.

The reproductive system not only has the potential to create new life; it can help rejuvenate the life that one already has. Our sexual energy is the key power in the body for rejuvenation as well as it is for birth, growth, and reproduction. Without being able to harmoniously access its power, other methods of rejuvenation may prove limited. Yet right use of sexual energy is not just a matter of outer practices, it requires an internal energy balancing, and a certain psychological and emotional maturity.

Part of the normal function of the reproductive fluids is to nourish the body, mind and nervous system and to sustain them from within. In Ayurvedic and yogic terms this means to serve in the development of Ojas, our core vital fluid reserve which is the essence of the reproductive fluid and the endocrine system in general. Depletion of our sexual vitality can cause nervous exhaustion, weak immunity and promote the aging process, reducing overall longevity and compromising greater well-being. This is particularly true in the case of Vata type individuals in whom an airy and nervous energy prevails, as for Vata,

171

the amount of the tissues, including the reproductive fluids and Ojas, tends to be less and can be more easily depleted.

On the other hand, suppression of our sexual vitality can also weaken its power. It can lead to deep seated unhappiness and frustration. It can breed anger and violence, particularly in men, more often creating depression and anxiety in women. Or it can simply render our energy weak and unable to renew itself.

As we age, the sexual drive naturally tends to diminish at an outer level. This need not be resisted. However, at an inner level, the same energies continue and one can work with them as psychological and spiritual forces in perhaps more powerful ways. One needs to get to the creative essence of the sexual drive as a power of consciousness in order to use it has a healing force.

Ayurveda has always linked rejuvenation (rasayana) therapy with therapies to improve sexual vitality (vajikaranas) often called aphrodisiacs. Often both are taught together. This is not simply to help us remain sexually active into old age, but to teach us how to use our sexual vitality to regenerate body and mind. Classical Yoga usually emphasizes *Brahmacharya*, preserving one's sexual vitality, as a means of developing a higher energy of awareness. Brahmacharya is not merely celibacy but requires using directing the sexual vitality into the nervous system and mind to sustain a higher energy.

Shiva and Shakti as One

Our happiness and well-being depends upon balancing the male and female or masculine and feminine energies within us. This is not merely an issue of becoming sexually neutral as it were, neither male nor female, or androgynous. It means allowing both our male and female energies their full and interrelated expression.

Here one is reminded of the Hindu image of *Ardhanareshvara*, meaning God as half male and female, which portrays both Shiva and Shakti in one body. The right half of the body is distinctly male or Shiva and the left half is distinctly female or Shakti. This is very different than depictions in which a deity is depicted in such a way as one does not know whether the figure is male or female! *Ardhanareshvara* shows the complete development of both male and female energies without their confusion, yet in a way that is complimentary rather than competitive or conflicting.

Each one of us has within ourselves both male and female energies, with the male or Shiva energies prevailing on the right side of the body and the female or Shakti energies on the left. Our energy shifts from one side of the body to the other in the course of the day as the breath shifts from the right to the left nostrils. This corresponds in an inverse way with the right nostril and right body corresponding to the left brain, which is more masculine in function, and the left nostril and left body corresponding to the right brain, which has a more feminine nature.

Each one of us is also born male or female (with a few exceptions) in our outer physiology and psychology. We hold that particular sexual energy in our outer form and expression and should strive to develop its higher qualities and spiritual attributes. Yet the energy of the opposite sex dwells within us at a deeper level, as well as forming the basis of our outer relationships. We not only seek that complementary energy externally, we also seek it internally.

We need to harmonize our sexual energy, honoring both male and female forces as sacred, so that we can access the state of unity that holds the best of both the male and female aspects of nature, and allows each its full expression. We need to honor the sacred aspects of both the cosmic masculine and feminine forces, not to reject either force as inferior. One important way to do this is to honor the Divine as both male and female, father and mother, brother and sister.

Yet this duality of forces is more than just a sexual, emotional or human formation. It requires recognizing the cosmic duality of Shiva and Shakti that is behind not only the sexual duality in our biology but all the dualistic forces of nature, like Sun and Moon, fire and water. Immortality requires connecting to these two great cosmic powers and their influences that are active in all spheres of existence.

To unite both the Shiva and Shakti, male and female, Agni and Soma forces within us is the key to rejuvenation of our entire being.

Their child is the immortal Prana that takes us beyond the limitations of body and mind. To accomplish this process requires that we honor the two great powers in all their manifestations. Working with fire and water and other natural forces helps us do this, not simply analyzing our love lives!

Connecting to the Cosmic Forces of Shiva and Shakti

At an outer level, Shiva represents the male, fiery and active energy, while Shakti is the female, watery and receptive energy. However, at an inner level of our functioning, which is the basis of yogic alchemy, the feminine Shakti force awakens and becomes fiery and active, while the masculine Shiva energy is internalized and becomes calm and inactive, lunar in nature. Shakti develops into Kundalini or the ascending power of consciousness. Shiva develops into Soma or the descending power of grace. *This spiritual role reversal of male and female energies is essential to any higher consciousness.*

The Shiva force gives us strength, steadiness, focus and expansion. The Shakti force affords us receptivity, pliability, adaptability and creativity.

• Awakening the Inner Shiva Energy

The higher male energy is developed by connecting to the Shiva energy or cosmic masculine force. This requires developing self-control, calmness, steadiness, strong will power, fearlessness, daring, friendliness, clarity and compassion, with coolness of mind and non-violence. You can use the simple bija mantra *Om* to awaken this Shiva energy or mantra *Om Namaḥ Śivāya!*[79]

• Awakening the Inner Shakti

The higher female energy is developed by connecting to the Shakti energy or cosmic feminine force. This requires developing the ability to nurture, to support, sustain, love and care for, along with receptivity, faith, creativity, grace, devotion, gentleness and kindness. You can use the simple bija mantra *Aim* to awaken this energy or the mantra *Aim Paraśaktyai Namaḥ!*[80]

Of these two forces, the Shakti force plays a more crucial role in revitalization and rejuvenation, which depends upon a deeper level of receptivity and nurturing. Shakti is connected to the healing forces of the universe, particularly the powers of earth, water and space, the feminine elements. This 'Shakti of rejuvenation' or *Rasayana Shakti* is necessary for any other rejuvenation practices to really work. We should strive carefully to awaken it. There are special pranayama and mantra practices for both developing and balancing these two energies. We will discuss these later in the book, particularly through alternate nostril breathing to balance the solar and lunar aspects of this duality.

However, we must remember that the terms Shiva and Shakti are indications of universal powers that transcend all names and limitations. Throughout the ancient world and in all traditional cultures we find a similar worship of the cosmic male and female forces through fire and water, the standing stone and the ring stone, the pyramid and the altar, the mountain and the valley, and many other natural symbolisms. It is this reading of the cosmic forces that we need to learn, not simply attaching them to the names and forms of one culture or another.

Sexuality and Love

Sexuality is not a mere biological force to manipulate at an outer or physical level. Sexuality is connected to the mind, the heart and the deeper energy of love that is immortal. It is the root of all our emotions, and reflects the prime power of love and attraction, the bliss or Soma from which the entire universe arises.

The reproductive fluid is the primary Soma formed from the physical body and its tissues, the most refined essence of our bodily fluids. Yet the reproductive system is connected with more refined forms of Soma, ultimately with the energy of universal love within us. We cannot mechanically control our sexual energy, much less suppress it in order to live longer or be healthier. We need to develop the love energy working behind it and turn that in a spiritual direction through developing devotion and compassion.

Tantric Yoga contains special practices of sacred sexuality. These should not be confused with popular modern Tantra and its self-indulgent orientation, its free sex approaches involving multiple partners, including casual sex with people one does not even know! Traditional Tantra turns sex into a sacred ritual, which is its true role in life as a union of the two primary forces of the universe, in order to liberate the spiritual energy behind it. This involves honoring the partner as a manifestation of the deity, with respect, commitment and consistency.

Another option is to develop Bhakti Yoga or love for the deity. This can be used to sublimate the sexual energy and remove any need for a physical partner. One can chose whatever aspect, manifestation, form or relationship with the deity that has the greatest power to inspire one on the level of the heart. The key to rejuvenation is to strengthen the reproductive system and its creative energy and turn it within through aligning it with the heart. This is to connect it with a higher force of love and creativity.

Food and Herbs for Strengthening the Reproductive System

Ayurveda has an entire class of special foods and herbs for strengthening the reproductive system and promoting longevity (vajikaranas), including many listed previously in the book for rejuvenation of body and mind. There are a number of animal products like eggs, fish and shellfish, as well as various types of meat, which can nourish the reproductive fluids, but may not promote rejuvenation because their energy is heavy. Garlic and onions are often viewed in this light as well. They have irritant properties and though they build the reproductive fluids can also cause us to unnecessarily discharge them.

For rejuvenation, certain sattvic (vegetarian and non-irritant), cooling, moistening and nourishing foods are better, especially dairy products, seeds and nuts, root vegetables, natural sugars and fruits.

SATTVIC REJUVENATIVE FOODS FOR THE REPRODUCTIVE SYSTEM
Milk, ghee, butter, yogurt, sweet cheeses, almonds, cashews, pistachios, sesame seeds, sweet potatoes, asparagus, mung beans, urad dal, kulattha, dates, raisins, figs, bananas

Ayurveda's aphrodisiac or vajikarana (vigor promoting) herbs are closely related to the rasayana or rejuvenative herbs and many herbs have both properties. Yet those vajikarana herbs that are sattvic and non-irritant are best for rejuvenation.

SATTVIC REJUVENATIVE HERBS FOR THE REPRODUCTIVE SYSTEM
Ashwagandha, bala, shilajit, amalaki, shatavari, vidari kand, white musali, black musali, kapikacchu, gokshura, saffron, nutmeg, pippali, cloves, rose, aloe vera, licorice, lotus seeds, water lily seeds[81]

Of these herbs shatavari, amalaki, saffron, aloe vera and rose are particularly good for women. Ashwagandha, bala, vidari kand, white musali and kapikacchu are particularly good for men.

Your Inner Ecology: Rejuvenation, Environment and Life-Style

Rejuvenation rests upon a particular life-style. It is not a short-term therapy or something that can be achieved through taking a few medications. In fact, our life style should always be rejuvenating, even if we want to experience ordinary happiness and well-being.

One of the great problems in the modern world is that most of us are following highly stressful, if not toxic and disturbing life-styles. This includes not only our dietary habits but also our work, entertainment and associations. We have little time for ourselves and our personal well-being. Sometimes clients tell me that they do not have the time for the Yoga and Ayurveda practices that I recommend to make them healthy. My answer is: "Does this mean that you have the time to be sick?" Clearly our health and well-being is the most important factor that we have in our lives, without which we cannot do anything else. Medical expenses are our biggest expense, particularly as we grow older. To create a healthy tree, one must first nourish the root. The root of our lives is our life-style. If we don't create a long-term wellness sustaining life-style for ourselves, nothing else that we do can be successful.

We should follow the diet, herbs, exercise, life-style and spiritual practices that promote our overall well-being. In addition, we need to engage in special periodic renewal and rejuvenative practices, which require a supportive environment and a favorable time of the year. We must create the matrix or field for rejuvenating energies to be able to flow and develop, so that we can sustain them through the rest of the year.

Climates and Seasons for Rejuvenation

For rejuvenation practices, certain times and places, seasons and climates are preferable, though we can also modify the environment in the buildings where we live and work. The main outer enemies of rejuvenation are cold, wind and dryness. Excessive heat or moisture is also not good. Warmth, moistness and still air are helpful.

Timing of rejuvenation practices is particularly important if one does not live in a good climate for rejuvenation. Relative to the seasons in temperate climates, the best time for rejuvenation therapies is during the late spring to mid-summer, which is April to July, when Nature is undergoing growth and expansion. May is usually the best month in most places. Autumn is a time for tonification or building up bodily bulk and strength as a preparation for the challenges of the winter season. This can aid in rejuvenation, but does not carry the revitalizing prana that prevails in the spring. Yet spring is also a time of purification and we need to cleanse the body from the toxins and stress of winter before being able to energize it at a higher level.

Probably the best geographical areas for rejuvenation are tropical locations where there is adequate but not excessive warmth and moisture, and not too much wind. This usually requires a slight elevation in the hills and mountains, not the dense heat of the jungle, low lying tropical areas or locations on the sea. This is usually an altitude of fifteen hundred to four thousand feet depending upon the area. One can follow rejuvenation practices in these areas almost any time of the year; though the spring is better to the extent that season may exist in the tropics. One should avoid the rainy season, particularly when the rains are heavy or frequent, or winds are high, and start rejuvenation practices after the main rains have ended.

Tropical streams, lakes and pools have strong rejuvenating powers, as do the tropical plants, flowers and fruit. Yet one must be careful with the beach, as the wind and the ocean waves can absorb or take away one's energy. The ocean has a magnetic energy that can draw our energy into it.

Tropical islands like Hawaii that have such moderate elevations are particularly healing, where there are mountains and hills by the sea to draw the prana down. Yet there are many such locations in Central and South America, Africa, Southeast Asia, Australia, the Pacific Islands and other parts of the world, which have hills by the sea or inland.

The Himalayan foothills or some of the hill and mountain regions of South India are particularly good in this regard. Such hill and low mountain locations in temperate regions can be good for rejuvenation, but during the appropriate seasons of late spring and summer.

Mountain elevations are particularly good for rejuvenation of the mind. At high elevations, the Sun is stronger and the sky more blue bringing in a powerful healing prana for the mind and heart for expanding awareness. In the mountains, the elements of air and space have a special rejuvenating power for our consciousness. That is why yogis and mystics often retire into the mountains. However, such mountain climates are usually not favorable for rejuvenation in the fall and winter, and are not always helpful in the case of Vata dosha individuals who suffer from lightness and dryness and need strong physical rejuvenation. In addition, care must be taken to avoid too much sun or wind in mountain regions, as the sun can take away our energy quickly in these areas. In general mountain regions around three to eight thousand feet are best for rejuvenation of the mind, as higher altitudes tend to be too harsh.

Relative to the seasons, besides spring, the middle of winter around the winter solstice can be a helpful time for rejuvenation of the mind, which can benefit from the energies of introversion and inaction prevalent at this time, provided one avoids exposure to the cold and wind. Our inner prana is awake in the winter and we can use that winter rest of our outer faculties to allow it to regenerate itself.

In general, too much sunshine and sun bathing is not good for rejuvenation practices, though a certain amount, half an hour up to an hour a day in some instances can be helpful. The Sun can take our prana away if we expose ourselves too much to it, though it can give us prana if we take the right amount of it. Air conditioners, however, can be depleting as well as being too close to heaters or fire sources.

Yet one can create a rejuvenation climate in various locations wherever nature is strong, where there is some degree of moisture and where the rejuvenation rooms and accommodations are properly built. One can design a special rejuvenation hut or room to mitigate against negative outer climate factors. A rejuvenation room should not be exposed to cold, wind, sun, heat or other strong environmental influences. In this way special rejuvenation gardens, accommodations, Yoga and Ayurveda spa centers can be created that can compensate for negative environmental influences, which are hard to entirely avoid. Ashrams and Yoga retreat and sadhana centers can provide such accommodations as well.

Rejuvenation Environment in the Home

One can prepare one's own home to aid in rejuvenation practices. After all, the home is where we are located most of the time. After time spent at special retreat centers, rejuvenation should be continued at home in order to sustain its best results. But there must be peace and quiet in the home, including a good natural home environment for this purpose. If the home is a place of conflict or disturbance, it cannot be helpful in healing body or mind.

It is important to keep certain plants in the house or treatment area that promote rejuvenation and longevity. These include aloe, holy basil (tulsi), hibiscus and tropical fig trees (ashvattha, udambara, Bengal fig). Flowers in the house are very important for a healing environment including marigold, lily, rose, gardenia, jasmine and other flowers with sweet and stimulating aromas. Some can be grown in the house if possible, or in the garden, or bought as cut flowers. We should learn to bring in and adorn our home with the beauty of nature.

The burning of incense in the house is very helpful, particularly gentle aromas like sandalwood, jasmine, rose, champak or loban. The burning of ghee lamps is also very important, or lamps with sesame or mustard oil, or fragrant candles. Water should be present in the house in the form of fountains, basins or other structures.

Performing regular puja or devotional worship in the house using flower offerings helps immensely, as does maintaining a meditation room that is not used for other purposes. It is best to make one's entire home a temple but at least a special sacred room and altar should be maintained. One's bedroom should be a place of peace and be open to the light of the sun. The home overall should be well ventilated and allow fresh air to come in.

Rejuvenation, Rest, Relaxation and Sleep

Rejuvenation requires a reduction of both physical and mental movement. Ayurvedic rejuvenation therapy involves placing a patient in a special rejuvenation hut and avoiding all activity during the process of treatment. Less radical measures can be taken up for those not ready for this, but a reduction in physical activity and mental stimulation is essential for all forms of rejuvenation.

Every day we undergo a mini-death and rebirth. This is the process of sleep. The state of deep sleep provides us our natural daily rejuvenation that we cannot live without. In deep sleep we return to the original Prana of the soul and experience our connection with the Divine Mother. If we have a good deep sleep we awake fresh, renewed and revitalized for another day. If we fail to achieve a good deep sleep we awake drowsy, tired, irritable or even disturbed and disoriented.

Rejuvenation requires adequate rest, relaxation and sleep. Many of us today are sleep deprived. We travel too much, over stimulate the mind and senses, and keep odd hours that go against our biological rhythms. Even if we sleep enough hours, our sleep is disturbed by agitated dreams and is not entirely restful. Cultivating deep sleep is an important aspect of rejuvenation therapy.

Yet even better than ordinary deep sleep is the wakeful deep sleep that arises through meditation. This can be developed through special meditation practices or learning the art of *Yoga nidra* or yogic sleep. Rejuvenation of the mind requires sustaining this deeper restful wakefulness. It is helpful for the body as well.

Yet too much sleep, particularly sleep during the day, reduces our longevity and can promote the toxins in the body. It increases Kapha dosha and creates heaviness in body and mind. It is important to take our main sleep during the prime hours of midnight to five AM. However, short afternoon rests can be helpful during rejuvenation therapy, particularly for those whose energy is particularly low, like many Vata types.

Rejuvenation also requires relaxation. True relaxation, however, is not simply a relaxation of the muscles of the body. A deep relaxation of the nervous system is required, which means turning our awareness, focus and attention within. This depends upon being able to surrender to the Divine presence within and around us, whatever name we wish to call it by, opening to the sacred nature of all life. It means letting go of the ego and our need to control things and letting things and people be what they are.

Yoga asanas can help us relax and are designed primarily for this purpose, particularly sitting poses, but can only work if combined with peace of mind and turning our energy within. Otherwise, asanas like other exercise forms can stimulate our nerves and senses and disturb us further if we approach them with too much effort or movement.

Ultimately, rejuvenation of the body depends upon letting go of body consciousness – forgetting that we are the body – and letting our awareness return to pure light which is its true nature. When we let go of body consciousness, we relax our ego grip upon life as a whole. We de-tense the body as it were. We remove our toxic thoughts, emotions and urges that disturb the body's natural harmony. Our body is a marvelous instrument that we must respect. Its own natural intelligence can heal and rejuvenate us. But we must move our awareness within to allow nature to do its magic with the body, letting it become a divine instrument.

Conserving our own Nature

Most of us now recognize the need to conserve the natural resources in the world around us. Yet we also should strive to conserve the natural resources within ourselves, which means our own vitality and awareness, and the cosmic powers that are behind our own soul. This is not an abstract matter but requires reducing unnecessary stimulation and irritation to our mind and senses, avoiding emotional reactions, and reducing unnecessary movement and activity. We must learn to conserve our vital energy and hold it deep within, not as a selfish hoarding but as an offering to the immortal consciousness at the core of our being. We must make sacred the elements within us: the earth, water, fire, air and space of our bodies and mind. Our body itself should become a temple for Yoga and meditation.

Begin by reducing unnecessary activity in your life, including unproductive and disturbing forms of entertainment. You can also reduce unnecessary possessions around you. Remove clutter from both your home and your mind. It is simplicity that allows us to renew, not excess baggage, which can only weigh us down. Learn the simple art of living, which is the art of simple living – life in harmony with the cosmic life and light, not to be at the beck and call of social distractions. More importantly, learn to conserve your mental energy by avoiding unnecessary thought, worry, anxiety or anger. Learn to honor the Divine presence within your own heart that is your true Self and being.

Yet it is not just a matter of preserving our energy, we must preserve our integrity as well. This requires being true to ourselves and not throwing ourselves away upon the outer world and its enticements. Stand in your true Self and you are greater than the entire world, greater than all time and all circumstances. Learn to conserve your own Self, which is to live in harmony with your inner being, not letting yourself be dominated by the world and its agitation. Then you will never find yourself exhausted or defeated.

Preparing Yourself for Soma: Preliminary Purification and Pancha Karma

We all seek rejuvenation but the question must first arise whether we are ready for it. Special rejuvenation practices require preparation in diet and life-style, extending to weeks, if not months before any strong rejuvenative practices are attempted. Even milder rejuvenation procedures have prerequisites. For true rejuvenation to occur, the disease and decay causing toxins and doshas should first be removed from the body. Such purification practices are essential to promoting longevity and countering the aging process, as well as for creating the foundation for rejuvenation practices to be effective.

To purify ourselves of disease causing toxins requires strengthening our digestive fire or Agni in order to burn them up. It can be aided by fasting or the use of special herbs and spices to increase Agni. This is a procedure called *Shamana* or palliation in Ayurvedic medicine. Secondly, it requires draining the toxins out of the bodily tissues and removing them from the body. This is a procedure called *Shodhana* or purification.

The Digestive Fire and Rejuvenation

One must balance and rejuvenate one's Agni in order to proceed with other detoxification or rejuvenation practices, particularly taking rejuvenating diet and herbs. Otherwise they will not be adequately digested and assimilated. What causes disease and aging is not simply the types of food we take but the condition of our digestive fire when we are eating. The digestive fire has four states:

1. High: excess appetite and quick digestion, most evident in fiery or Pitta types

2. Low: low metabolism and slow digestion, most evident in watery or Kapha types.

3. Irregular: variable appetite and digestion, most evident in airy or Vata types.

4. Balanced digestive fire, indicating health and well-being.

Weakness of the digestive fire is indicated whenever we have a pronounced tongue coating and bad breath. It is an easy condition to self-diagnose. Look at the condition of your own tongue and you will see the state of your digestive system.

There are certain spices that have the power to help digest our foods even when our Agni is weak or low. These are the hotter type of spices like cayenne and chilies. While these are usually not used during rejuvenation therapy because they can create excess heat in the body, they are very important for the preliminary detoxification that precedes rejuvenation as they help burn up toxins. Most common in this regard is the Ayurvedic formula Trikatu, which consists of dry ginger, black pepper, and pippali (long pepper). It is best for low Agni, such as in common in Kapha types. Other similarly useful hot spices include mustard, horseradish, cayenne, garlic and asafoetida.

There are many aromatic spices that help enkindle or revive our digestive fire when weak. These are more commonly used in rejuvenation therapy, as hot spices can also burn up one's Soma. These include cinnamon, cardamom, fresh ginger, cloves, cumin, coriander, fennel, basil and turmeric. These spices can be taken with foods, before meals, or as herbal teas during the day to keep the digestive fire normalized. Warm water and spice teas are our best beverages to sustain our digestive fire, not cold water, ice water or soft drinks.

Asafoetida (hing), particularly in the form of the compound *Hingashtak*, is particularly good for Vata caused nervous or irregular Agni. For Pitta caused weak Agni, mild spices and bitters are indicated like coriander, turmeric, gentian and amalaki.

In addition, the practice of fasting can be a good preparation for rejuvenative therapy. For this, Vata types do best with only three to five days of fasting, Pitta types up to a week of fasting, and Kapha types for more than a week. Yet one must develop some experience fasting and not attempt long fasts immediately. Shorter fasts should precede longer fasts for those not used to fasting. After fasting a light diet of pure vegetarian foods should be taken, like kicharee, gradually working in heavier food items like root vegetables, nuts and dairy products. Such practices to clear out Ama and balance Agni may take several months before rejuvenation practices properly can begin.

Radical Purification and Pancha Karma

Besides restoring the power of our Agni or digestive fire, there are more powerful detoxification procedures in Ayurveda, notably the five practices of Pancha Karma. These are required for any radical removal of the doshas from the body. Anyone considering rejuvenation practices should first consider doing Pancha Karma, which is traditionally regarded as the basis for rasayana or rejuvenation therapy. Many Ayurvedic centers provide Pancha Karma treatment and can be consulted for this purpose. Of these five, the first three practices are the most important for the body. Nasya, the fifth practice, is also important for the mind.

1. Therapeutic emesis (vamana) to remove excess Kapha and mucus upwards from the body from the stomach and through the mouth.

2. Therapeutic purgation (virechana) to remove excess Pitta and toxic heat downwards from the body from the small intestine and the rectum.

3. Therapeutic cleansing enemas (basti) to remove excess Vata or toxic gases in the body downward from the large intestine and the rectum.

4. Therapeutic blood purification (rakta moksha) to cleanse the blood, which classically includes blood-letting and is primarily for Pitta.

5. Nasya or nasal therapies to remove mucus and toxins from the head and sinuses.

These processes are facilitated by a preliminary period (usually at least one week) of daily oil massage (snehana) and steam therapies (svedana), which serves to draw the doshas from the tissues and organs in which they are lodged, into the blood and plasma and back to their sites of accumulation for their eventual elimination from the body.[82]

As long as the doshas are present in the body, rejuvenation is obstructed. However, many of the same results as Pancha Karma can be achieved through long-term diet, herbal and life-style procedures to eliminate the doshas. Such practices can also support the benefits of Pancha Karma.

- Spicy herbs like Trikatu, dry ginger, black pepper, pippali, mustard, cayenne, garlic, cinnamon and cardamom, strong pranayama and vigorous exercise for reducing Kapha.

- Bitter and blood-cleansing herbs like aloe, gentian, barberry, coriander and turmeric for reducing Pitta.

- Mild laxatives like Triphala and carminatives like cumin, asafoetida or basil for reducing Vata.

Hatha Yoga Purification Measures

Hatha Yoga has its *Shadkarmas* or 'Six Purification Measures',[83] which are often used for such preliminary purification in Yoga before undergoing deeper spiritual practices. These methods include such difficult procedures such as swallowing clothes to clean the stomach or putting plastic tubes through the nose. They are sometimes attempted without specific diagnosis by a doctor or teacher.

Ayurveda does not quickly recommend most of these Shadkarma practices, with the exceptions of *Jala Neti*, clearing the nostrils with salt water, *Trataka*, gazing at a flame to cleanse the eyes, or strong pranayamas like *Kapalabhati*. Instead Ayurveda recommends its own process of Pancha Karma. The beauty of Pancha Karma is that it is based upon diagnosis of both the individual and the diseases they may have and is adjusted relative to age, location and season.

The *Hatha Yoga Pradipika* states that Shadkarma practices are mainly indicated for Kapha types who are overweight and not ready for pranayama.[84] Other types may not need them and in fact these practices may disturb Vata dosha. Any purification measures owing to their harshness should be performed only with discretion and proper guidance.

Pancha Karma and Rejuvenation

Traditional Pancha Karma therapies are followed by a period of re-juvenation or rasayana. Any strong detoxification therapy requires a follow-up procedure of tonification and rejuvenation. First, such therapies tend to weaken or deplete the body, which then must be revitalized. Second, the purified body is an ideal place for such rejuvenation therapies to work. Modern Ayurveda has arguably put too much emphasis on the detoxification side of Pancha Karma and has not adequately considered its rejuvenation side. As a general rule, however long the period that one receives Pancha Karma or any strong detoxification therapy, one should take twice as long afterwards for tonification and rejuvenation.

Any detoxification therapy should be viewed as a preliminary practice for rejuvenation, not as an end in itself. The main exception is that when toxins are deep seated or not completely eliminated by the application of detoxification therapy, additional detoxification practices maybe required before any real tonification or rejuvenation can proceed.

The Colon and Rejuvenation

The colon is a little understood and appreciated organ, mainly regarded as an organ of elimination. According to Ayurveda the colon is also an important organ of digestion and assimilation. It is in the large intestine that the prana or life-force is absorbed for the food that we have eaten. This prana is taken in along with the air and ether elements from the food, which serves to nourish the life-force, the senses and the mind, as well as to sustain the immune system and aid in reproduction. The colon along with the lungs and skin is a prime site for taking in prana, which three systems are all closely related.

Ayurveda regards the membrane of the large intestine as having a special role in absorption.[85] It takes the life-force from the food and transfers it to the bone tissue, where it serves to nourish the deeper tissues of nervous and reproductive tissues. If our digestion is normal, we will absorb the life-force from our food. If it is abnormal, we will

189

take in the negative waste gases, which will be absorbed into the bone tissue and cause many problems. Hence arthritis and most bone diseases relate to malabsorption in the colon. Nervous and reproductive system disorders usually have their origin here as well.

Weakening of colon function occurs with aging. It also occurs with excess sexual activity or diseases of the reproductive system. With age the downward moving energy in the body (apana vayu) becomes increased. This is nothing esoteric. It is simply the long-term effect of gravity and the entropy of our system to return to its constituent elements.

While this downward moving energy is necessary to allow for such functions as excretion, urination and reproduction, in excess it drains the positive and upward moving energy from our body.

Maintaining a healthy colon is an important support for any rejuvenation practice. First one needs to work on the colon through the diet. This requires proper fiber in the food. There are many new forms of fiber, some artificial in their nature, some combining herbal with artificial ingredients. Generally psyllium husks are the best or the powder made from it. Other good quality fiber comes through greens, whole grains, fresh fruit and root vegetables.

Many people take laxatives to stimulate colon function that deteriorates with age. However, most laxatives do not improve assimilation in the colon, nor do they strengthen its tone. While laxatives can artificially empty the colon, they cannot guarantee right absorption within the colon. We tend to associate poor colon functioning with constipation, and its treatment with laxatives. Most laxatives, particularly stronger purgatives, promote long-term constipation, however effective they are short-term. This is because they are mainly irritants. For this reason many people, particularly the elderly, become laxative dependent, and the colon gets weaker.

Colonics are a popular detoxification measure and sometimes ascribed with rejuvenating powers as well. However, they are mainly useful for short-term detoxification according to Ayurveda. The use of colonics can also weaken the colon and impair longevity, particularly for those who are suffering from cold, dryness, debility or lack of body weight. They should be used with caution and short-term duration particularly for Vata body types or anyone in whom the body weight is low.

All strong bitter laxatives are to be avoided during any rejuvenation process. This includes rhubarb root, aloe and senna, and formulas based upon them. These can actually promote the aging process as they aggravate Vata and can weaken the long-term tone of the colon. Again they are mainly for detoxification.

Most oily laxatives, like castor oil, though not specifically contraindicated during rejuvenative therapy, are not themselves rejuvenative, as being a bit heavy in energy they can have a congesting effect upon the body. Bulk laxatives like psyllium or flaxseed are not specifically rejuvenative, though they can be helpful during the rejuvenative process as well and are the best laxatives for rejuvenation therapies.

There are special herbs that can help rejuvenate the colon, that work to restore its tone and proper function. The main such Ayurvedic formula is called Triphala, which we have discussed a bit already. The main laxative agent in Triphala is haritaki, which can be used by itself as a laxative. Haritaki helps tighten and strengthen the tone of the colon. Amalaki aids in the lubrication of the colon and protecting its mucus membranes. Bibhitaki stimulates the production of mucus along the linings of the large intestine. Amalaki can be used by itself in mild conditions of chronic constipation.

The aging process causes us to lose our power of absorption of food, water and nutrients in the digestive tract. To counter it there are certain herbs that improve absorption. This is usually an issue opposite that requiring the use of laxatives. In fact, excess use of laxatives and colonics can weaken the tone of the colon or promote excess elimination.

In such instances certain astringent taste and absorption promoting herbs are required. Most helpful in Ayurveda is bilva or bael, a tree sacred to Lord Shiva, which is an excellent intestinal rejuvenative and astringent. Other such helpful herbs include fennel, nutmeg, cardamom and ginger.

Danger of Over Detoxification

Most of our natural healing business operates in what could be called a high detoxification mode. Much of this is understandable as our general population is overweight, with a high level of fat, mucus and toxins in the body which should be reduced. Yet detox is also something easy for us to get into as a kind of fad or marketing strategy. We like quick fixes and radical and strong programs are appealing, promising to correct our health problems with a short fast or quick cleanse of one type or another.

Weight reduction programs of various types proliferate everywhere. Yet there are many detoxification programs through colonics, juice fasts, fasting from food altogether, strong exercise and workout regimens, liver cleanses, kidney cleanses, sweat lodges, saunas and hot tubs. Every month it seems some new cleanse or detox regimen, herb or food is being highlighted. We seem obsessed with these cleansing procedures. Yet do not always recognize that such strong detox measures require the right preparation and the right type of constitution to handle them.

We are even inclined to look at any rejuvenation therapy as a kind of crash course that we can get over with quickly in a week or two, so that we can return to our ordinary life style with renewed energy and zeal. Yet rejuvenation takes time. Even radical or stronger rejuvenation programs take at least two weeks and generally more than a month to have strong effects. But more important is our long-term life style. The most important thing is to maintain a sustainable, renewable and rejuvenating life-style in terms of our basic living habits of diet, herbs, exercise, work and recreation. We should not forget this principle as we go over all of our healing options. Even if we take up some rejuvenation practices, we should make sure that our way of life continues in a modality of conserving, internalizing and spiritualizing our energy.

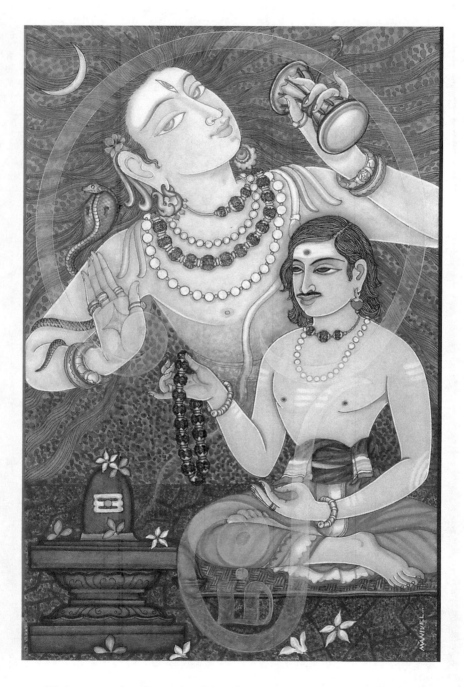

Shiva as the Lord of Yoga and His Worshipper

PART III

Soma Yoga

Rejuvenation of the Mind and
Heart Through Yoga and Meditation

He knew that bliss is Brahman. From bliss all beings arise. By bliss all beings live. To bliss all beings return. That is the wisdom of the sage Bhrigu, son of Varuna, which is established in the supreme ether.

Taittiriya Upanishad III.6

They think they have drunk the Soma after they have crushed the plant, but of the Soma that the seers know, no mortal ever drank.

Rigveda X.85.3

YOGA AND INNER REJUVENATION

Yoga is the calming of the disturbances of the mind. Then there is a dwelling in the Self-nature of the Seer.

Yoga Sutras I.2-3

The greater part of rejuvenation is not of the body but of the mind and heart. It is of little value to have an old mind in a young body or to renew the body but keep the mind tied to the past and its compulsions. Yet most of us are more concerned about rejuvenating the body than we are about rejuvenating the mind. In fact, we often want to rejuvenate the body and prolong our lives in order to continue the same old mental and emotional patterns that are wearing us out and causing pain to others as well! We want to keep the ego and its drives for power, success or pleasure going on longer and avoid the questions that the impermanence of life poses for us. On the other hand, one can renew the mind and heart, even as the body ages and dies, with death itself becoming a doorway to an inner immortality. One can make the mind younger even as the body inevitably decays.

For any successful rejuvenation process to occur, we must first have the right attitude, which means clarity as to what we are seeking. The goal of any authentic rejuvenation therapy is not merely longer life or improving physical health but making us into better, more aware and more helpful human beings. This requires that we align ourselves with the cosmic forces of vitality, creativity and bliss, which are beyond the control of any individual or group, and cannot be developed mechanically or by force. It means that we must seek to transcend ourselves and our time bound urges for what is meaningful in the world of eternity.

Rejuvenation rests upon an inner surrender to the forces of immortality, which occurs at the level of the heart. It is not something that we can buy with the right amount of money, nor is it something that we can arrive at through the right herbs or drugs, nor by doing the right techniques or practices, however helpful these may be as support factors. We must first have an inner openness to the source of life in the heart, which means the willingness to let go of our outer attachments and embrace the greater universe of consciousness, beauty and delight.

Physical rejuvenation is merely a preliminary step towards mental rejuvenation, which includes revitalizing our emotions and senses. Yet mental rejuvenation must be understood in the proper manner as well. Rejuvenation of the mind is not simply a matter of restoring our normal mental faculties of reason, memory or perception. Rejuvenation of the mind is only possible by connecting our minds with the forces of immortality that are inherent in consciousness itself. It is not about continuing the mortal mind with its personal and social compulsions, its information, opinions and beliefs.

Rejuvenation of the mind requires a spiritual practice, what is called *sadhana* in Sanskrit, which means following a spiritual path on a daily basis in which the mind is gradually merged into a higher awareness. To take the mind beyond death requires dying to the mortal mind and awakening to our higher or true Self beyond our habitual thoughts and bodily identity. The ordinary mind itself with all of its memories is our mortality and cannot take us beyond death. We must awaken a higher intelligence within the mind that is aligned to our immortal consciousness, what is called *buddhi* in Sanskrit.

Factors of Psychological Aging

If we want to rejuvenate ourselves and experience each day as the first day of creation, as it were, we must first rejuvenate the mind. This includes clearing our senses from their habitual reactive patterns and awakening a higher prana or life-energy that is connected to greater energy of the universe, not just to the changing trends of our human society.

In this regard, we can easily discriminate between an old mind that is taking us towards death and decay and a young mind that is connected to nature's powers of renewal. An old mind is a mind trapped in its burden of memories, attachments and traumas, unwilling or unable to let them go. The mind, like the body, is also undergoing its aging process, its entropy, which includes a tendency to decay. The longer we live, the more memories we tend to hold and carry in our minds. Psychological aging is born of this taking in and holding of negative emotional patterns, fears and desires. These may be hurts, insults, achievements, enjoyments or simply inertia. Senile dementia, for example, involves being so trapped in the past that the person cannot be truly aware of the present. It is a mind that has lost its capacity for renewal, which exists in the present moment, not in the past.

It is the ego – our sense of the me and the mine – which causes the mind to age, making it rigid, opinionated and incapable of change and adaptation. The power of our ego is the measure of our mental aging. A strong ego, in spite of its pride, arrogance or vanity, hides mental decay, an inability to be open to life that is not centered on itself or its identifications. An innocent mind and heart, on the other hand, naturally renews itself in the beauty and power of the present moment. It has no self-concern or self-fixation and can allow the new, the beneficent and the unexpected, which life brings us every morning, to enter into it without resistance.

Our burden of memory reflects an inability to understand and absorb our experiences in life, which can be described as a weakness in our power of mental digestion. Our mental digestion gets impaired by the opinions of the mind and we build up mental toxins or *ama*,[86] the residue of undigested experiences which clog the channels of the mind, the heart and the nervous system. These undigested experiences form karmic patterns or *samskaras* that limit our actions and cause us to repeat negative behavior, in a constricting web of time, birth and death, which includes past, present and future lives. The mind like the body begins to age and becomes rigid, losing its power of flexibility and movement.

Mental aging occurs through the blockage of our channels of perception by old ideas, emotions, opinions and beliefs. It prevents us from seeing things fresh and direct, like the vision of a child. The old mind is trapped in its burden of the familiar. In fact, the accumulation of preconceptions causes the mind to age. When we become too familiar with life, we lose the beauty of life, in which there is always something beyond what our mind's habits are willing to see.

One of the main causes of mental aging today is our addiction to the mass media and the taking in of artificial media based impressions. These artificial impressions born of technology (like junk food) cannot be fully digested and tend to wear the mind down. They do not contain the Prana of nature but project various human currents of agitation. They are like drugs and disrupt the organic functioning of the mind. They make the mind more reactive, more capable of being disturbed and controlled by commercial or political interests. The media not only pushes our buttons but also creates more buttons in us that it can push. The result is that our minds remain externally oriented, caught at the surface of our being far from the inner wellsprings of happiness and eternity. Mental rejuvenation requires that we turn the media off and connect with these inner sources of vitality born of our mind's connection to the deeper consciousness within us.

Our psychological age is also reflected in how we breathe, whether the breath is deep or shallow and whether we are aware of our breath or not. The deeper and more conscious the breath, the more prana we have in the mind. Also important in this regard is the type of emotions that we hold in our breath. Most of us restrict our prana by how we breathe, creating a certain emotional tension in the lungs and heart. We hold negative emotional patterns of fear, anger and attachment that weaken our vitality and limit our awareness in our very breathing process, circulating forces of decay and fragmentation with us. Without learning to ally ourselves with the cosmic breath and greater life-force of nature, our ability to heal and rejuvenate ourselves will also be limited.

Another factor of psychological aging is the aging of our five senses. This has two aspects as outer and inner. Outer aging of the senses is easy to determine with the decline of our sensory power, particularly the eyes and ears, whose acuity diminishes as we get older. It extends to our five motor organs with a decline in our powers of manual dexterity, physical movement and speech. Inner aging of the senses, on the other hand, is reflected in the rigidity of our patterns of sensory usage. It reflects the orientation of our senses, not simply their functionality. We look at things in an old way, with old eyes and ears, noting only the familiar and the known, confirming our set ideas about the world, other people, or ourselves, rather than perceiving the new and the magical.

A significant part of rejuvenation depends upon our ability to revitalize our senses, which themselves bring in revitalizing Prana. This is not a matter of merely purchasing better video or audio equipment. It requires both developing a greater sensitivity to the patterns of nature outwardly and an ability to turn our senses within to contact the inner world of consciousness. It means becoming masters of our sensory instruments, which have wonderful capacities, not being driven by them for superficial entertainment or distraction. Once the inner senses are open, like the third eye, even if our outer senses lose their acuity, their inner beauty and vitality will continue to grow.

Yoga as a Rejuvenation Therapy for the Mind and Heart

Ayurvedic medicine applies classical Yoga as its primary rejuvenative therapy along with the appropriate diet and herbs. By Yoga here we do not simply mean Yoga asanas but all eight limbs of Yoga, particularly pranayama and meditation, as grounded in devotion and Self-knowledge. A comprehensive and integral Yoga is the best thing that we can do to rejuvenate both body and mind, and also to connect with our inner immortality. Yet this requires a full practice of Yoga from a yogic life-style to deep meditation. Merely performing Yoga poses will not be enough, though it can be a good place to start.

In fact, Yoga is more aimed at inner rejuvenation of the mind and heart than at the outer rejuvenation of the physical body. This is because rejuvenation of the body requires physical factors of diet, herbs and massage, such as Ayurveda teaches us. Inner rejuvenation rests upon pranayama, mantra and meditation, which is the main focus of classical Yoga.

Yet Yoga as an inner spiritual practice is not just another thing for us to do. Real Yoga requires changing how we view both self and world, moving from action and doing to being and awareness. We wear ourselves out in life through excess action and stimulation. Rejuvenation is not another form of practice, preoccupation or entertainment that we can add to those that are already depleting us. It occurs not by doing more but by doing less and being more, resting in the forces that endure.

The greatest powers of rejuvenation reside in stillness, silence and space. The difficulty is reaching that natural stillness, which cannot be arrived at by ego effort or outer action. It requires a special turning in of the mind and heart, a merging of our outgoing urges back into the inner core of love and wisdom that is our true nature and home.

Yoga works through seeking the still point of balance on all levels, whether through the body, senses, mind or heart. In all that we attempt in the search of rejuvenation and immortality, we should not forget this need for space, stillness and surrender. We cannot rejuvenate ourselves. The active and motivated ego is the very inertia of mortality. We can allow rejuvenation to occur, however, if we learn to align ourselves to the forces of nature and higher consciousness that pervade us on every side. Every moment and every place provides such an opportunity if we become receptive to the greater cosmic energy and awareness.

Rejuvenation requires a certain inner silence, a silence of mind. When the mind is chattering or revolving in its habitual patterns, a friction is created that causes it to decay. Similarly, rejuvenation of the mind requires space. The mind is a kind of space or openness that if filled or cluttered with thoughts, emotions or sensations, gets weighed down and depleted.

- What regenerates the mind is calm and peace of mind, best developed through meditation. It involves cooling, slowing down, concentrating and stabilizing the mind, so that we can find contentment, happiness and serenity in our own nature.

- What regenerates the heart is love, which is best developed through devotion. It involves opening the heart to our relationship with the Divine, sacred and cosmic, going beyond our human fixations to a reverence for all life.

- What regenerates the prana is the unitary prana developed through pranayama, deep slow breathing in which our awareness is directed within.

- What regenerates the senses is a reduction of outer sensory stimulation, making our senses more sensitive to the subtleties of nature, and open to new ways of seeing beyond the conditioned reflexes of our opinions and beliefs.

The following chapters will deal with these factors of the rejuvenation of the mind, heart, prana and senses.

THE YOGIC SOMA AND HOW TO PREPARE IT

Within the thousand-petal lotus of the head is the pure full Moon, without the mark of a hare, flashing with a delightful water, smiling with the supreme rasa (juice) increasing moisture.

Description of the Six Chakras 41[87]

Classical Yoga can be described as the cultivation of Soma as the inner nectar of bliss, ananda and immortality. It is not a mere outer practice or exercise but rests upon a deeper inspiration and aspiration to the highest. Yoga or union in any form brings about a flow of happiness or delight, which is Soma, once that union is achieved.

When the individual soul and the Supreme Being unite – which is the highest Yoga or union – there is the greatest Soma flow, which opens all the knots of the heart and floods the *nadis* or subtle channels with bliss. Unless our Yoga practice has a Soma to it, it has not yet entered into the real field of Yoga or union, in which the inner connections occur that link us with all things in the universe. Such practice will eventually dry us out, both at outer and inner levels, if we do not cultivate a flow of Soma behind it.

Classical Yoga through the teachings of Patanjali in the *Yoga Sutras*, which reflects yet older traditions,[88] is defined primarily as *samadhi*, a state of bliss in which the inner nectar flows.[89] The subject of samadhi or its related term *samyama* (which combines dharana, dhyana and samadhi) is the main focus of the great majority of *Sutras* or axioms in the text. Vyasa's classical commentary on the *Sutras*, the oldest available, defines Yoga as samadhi.[90] The eight limbs of Yoga can therefore be regarded as the eight aspects of samadhi. Samadhi meanwhile can be defined as the flow of Ananda or the inner Soma through the mind and heart to all aspects of our life and being.

Patanjali mentions *Dharma Megha Samadhi*, as the ultimate goal of Yoga, the basis of liberation of the Spirit or *Kaivalya*, in which the rain of Dharma or higher truth removes all negative tendencies in the mind and replaces them with pure wisdom and sheer joy.[91] That rain cloud of Dharma is the same as the Vedic descent of Soma, which is the Divine rain, the blissful power of the Vast Truth, *Ritam Brihat,* in the Vedic mantras.[92] It reflects the *Ritambhara prajna,* the wisdom that carries Ritam or the higher truth in the *Yoga Sutras.*[93]

All primary branches of Yoga, which have considerable diversity in their approaches, aim at the unfoldment of our inner Soma or power of bliss, love, peace and truth according to different angles.

- *Raja Yoga,* such as taught in the *Yoga Sutras,* rests upon the Soma of samadhi to calm the mind and connect us to the Purusha or being of bliss within.

- *Hatha Yoga* rests upon the Soma of Prana to awaken our internal energies and nourish them with delight.

- *Bhakti Yoga* or the 'Yoga of Devotion' rests upon the Soma nectar of devotion (Bhakti Soma) to unite us with the Divine within.

- *Jnana Yoga* or the 'Yoga of Knowledge' rests upon the Soma nectar of knowledge (Jnana Soma), the direct perception that distills the essence of truth from all that we see.

- *Karma Yoga* or the 'Yoga of Service' rests upon the Soma nectar of selfless action, in which we find happiness in the happiness of others.

- *Tantric and Kundalini Yoga* requires the descent of Soma from the crown chakra for the Kundalini to arise from below and unite with.

- *Vedic Yoga,* through Vedic mantras, requires making the Soma of mantra flow within us through its rhythmic meters (chandas).

- *Laya Yoga* can be defined as merging into the Soma of the sound current or Nada.

Though Soma is contained in all things, it must be extracted as the inner essence or vital energy, which requires a deeper discernment, concentration and focus. Yoga practice exists to prepare and extract the Soma within us and in our interaction with the greater universe. Yoga is the 'alchemy of Soma', the fruit of which is abiding in our own immortal essence. Without an inner flow of Soma, there is no real Yoga, one could say. So to cultivate Yoga in any form, one must understand the importance of Soma and learn how to extract it. Even each asana or Yoga posture has its own Soma, the sense of delight, peace or well-being one feels in properly performing it.

Soma and Kundalini: The Inner Alchemy of Immortality

Yoga is an art and a science of balancing and transforming our life energies so that we can return to our unitary essence in pure consciousness. However, we need to understand the nature of these subtle forces in order to be able to relate to them properly. Otherwise our Yoga practice may not produce Soma or the nectar of bliss, but may have little spiritual effect or perhaps disturb us even further.

According to Yoga philosophy, particularly in Tantric texts, there is a secret force of the higher evolution of consciousness hidden deep within our psyche. This is the *Kundalini Shakti* or serpent power that lays dormant at the base of the spine and root chakra. This Kundalini Shakti is described as a higher power of Prana and Agni, a kind of subtle electricity that can be awakened to energize us at a much more powerful level of awareness and perception. Many traditional Yoga lines, particularly of the Tantric variety, aim at arousing the Kundalini Shakti from the root chakra, to ascend through the central channel of the spine or *Sushumna* and unite with the Soma principle of Shiva in the crown chakra for the gaining of Self-realization.

The ascent of the Kundalini Shakti through the chakras – and the complimentary descent of the Soma Rasa or Soma nectar – results in the realization of the immortality of pure consciousness, the *Atman* or *Purusha* of Vedic philosophy. This is the way of traditional Kundalini Yoga as outlined in Hindu Tantric texts.[94] It is alluded to in many Yoga texts and explained as the prime practice of Hatha Yoga as well as in the *Hatha Yoga Pradipika*.[95] However, we should not take the process literally as a movement within the physical body. It is an energetic alchemy that can vary in the details of its unfoldment in different individuals. Yet it does have certain guidelines.

The crown chakra, yogically known as the 'thousand-petal lotus', holds the main energy of Soma in the subtle body. In Tantric Yoga, the crown chakra is associated with Soma or *Chandra*, the Moon, and the mind, which are all related. The root chakra is the earth altar that holds the energy of Agni or fire.[96] The inner process of Yoga consists of the ascent of the Kundalini Fire from the root chakra and the corresponding descent of the Soma nectar from the crown chakra, in which the various chakras along the way become opened. It is not just a matter of developing the Kundalini Shakti force but of also developing the Soma force.[97]

Kundalini and Soma

Without the proper prior preparation of the Soma or nectar in the crown chakra, the Kundalini fire can overheat and burn up the nervous system, depleting our Soma and even reducing our longevity. *That is why for anyone who seeks to develop the Kundalini, developing the corresponding Soma is imperative.* In fact, if one develops the Soma above, the Kundalini will naturally arise to partake of it. No other effort, action or practice may be required. On the other hand, if one seeks to develop the Kundalini and has no inner Soma, the Kundalini will be irritated, not awakened. We must remember that *Kundalini awakens in search of the Soma.* To awaken it without Soma is to awaken a serpent but have nothing to feed it. Meanwhile to awaken the Kundalini in a positive manner, we must also stop seeking the outer Somas. It is the outer Somas of sensory enjoyment and ego imagination that keep the Kundalini asleep.

The proper awakening of the Kundalini provides a tremendous energy and inspiration, a vast widening of the consciousness, and can aid in deep healing, rejuvenation and longevity. Yet as a powerful electrical force, Kundalini can be difficult for the nervous system to handle, particularly in the case of practitioners who are not adequately prepared to handle its powerful currents. We must be able to endure and sustain the awakening of its power, which requires the necessary Soma, calm and peace.

There tends to be an overemphasis on Kundalini in modern books on Yoga and the chakras, which rarely emphasize the necessary preparation for arousing this powerful force or the necessary factors for keeping it in balance, once aroused. There is a naïve thinking that one can manipulate the Kundalini mechanically by personal effort, through certain asanas, pranayamas, bandhas, mantras or yoga kriyas, largely of a physical or mechanical nature, as if it were little more than a matter of technique to get it to move.

The role of Soma in the awakening of higher consciousness is probably more important than that of the Kundalini, though it is a secret not easily found. If one's Soma is not first protected and prepared, the rising of the Kundalini can have side effects or fail to occur altogether. If our Soma or inner mind is pure, the Kundalini will naturally arise to receive it and will do so with grace and gentleness.

Kundalini, we must remember, is a force of the non-ego and for the ego to try to manipulate it will only serve to inflate the ego, taking it eventually to a point where it is likely to break and disturb the nervous system. Kundalini is a force of nature like lightning that is beyond our personal control or our ability to predict. To safely arouse the Kundalini requires the right life-style, emotional balance and power of concentration. In fact, if one has the right preparation, particularly the inner Soma to attract it, the Kundalini will arise in a gentle and harmonious manner. Kundalini is a sacred spiritual force, a power of the Goddess that we must approach with reverence, respect, devotion and humility.

To allow the Kundalini to arise in the best possible manner, we must first prepare our Soma. This means developing the cool, content, meditative mind of the crown chakra or lotus of the head. It requires that we ourselves, particularly our psychological natures, become the Soma and allow ourselves to be purified and consumed by the higher forces. As a power of fire, Kundalini requires our own internal purification or tapas. We must be willing to burn up our own ego in the Kundalini fire, which occurs in the lower chakras where both the ego and Kundalini dwell.

Kundalini as the Shakti naturally seeks out this detached Shiva energy or Soma, which is her lord. If an undetached motivation awakens her, she will not be happy. The yamas and niyamas of Yoga help purify the Soma, as do the other limbs of Yoga, if applied in the right manner, notably pranayama, mantra and meditation.

We must learn to breathe in the Soma, which occurs through the third eye, when the mind and breath are calm and balanced. This happens when our mind has no burden of memory and our emotions have been transformed into devotion. This unitary breath is the basis of both Soma and Kundalini, which are the water and fire aspects of this primal Prana or air energy. When the Soma in the crown chakra fully develops it overflows and descends to purify the body and to collect in the ocean of the spiritual heart that is its final abode. That is why Soma is closely connected to the heart as well.

Soma and the Subtle Body: the Five Koshas

The five sheaths or koshas, which represent five layers of our being, are a common yogic teaching going back to the *Taittiriya Upanishad*.[98] Each of these five levels of our nature has its own form of Agni or fire, which is its essential energy. Each has its equivalent form of Soma, which is its main fuel. Agni is the eater or enjoyer, while Soma is the food or substance enjoyed.

- At the physical level (Annamaya kosha), the digestive fire (Jatharagni) is the Agni, and the food and drink we take in through the mouth is the Soma. Higher physical forms of Soma include special rejuvenating foods, beverages and herbs that can revitalize the body, brain and nervous system.

- At the pranic or vital level (Pranamaya kosha), Pranagni or the vital fire is the Agni and our vital enjoyments of exercise and activity are the Soma. Higher Pranic forms of Soma including pranayama practices that can revitalize our internal Pranas and balance their energies towards transformation.

- At the level of the outer or sensory mind (Manomaya kosha), the mental fire is the Agni and our various sensory enjoyments are the Soma. Higher mental forms of Soma include mantra, visualizations and meditations that bring in a higher level of experience into the mind.

- At the level of the inner or discriminating mind (Vijnanamaya Kosha), the Buddhi or discriminating intelligence is the Agni and the various principles, beliefs, ideas or dharmas that we pursue in life are the Soma. Special types of Soma for the higher mind include meditation on truth, unity, bliss and harmony.

- At the level of the soul (Jiva or Anandamaya kosha), our inner consciousness (Chitta) is the Agni, and our entire life experiences and memories are the Soma. Special types of Soma for it include the practice of Self-inquiry in which we digest our life-experiences, burning up our Samskaras (internal karmic tendencies) and turn them into pure awareness, or Self-surrender, in which we surrender in devotion to the Divine within us.

- Through these five sheaths, the soul takes in substances, impressions and ideas from the external world and extracts the nectar of Ananda from them, just as a bee gathers pollen from various flowers and turns them into honey. The ultimate result is the essence of our experience that becomes the Anandamaya or 'Soma Kosha', in which our karmas and samskaras are held and through which we can experience a deeper bliss from Yoga and meditation. Moving through and beyond the bliss sheath one can access the pure bliss of Brahman or the Absolute.

The subtle body can be called our 'Soma body' as it provides means of enjoying Soma bliss through samadhi or unitary consciousness.[99] Learning to access this 'inner Soma body, particularly its summit as the crown chakra, is the key to real happiness. Compared to the subtle body, the physical body is gross and heavy and does not provide much by way of real enjoyment, much less bliss. The physical body is more a vehicle of work or karma than of enjoyment, which enjoyment is largely experienced after death when the subtle influences of our karmas come out.

Yet besides this prime Soma of the crown chakra, each chakra of the subtle body has its own Soma, relative to the specific forms of the five elements, five sense qualities, five sense organs and five motor organs that it rules. Each chakra as it is opened grants us the inner or cosmic Soma that relates to it. We must learn to use the Soma of each chakra in a sacred way as an offering to the Kundalini fire for it to rise properly. This requires honoring the senses, organs and elements that each chakra relates to, giving up sensory indulgence for a spiritual refinement of the senses as tools of worship and meditation. Rejuvenation begins with strengthening the earth and water chakras and their powers, including their Somas, as these elements are the foundation of our physical life.

SOMAS OF THE CHAKRAS

Root Chakra	Earth, aroma and texture based Somas
Sex Chakra	Water, fluid and taste based Somas
Navel Chakra	Fire, light, color and sight based Somas
Heart Chakra	Air, energy, touch and movement based Somas
Throat Chakra	Space, sound and music based Somas
Third Eye	Mind, thought and perception based Somas
Crown Chakra	Consciousness, meditation and bliss based Somas

The Sushumna as the Soma Channel

To access the chakras and their Somas, as well as to awaken the Kundalini, we must first energize the *Sushumna*, bringing the prana into the central channel of the subtle body. If the Sushumna is not energized then we cannot directly access the chakras, whatever else we may do. All the chakras are connected to and can be regarded as an expansion of the central channel or Sushumna of the subtle body, which is our inner space or void. The chakras can only be opened by an expansion of that inner space of awareness, not as mere physical locations, emotions or personal powers.

Sushumna means 'what is very blissful'. It is our inner space in which the Soma can flow. Higher Yoga practices require opening the Sushumna or central channel of the subtle body. Otherwise neither Kundalini can arise nor can the Soma descend. This opening of the Sushumna in turn requires releasing the knots of the heart, letting go of our deep seated fears, desires, anger and attachment. Without developing our inner Soma, there is no space for the higher energies to move within us. To reach that inner space requires the unification of the dualistic energies inside us, which are mirrored in the duality of our breath, thoughts and emotions. We must go beyond inhalation and exhalation, attraction and repulsion, like and dislike.

Soma is the key to all higher Yoga practices, the magic, the nectar and inspiration that allows them to work – and the flow of grace that takes us beyond personal effort. Learning this yogic alchemy of Soma is the true immortal art. It not only revitalizes the body but also creates within us a consciousness that can endure beyond death.

The Arising of the Shiva or Purusha Energy

Along with the ascent of the Kundalini, there needs to be a complementary ascent of the soul, an arising of the Shiva consciousness, which is part of the awakening of the Purusha or higher Self. This is experienced as an ascent of calm and expansive force, around which the Kundalini spirals and is held. This rising Shiva energy, symbolized by the *linga* or pillar of Shiva energy, affords stability to the mind and nervous system. This ascending Shiva force rises to reach the immutable immortal Shiva force in the head. Yet it is also like the power of a mountain. It is on that mountain of Shiva that the Soma can be found.

Like Kundalini, with which it is connected, this ascending Shiva energy is fiery. It needs to be continually cooled through pouring the water of Soma over it. The ascending Shiva energy is also called the *Hamsa*, which means both the Prana and the bird of the soul. It flies upward with the breath as it were. Hamsa is also the bird that dwells on the lake of the Soma. As the higher spiritual fire and light energy arises within us, whatever name or form we give it, we must learn to bathe it with the descent of water and grace which is Soma. This bird of Soma becomes the eagle of higher perception as the flow of Soma cleanses the doors of our perception and opens us up to the vision of all things as infinite and eternal.

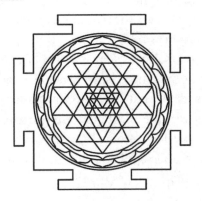

Sri Yantra, the Supreme Soma Meditation Teaching

The main Tantric Soma Vidya or way of Soma knowledge in Raja Yoga is the *Sri Chakra* and *Sri Yantra*, which is identified either with the chakra system as a whole or specifically with the thousand petal lotus of the head and the spiritual heart. The yantra has five downward pointing triangles and four upward pointing triangles. It has forty-three angles representing the 27 lunar Nakshatras and 16 Kalaas or digits of the Moon. Its central point or *bindu* is represented by the mantra *Om Īm Īm*.

The Sri Yantra is closely associated with the worship of the Goddess Tripura Sundari in Shaivite thought and with Lakshmi in Vaishnava thought. It is energized by the Sundari mantras mentioned later.[100] Any Soma based practice should consider the worship of the Sri Yantra, which however is a vast subject in its own right.

THE YAMAS AND NIYAMAS OF YOGA: CONSERVING YOUR INNER SOMA

Yoga is said to be the *Moksha Dharma* or 'way of liberation' of the Spirit, our highest Dharma beyond the outer values of vocation, wealth or enjoyment. We could say that Yoga is our 'Soma Dharma', our inner duty to seek immortality, not for our human personality but as part of the universal movement. Our Dharma consists of our primary activity in life, which is most often allied with our vocation. Our Dharma reflects the prime principles, attitudes and actions we apply. Soma also has its own Dharma or way of life to support it. In order to be able to take in the inner Soma, we must have a life-style or Dharma that can sustain it.

Most of us waste our Soma or bliss in life through pleasure, sensation and entertainment rooted in wrong values and an unspiritual life-style. Each one of us has a certain amount of Soma, delight, or happiness that is open to us karmically. But we are quick to expend, if not waste it, which leaves us without Soma or in a state of suffering or debility. For inner rejuvenation, we need to know how to conserve our Soma and let it naturally grow and expand.

Developing the inner Soma requires a kind of gestation as it were, just as gestation in the womb is necessary for a new child to be born. We must learn to hold our Soma within us, becoming a Soma vessel ourselves. This Soma building process requires refining our nature, becoming more sensitive, aware and perceptive, patiently developing a deeper feeling and knowing. We must search out the Soma in our lives as a great spiritual adventure, unfolding our higher potentials and capacities with steadiness and determination.

During this period of gestating our Soma, we must hold our energies within and cultivate a higher Soma-bearing life-style, which is also the life-style of Yoga as defined in the yamas and niyamas of Classical Yoga. The five yamas beginning with ahimsa are the attitudes that enable us to conserve our Soma. The five niyamas beginning with tapas are the practices that enable us to purify our Soma.

THE FIVE YAMAS

Ahimsa or Non-harming

The flow of Soma is only possible when we are firmly rooted in *ahimsa* or not wishing harm to any creature. Rejuvenation rests upon removing the energy of violence, hatred and death from our own bodies and minds. Such an energy of violence first harms ourselves, upsets our physiology and psychology, and sets in motion the processes of friction, decay and agitation within us.

However, true ahimsa is not a simple matter of avoiding overt aspects of violence, which even a coward can do. Ahimsa requires removing harm from our thoughts, which means not thinking ill of anyone, and instead honoring the Divine presence and sacred reality within all. Ahimsa begins with eliminating harm from our speech, which means stopping negative gossip about others. Most of us cause far more harm in the world with our words than with anything outwardly that we may actually do. Of course we can and must oppose wrong ideas and actions in the world, that is part of our duty to truthfulness, but we should not send negative energy to harm the person who we think represents such wrong views.

Ahimsa is not simply something that we do for others; it is also something that we do for ourselves. Not wishing harm to others involves removing harm from ourselves. When the negative energy of harm and death is removed then the positive energy of immortality or Soma can develop within us. This means that we should not think ill of ourselves, or we will cause harm to our own being. Violence against oneself, the ultimate expression of which is suicide, is promoting the death process within us. To affirm our deathless Self is perhaps the best attitude of ahimsa.

Satya or Truthfulness

The inner Soma is the bliss, happiness and delight that arise from eternal truth. Only what is true never passes away; falsehood can never endure. The outer Somas of the body and senses are forms of Maya or illusion, resulting from a pursuit of transient desires and surface images. Yet real truthfulness is not simply a matter of correct information or of telling what is factually accurate. *Satya* means holding to the eternal truth, which is the source of immortality. This requires letting go of the transient truth and trivial information that confuse the mind, cultivating deeper principles, spiritual study and meditation instead. It means being truthful with ourselves and learning to place the truth above all else.

Brahmacharya

Brahmacharya is a key concept of Soma and rejuvenation overall. Often it is translated as celibacy, but it means more than that. Brahmacharya means taking one's creative energy into Brahman or the Divine. It does not mean merely suppressing sexual function, though it does require control of the sexual organs. It means developing a higher creative energy beyond procreation. Brahmacharya means holding our Soma or sense of enjoyment in our inner search for higher consciousness. This moving in Brahman should replace our moving in Maya or the world of illusion.

Asteya or Non-stealing

To gain our own inner Soma, we must stop trying to take or expropriate the Soma of others, which includes their property, reputation, associations and achievements. The Soma of another can never bring us happiness or delight; in fact, it will always become a poison for us. This is the importance of non-stealing as factor of longevity. It also means that we should stop comparing ourselves with others and seeking what they have. Ultimately, we do not own anything and are merely pilgrims in this world. Asteya also implies giving up a commercial view of reality and not taking advantage of others in the business realm.

Aparigraha or Non-coveting

To hold our inner Soma, we must stop being jealous, envious and coveting what other people have or what we would like to get from them. For this it is not enough simply to avoid taking or holding to material objects. We should not hold to things in our mind and should live a simple life in which we are not weighed down by possessions. We should surround ourselves with positive energies, not with the weight of desires and expectations.

THE FIVE NIYAMAS

Tapas

Tapas is the basis of *Kriya Yoga* in classical Yoga, the 'Yoga of action' designed to prepare the body and mind for samadhi. Tapas means the application of heat and includes self-discipline in all its various forms. In fact, all the yamas and niyamas can be regarded as types of tapas, which also refers to various vows and observation. Yoga practice overall can be defined as tapas, which is often a synonym for Yoga in Sanskrit literature. In the *Vedas*, tapas is the means through which the entire universe is brought into existence. Tapas is the inner orientation of Agni or our flame of aspiration that readies our inner Soma. The real practice of Tapas requires preparing our inner Soma, which implies ceasing to seek Soma from the outside. We must learn to prepare our inner Somas. This requires ripening and cooking ourselves.

Tapas implies self-control, not in the negative sense of trying to suppress ourselves but in the positive sense of mastering our own faculties and energies. It means not being controlled by others or by impulses and desires coming to us from the outer world. Tapas is the power that arises from patient observation and turning within. The highest types of tapas involve pranayama, pratyahara, mantra and meditation.

Of these ten principles, tapas is probably the most important. It is the inner fire purification that prepares us for the real Soma to come forth. Tapas, svadhyaya and Ishvara pranidhana are the threefold basis of Kriya Yoga, which is the means of purifying and preparing our inner Soma of samadhi.

Svadhyaya

Svadhyaya or 'self-study' means learning to know our unique essence or inner Soma, which implies understanding the elements, doshas, gunas and karmas at work within ourselves. We need to discover what our Soma is and where it lies, including what yogic path we should follow. This implies how to connect to our 'inner deity' or *Ishta Devata* and our own unique Divine essence. As we study ourselves deeply we can determine who we really are and where our true happiness lies. Extracting our inner Soma requires introspection at a deep level. Such introspection is not book study, psychological analysis or self-criticism, but the search for our true nature beyond the factors of our outer existence.

Ishvara Pranidhana

Ishvara Pranidhana is surrender to Ishvara or the guiding Divine consciousness within us, which requires giving up of our fears, desires and aggression. It is said to be the best means to samadhi, which is the flow of Soma through our minds and hearts. From Ishvara as the cosmic lord comes a continual flow of Soma as love and wisdom through the Divine Word *Om* and primal sound pervading the universe. By surrendering to the Soma of grace, our inner Soma rapidly increases. The grace of the Divine Soma is always there for everyone, but if we are unwilling to surrender we cannot experience it.

Saucha

Saucha or purity is above all about purifying our Soma. This means purity of body, speech and mind, including purity of diet, sensory impressions and behavior. It implies knowing how to bathe ourselves with higher energies and frequencies that remove toxins and impurities from within us.

Actually, it is the inner flow of Soma that is the real purifying force for the mind. It is the flow of Soma, the flow of the mind's own deeper love and inspiration, which cleanses the mind of negative emotions and crude ego drives. The *Vedas* commonly laud Soma as *Pavamana*, the great purifier,[101] for this reason. Only when we regularly bathe ourselves in that inner Soma current will our hearts become clean and our minds become clear.

Santosha

Santosha or contentment is all about conserving our inner Soma. It is perhaps fitting that the yamas and niyamas end with this Soma principle. Soma grows when we cultivate contentment and are at peace within, regardless of what may happen to us externally. This does not mean that we should become complacent and make no efforts, but that our efforts are born of an inner inspiration, not of an outer restlessness, agitation or seeking. We should ever hold to an inner contentment, which allows us to act wholeheartedly and do our best.

Contentment is one of the main attitudes required for the practice of Yoga and is also essential for longevity or rejuvenation. As we age our minds tend to become more critical, harsh and negative, particularly as we have experienced so much of the fallibility of human nature. However, we must remember that a negative mind tends to breed a negative body and cause disease as well.

True meditation is a cultivation of contentment. True detachment is born of inner contentment, not of trying to give anything up. Contentment is the very nature of awareness in which we rest in the beauty of life and perception that is there for us at every moment.

Yamas and Niyamas and the Three Gunas

The yamas and niyamas are designed to promote a sattvic or pure life-style within us and to counter the negative gunas of *rajas* (disturbance) and *tamas* (inertia).

Yoga depends upon the development of sattva guna, the quality of peace, harmony, non-violence, truthfulness and devotion.

Rejuvenation similarly depends upon sattva guna, particularly for rejuvenation of the mind. Rajas causes friction and agitation in body and mind that ends up exhausting us. Tamas causes decay and debility and increases the rate of aging and mental decline. Sattva is born of self-control, reduced activity and heightened awareness, through which rajas and tamas are controlled.[102] We should not forget or underestimate the role of sattva guna in all higher healing and yogic practices.

Asana and Rejuvenation: The Healing Power of Physical Stillness

Without knowledge, Yoga cannot provide liberation. Yet without Yoga, knowledge cannot provide liberation. Thus both Yoga and knowledge should be practiced together by those aspiring to liberation.

Yoga Tattva Upanishad. 14-15

Proper exercise overall helps us become healthier and live longer, particularly activities like walking and hiking that take us outdoors and into nature. Running and jogging can also be helpful, but require the right preparation and nutritional support.

Ayurveda defines exercise relative to the three doshic types. It holds that Kapha types need strong exertion that promotes profuse sweating in order to move the excess Kapha out of the body. Pitta types need moderate exercise but ending in a cooling and relaxing rest. Vata types need only gentle and warm exercise to the point of moisturizing the skin with mild sweating. They should avoid exhausting themselves and rest well afterwards.

Yoga asanas, however, are not just another form of exercise. They are a means of drawing our energy within for deeper meditation practices. Classical Yoga recommends Yoga asanas for releasing tension from the body and allowing the inner Prana to flow. It is not simply an issue of a good workout but of preparing the body to receive a higher awareness. Ayurvedic rejuvenative practices are connected with Yoga asana more so than with ordinary exercises, though these can be helpful as well. This is because rejuvenation requires slowing down our metabolic processes and drawing them inwards to the universal Prana.

We wear out our bodies through wrong movement or lack of movement. Most of us today do not move enough physically and follow a sedentary life-style that can block, depress and reduce our energy.

However, even those of us who do exercise regularly often do so in a way that is forceful or disturbing, causing more friction, wear and tear on the joints and organs, rather than developing calm and healing energies.

Exercise overall, particularly with force or speed, has a depleting effect that can be purifying but is seldom rejuvenating. Strong exercise in Ayurveda is usually part of a detoxification therapy and works mainly to reduce Kapha dosha, while increasing Vata and Pitta. Rejuvenation requires a building and revitalizing approach to exercise that is more allied with the conservation of energy than with its expenditure.

Gentle, steady yet firm Yoga asanas are the ideal rejuvenative exercise, bringing stillness, peace and deep relaxation to the body, mind and nervous system. This calming approach to asana should be differentiated from the energetic and movement based Yoga styles that dominate the Yoga scene today. Asana approaches emphasizing power and movement, as well as employing heat, are purifying or detoxifying in nature, more appropriate for the youth or for Kapha dosha, but not usually recommended for rejuvenation. Rasayana based asana is a slower and more internalizing practice for those who are older or those whose bodies are already purified. It is more restorative in nature.

Yoga asana, we should note, is not only about developing flexibility in the body but also developing stillness. Those who are flexible may not have this inner stillness, while those who have it, may not be flexible in every part of their bodies. Stillness has the power to heal the body and to awaken a higher energy and awareness in the mind. Such a yogic stillness, however, is not an enforced stillness born of personal effort but a natural stillness born of deep relaxation. To arrive at that stillness we must first let go of any disturbances and agitation in our body and any aggression in the mind. This may initially require movement to break up deep seated tension. But movement should not be the goal or end of the practice. We should learn to move into stillness, which is to slow down in body and mind.

Each asana, we should note, has its own Soma, rasa, delight or particular enjoyment. Yet this 'Soma of the asana' is usually best revealed when one holds the pose in a gentle way with a concentrated mind and prana. Once the Soma is flowing in the asana, the mind, heart and prana are united and there is an inner dynamic energy in a state of equipoise.

Importance of Inverted Poses to Counter Gravity: Apana and Udana

The aging process is promoted by the downward moving air or apana vayu that is connected with the force of gravity. Gravity and time literally pull us down in life, causing our posture to slump, our internal organs to sink, our energy to decline and our minds to get depressed. Increased apana results in the accumulation of waste materials in our tissues and loss of digestive power, weakened immune system and increased lethargy and sleep.

Rejuvenation is developed through promoting the positive energy of udana vayu, the form of prana that moves upward, which counters gravity and allows our spirit and mind to ascend, which is opposite apana vayu in nature. Developing the positive energy of udana, which is our own higher spiritual evolution, cannot be done mechanically, and is not simply a matter of promoting udana vayu in the ordinary sense, which is merely being active in our speech and sensory activity. This higher form of udana vayu requires spiritual aspiration, aligning ourselves with the ascending energy of consciousness, not merely the personal effort to achieve.

The simplest approach to asana practice in order to promote longevity is the use of inverted poses. Inverted poses are very powerful for reversing apana vayu and for strengthening udana vayu. They are the first consideration for rejuvenation based exercises. Yet inverted poses are also strong in nature and can disturb us if done too quickly or forcefully. Mild and gentle inversions should be emphasized in the first phase.

The headstand is the strongest of the inverted poses, and has the most radical power of revitalizing the mind and promoting udana vayu, but requires the proper preparation or it can have side effects. This includes the appropriate strength of the neck to sustain it. The headstand radically increases Agni but can deplete the Soma if it is done too quickly or with too much force. Its effect is more purifying.

The shoulderstand is safer and serves to guard the Soma in the region of the soft palate. The shoulderstand connects with the *Jalandhara Bandha* or the chin lock, which is specifically used to protect the Soma. The shoulderstand is probably the best of the inverted postures for rejuvenation. Yet there are many other inverted postures connected, forward bends or backward bends or prone positions, which also have their value. Standing poses and sitting poses can also help stabilize apana vayu.

Moving from the Periphery to the Center: Vyana and Samana

Aging also involves an outward movement of our energy in which we gradually lose our internal focus and point of balance causing our vitality to disperse and dissipate. Our activity seeking enjoyment and success in the external world causes our energy to go outward, which leads to eventual fragmentation, disintegration, and entropy. Whenever we place our center of gravity, value or meaning outside ourselves, we lose ourselves and must fall over! This outer dispersion of energies can be described as too much vyana or outward going vital energy and a loss of samana or inward moving energy. Excess vyana or extroverted action causes us to lose our inner balance and coherence or samana.

One should perform asanas that exercise the exterior joints and limbs first in order to draw the energy within, ending in a firm sitting pose, centered in the navel. Sitting poses develop a higher energy of samana, which promotes overall peace, balance and concentration, but any adverse vyana should be released first. Sitting poses, once achieved naturally, are ideal for rejuvenation practices of pranayama, mantra and meditation. Samana leads to balance (samatva) and to samadhi.

Sitting Poses and Rejuvenation

Success or siddhi in Yoga asana practice is determined by one's ability to comfortably hold a sitting pose for at least thirty minutes, without movement, pain or disturbance, or wandering of the mind and senses. It is not measured by one's ability to perform complex poses or make gymnastic like movements. In fact, the term asana in Sanskrit means a seat and implies seated postures as a preparation for meditation. Through sitting we can return the body to stillness and open up the potential for stillness of mind as well.

Sitting poses are the best asanas for rejuvenation, particularly the lotus pose and siddhasana, which center us in the navel and allow us to hold our energy within – provided of course that we arrive at this stillness through letting go, rather than as a holding type effort. A gently sustained seated pose promotes deep relaxation without causing sleep or drowsiness.

Sitting poses sustain a transformative samana vayu in the body and mind, allowing us to be both grounded and centered, with our energy ascending. They allow all the knots of the heart to be released, the body to be let go of, and the inner vision to awaken. They still the disturbed movements of the body and the Prana and help us let go of fear and anxiety as well as anger and aggression. Yet one may need to do other asanas to first release any negative energy or stress. For this even standing poses like the tree pose that promote balance can be helpful. One must have Samana in one's life and emotions, which means balance, steadiness and fearlessness.

If you want to rejuvenate your body and mind, your must first learn how to sit. This is not a matter of achieving some ideal Yoga pose, but of being able to forget your body. You can begin with any comfortable sitting posture that you can easily assume, even if it requires using a chair or some other form of back support. When the urge to move arises, draw your breath, focus and awareness to the navel, the central focus of structure and energy in the body. Or you can do some pranayama or gentle stretches until you can comfortably return to a seated pose.

Balancing the Right and Left Sides of the Body

Yogic pranayama emphasizes balancing the flow of the breath between the right and left nostrils as a means of achieving the unitary prana necessary to develop unity consciousness. This is the basis of alternate nostril breathing or *nadi shodhana*. To facilitate this process, asana practice should similarly aim at balancing the energy of the body on the right and left sides. Most of us are right handed and so our energy tends to work more on the right side, while the left side of the body is undeveloped or holds tension born of lack of movement. To balance both sides of the body, usually more exercise, exertion and stretching needs to be done on the left side, with greater relaxation on the right side.

In Hatha Yoga, the practice of *Mahamudra* is usually used for balancing the right and left sides of the body, touching the tips of the fingers to the tips of the toes while sitting with one's legs extended, alternating between the right arm and leg and the left arm and leg. [103] The tree pose is also very good, alternating between standing on the right or left legs until steadiness is developed on both sides. But any set of balanced poses for the right and left sides of the body can be helpful working from standing poses to sitting poses. Twists can be very helpful in this regard, helping to balance the energy within the spine itself.

This right-left balancing consideration should be brought into overall asana practice if one aims at rejuvenation. In this regard, it is particularly important to develop steadiness, strength and stillness on the left side of the body, which corresponding to the lunar current is the Soma side.

The Three Bandhas and Rejuvenation

The three *bandhas* or 'locks' of Hatha Yoga – *Mula Bandha, Uddiyana Bandha, Jalandhara Bandha* – play an important role in balancing Agni and Soma, in countering the three doshas of Vata, Pitta and Kapha, and aiding in the rejuvenation process.

Mula Bandha is important for countering apana vayu, the downward moving Prana that time and the aging process cause to increase. At an outer level, Mula bandha involves gently contracting and drawing upwards the sphincter muscles of the anus. This helps reduce Vata dosha at its site of accumulation in the colon.

Mula Bandha outwardly consists of a gentle upward contraction of the anal muscles. It can be aided by placing the heel at the perineum. Yet true Mula Bandha consists of more than just contracting the muscles, which is but an outer aid. To be truly effective, it requires an actual drawing of the apana upward from the root chakra to the navel. This is more an act of will power and attention than a mere physical exercise. It requires reducing Vata dosha in one's life style, diet and behavior and controlling the lower chakras and bodily orifices, especially proper usage of sexual energy.

This drawing up of the apana can be facilitated by pranayama, drawing the breath up from the base of the spine on inhalation and releasing it through the navel on exhalation. One can contract the anal muscles on inhalation to facilitate this movement and release them on exhalation. At a meditation level, Mula Bandha requires that we ground our consciousness in the Earth, with the stability of a mountain, connecting the Earth with the cosmic being or Brahman that is immutable in nature.

Jalandhara Bandha is the chin lock at an outer level, used to hold and protect the Soma energy in the head, and related Kapha and Ojas energies. It consists physically of a gentle bending of the chin, often done after inhalation. It helps draw the Prana downward from the head and hold it in the region of the navel, facilitating Uddiyana Bandha. In this regard it is opposite and complementary to Mula Bandha, which works on apana.

Yet for Jalandhara bandha to have full benefit, one needs to keep the mind calm and head cool as well. This means controlling our senses, most of which are located in the head, and reducing their rate of stimulation. It also means stabilizing the udana vayu or upward moving air so that it does not move up adversely. Most importantly, it requires restraint of speech, to control our throat chakra at an inner level, which is not just avoiding speaking but reducing the mind's chatter.

At an outer level, Uddiyana Bandha, which means 'flying upwards', consists of drawing up and contracting the muscles of the navel and abdomen upward, generally after exhalation. It can follow after a churning motion to add more energy to it. It is used to stimulate Agni or the digestive fire as well as Pitta dosha that is related to it, and to take the Kundalini energy into the Sushumna.

However, Uddiyana Bandha also consists of more than just creating muscular strength in the navel region. It requires actually uniting the prana and apana in the navel and stimulating a higher force of Agni.

This means having first accomplished Mula Bandha to draw the apana up to the navel, but also drawing the Prana down from the region of the head, which is aided by Jalandhara Bandha. Though it is a holding of the abdominal muscles, this holding should be done by prana, not by the ego, or it will increase tension, not develop prana. At a meditation level, Uddiyana Bandha consists of directing one's awareness upward from the individual soul to the Supreme Self. It is aided by chanting *Om* inwardly and letting one's consciousness ascend on the mantra's current.

The three bandhas should be linked with a corresponding movement of Prana, a calmness of mind, a supportive life-style and reduction of the doshas. In fact, if one can move the prana, one may not need to do the physical bandhas at all. If one can practice the three bandhas simultaneously as a development of prana, the prana can move into the central channel or Sushumna. Jalandhara bandha holds the prana down, by cooling and concentrating the mind. Mula bandha draws the apana up, by preventing the prana from flowing out below through control of the sense and motor organs. Uddiyana bandha allows the united prana and apana to enter into the Sushumna, through stimulating Agni or the digestive fire at a deeper level of spiritual aspiration.

Asana and Ayurvedic Rejuvenation Considerations

Vata dosha accumulates in the bones and joints, particular along the spine, during the aging process. Removing Vata dosha from the bones is a primary therapy for health and well-being in old age. Asana overall aids in this removal of Vata dosha, but twists, particularly spinal twists are probably the best asanas to do so. Otherwise a balanced and gentle asana approach should be carried out, with forward and backward bends, inverted and standing postures, contracting and expanding movements, to create a massage like motion in the body, to balance the body right and left and above and below, so that Vata can be removed.

Special attention should be given to the lower back and lower abdomen and Vata dosha's site of accumulation in the colon, in order to discharge it from there. Mild inversions help with this also. Pitta's site of accumulation in the navel and Kapha's site in the stomach and chest should also be considered and the energy kept flowing freely through these locations.

One should combine asana practice with Ayurvedic oil massage for the best possible results. The oil also helps reduce Vata dosha, particularly sesame or almond oils. A rejuvenative diet is also helpful along with rejuvenative beverages to keep our tissues adequately hydrated. Asana by itself cannot release deep seated Vata without these support practices, as Vata requires nourishment more so than movement in order to reduce it. During strict rejuvenative therapies, no strong asanas should be performed. Mainly gentle sitting or prone poses are done, with an emphasis on rest.

Yet the promoting stillness in asana for rejuvenative purposes does not mean that movement based asanas or vinyasas do not have any place. They are part of the preparation for stillness and are purifying in nature. They increase circulation to help remove toxins from the body, particularly lowering any excess Kapha, but they must give way to postures that reduce movement for deeper rejuvenation to go forward.

Asana as Going Beyond the Beyond the Body

The real purpose of Yoga asanas is to take us beyond body consciousness by letting go of the stress and strain created by our attachment to the body. Asana should be a means of relaxing out of body consciousness, not of increasing it. This is also the view of the *Yoga Sutras* that links asana with a practice of discrimination and detachment.[104] Rejuvenation of the body occurs when we let go of body consciousness and allow a higher energy and awareness enter into it.

The body as a material formation has a heavy or tamasic nature. If we focus too much on it, there is a tendency to develop tamas in the mind as well. For this reason, we should approach asana with the support of sattvic yogic life-style practices, contemplation and meditation. We should treat the body as a sacred vehicle for spiritual practices, not as a tool for personal enjoyment or assertion. In this way we can use the body as a receptacle for a higher Soma in which a deeper calmness can enter into it. In Raja Yoga, we bring peace into the physical body so that the subtle body and higher consciousness can be experienced through it, which requires that it becomes passive and no longer dominates our attention.

Prana Rasayana:
The Immortal Breath of Soma

The Gods beginning with the Creator, Lord Brahma, devoted themselves to pranayama to counter the fear of death. Thus the yogi should also practice pranayama.

Hatha Yoga Pradipika II.39

The basis of life is the breathing process, which is the main motor that runs our entire organism. Life begins with the first breath and ends with the last breath. The expanding and contracting action of breathing not only connects us with the outer energy of life but also with the inner energy of life within our own hearts. It keeps our entire existence connected and in motion.

The life force circulating by the action of the breath is the main power that vitalizes and rejuvenates us every moment of the day. The secret force of life, including the capacity for rejuvenation, is hidden in the breath as its essential or core energy. We can learn to use this power of the breath or Prana Shakti for higher restorative and transformative purposes.

In this regard, *pranayama or yogic breathing is probably the most important rejuvenating practice that we can do on a daily basis.* Pranayama is more significant than diet, herbs and asana, though it works better along with these additional aids. Yet to be really restorative or yogic in effect, it is not just enough merely to increase the length or power of the breath. One must also learn to direct the breath and prana inwardly to the mind and heart. Rejuvenative pranayama implies a deep and slow breathing process allied with an internalization of energy and awareness. Such yogic breathing is not simply any deep breathing practice but a deep breathing with a spiritual intent, focus and motivation.

The breath is a unique biological force in that we can consciously direct it or let it flow in an unconscious manner without giving it our attention. We can breathe with awareness and intention, using the breath to alter, purify or energize our state of mind and heart. Or we can rest our attention away from the breath and let the breath do its own work of renewal without our interference.

However, Prana or life energy is much more than the breath as a physical force. The breathing process in the lungs in itself is but a pump that circulates energy in the body, driving the respiratory, circulatory and nervous systems in an almost mechanical fashion. This means that the breathing process is something that we can observe, just as we can observe the flowing of a river or the working of a motor. The breath is not our inner nature or the essence of our being. You are not the breath, which is but an instrument. You are that which breathes, which is the energy and awareness behind the breath. This inner Prana of the spirit is what allows the outer physical breath to occur. It enters the body at birth and leaves it at death, but itself never dies. We can use the physical breath to connect with the cosmic breath. This is the real art of breathing and yogic pranayama.

The breath propels the water or fluids in the body to move through the circulatory system, as the blood and plasma. Yet the breath first energizes the space in the nostrils and sinuses that connect with the brain. The breath also moves downward from the lungs to the navel, enkindling the digestive fire and setting in motion the process of peristalsis in the digestive tract by a reflex action. Through the power of Prana working through the breath all the systems of the body are stimulated and sustained.

The problem is that we associate the breath with life and think that if we stop breathing, we must die. Yoga teaches us how to calm the breath, including taking it to a deeper level of function where it is subtle or even silent, where we can reach a kind of deep relaxation or inner hibernation that can allow a higher consciousness to emerge. The agitation of the breath drives us but can wear us out and inhibit our longevity. The rejuvenative breath is not this ordinary breath of personal drives and assertions but taking the breath back to its origin in Universal Prana. It is the breath behind the breath.

Vayu and the Cosmic Breath

In the breathing process we partake of the Cosmic Vayu and Prana, the universal Spirit, not just the external air. It is not only oxygen or other chemicals that we breathe; these are but outer traces of something deeper. It is the spirit and life-force of the Earth and its atmosphere we take in, which in turn is linked with the Cosmic Spirit that pervades all space. In breathing we unite with the cosmic and terrestrial spirits and their interwoven tapestry. When we breathe with the awareness of our interaction with the Cosmic Spirit our breath naturally becomes a form of Yoga, or means of unification. Through the breath we can draw in progressively deeper aspects of energy and awareness, allowing our consciousness to ascend. Breathing is probably the most natural and accessible Yoga practice; *the breathing process is the primary Yoga of Life*.

If we look deeply at our physical existence, we see that we are but an embodied form of the atmosphere, a form of the Cosmic Vayu, temporarily confined within an organism. We are the spirit or air trapped in the body, sustaining its connection with its source through the breathing process. In breathing, we link back with our spiritual nature and origin and touch the Universal Spirit.

A deep part of us is always seeking to return to our spiritual home in air and space. We crave freedom, which is ultimately the freedom of movement of the wind. We are uncomfortable with the limitations of our body, senses or mind. Breathing is evidence of our bondage to the body, our spirit's fall into the density of matter, from which we long to escape. We can break that bondage of the breath only by energizing our breath beyond the body through unity consciousness, what is called samadhi in yogic thought. In the state of samadhi or meditative absorption, the outer breath becomes very subtle or stops altogether, while the inner breath of the cosmic prana takes over and sustains body and mind, lifting our spirit beyond time and space.

There are many forms of Vayu or the Cosmic Prana. We are most connected to the terrestrial Vayu, the vital force of our planet Earth. The terrestrial Vayu is the Earth Spirit. It has its own energy and intelligence that pervades all of life, infusing every ecosystem with its unique energy and movement. It flows in the wind, across the rivers, seas, mountains and plains. We are manifestations of that earthly Vayu or air as it seeks to return to its home or origin in the heavens.

Unfortunately, our current humanity is disrupting, polluting and destroying the terrestrial Vayu or life-spirit, which must have severe consequences for the well-being of all creatures and for the planet itself. This Vayu may react and seek to correct the behavior of human beings and remove the toxins brought into its sphere. We must learn to use our breath to connect to the Cosmic Spirit and the intelligence inherent in the atmosphere and use that to heal ourselves and heal our planet. We can use the terrestrial spirit or Earth Prana to link with the Cosmic Spirit that is beyond all limitation.

We can rejuvenate ourselves through the Cosmic Prana, drawing it into us through the ground, the streams and waters, the atmosphere itself, touching it in the light forms of the Sun, Moon and stars, and embracing it pervading all space. Yet to do this we must move beyond our ordinary breath and thought to a unitary flow of awareness.

It is perhaps a paradoxical principle: *we can only rejuvenate the body by giving it up, by going beyond body consciousness and returning to our nature as pure spirit.* The body itself is heavy and aligned with decay and death. It becomes denser and tends to sink down with the aging process. Pranayama helps us raise the body up and reduce the pull of gravity and decay upon it.

The Great or Immortal Prana

The Cosmic Prana does not simply lie on the outside, it also dwells within us. The Prana at the core of our hearts and that moving through the universal space is the same Prana. In that inner Prana we contain the entire universe, as well as all time and space.

The real source of Prana lies in consciousness, the deeper unitary awareness beyond the mind and senses. It is not a mere product of the breathing process, of the external air, or even the cosmic space. The more we can access that energy or vitality of awareness, which requires deep meditation, the more Prana that we have at an inner level, the more we are connected to the eternal.

This supreme Prana is honored as Lord Shiva in the Yoga tradition, the patron of the great Yogis, who grants all the powers of Prana, energy and awareness, including the ability to cross over death. That inner Prana is a power of peace, stillness, fullness, steadiness and transcendence. By contacting the inner Prana, we can bring the energy of immortality into all that we do.

Prana and Rasa

Rejuvenation or rasayana works through rasa, which means both 'fluid' and 'essence'. Prana itself is a kind of rasa or essence of the body. Yet Prana also depends upon the fluids or rasas of the body. This means for pranayama to be really rejuvenative we must link it with these higher rasas. On an outer level, this means to have adequate rejuvenating liquids and oils in the diet, including Soma herbs. On an inner level, it means to link our breath with devotion to the Divine and aspiration to the higher truth. We must learn to let go of negative emotions, any fear, anxiety, worry, anger or attachment we are holding in the breath and use the breath to draw in greater love and wisdom. We must hold to the inner breath of consciousness, not the outer vital drives of the ego.

The Need for Pure Air

Air itself can be a rejuvenative energy or rasayana and in fact should be. Yet this only true of certain kinds of air, not the air that most of breathe in our modern polluted cities and homes. It includes the air by the ocean, the air by mountain streams and the air of the forest – fresh air where there is space. There is no substitute for good air; any more than there is any substitute for good food or good water. Living in stagnant or polluted air is a major factor in disease and premature aging. The use of flowers, incense and fragrant oils in the home can help counter bad or stagnant air. We must make sure that there are rejuvenative forces in the air if we want to revitalize our lives.

Rejuvenation and the Five Pranas

Prana, which is not just the breath but vital energy overall, is divided fivefold according to its movement. We need to understand these flows and learn to work with them. Life depends upon the proper function and balance of the five pranas within us.

- Prana: inward movement through eating, breathing, taking in of sensory impressions, emotions and thoughts.

- Apana: downward and outward movement through elimination, urination, reproduction and immunity.

- Udana: upward movement through exhalation, speech, effort, will and motivation.

- Samana: contracting movement from the outside to the inside through digestion, assimilation, homeostasis and balance.

- Vyana: expanding movement from the inside to the outside through extension of the limbs and promoting peripheral circulation.

Prana as a light airy force naturally tends to disperse upward. Apana as an earthy force tends to sink downward. Uniting prana and apana, through drawing the apana upward and the prana downward, results in rejuvenation, creating life and fire. On the other hand, the two forces moving in opposite directions, the separation of prana and apana causes decay and death. We must learn to keep the prana flowing down into us and draw the apana upward. This is one of the key practices of Yoga.

We must also learn to draw our prana, which naturally tends to disperse outwards through vyana, to move and become centered within through samana. This is not to become stuck, stagnant or congested but to be grounded in the navel, which means to breathe into the belly. The navel is the main point of physical balance for udana and apana, vyana and samana, which connect to Agni or the digestive fire. However, the deeper spiritual prana and power of consciousness dwells within the heart. Unless that is brought down to the navel we may create more vital energy but not necessarily of a spiritual nature.

Prana and Longevity

According to ancient Vedic texts, we are given at birth a certain number of breaths as part of our human nature, just as we have certain structure and number of bones, limbs and organs. This total number of breaths is said to be 21,600 or about one breath every four seconds. We are given 100 years of such breaths.[105] Yet this is an average number, some people may have more or less depending upon their karmas.

This means that if we can slow down our breath, we can live longer. If we can stop our outer breath altogether and rest in the inner breath, like a state of hibernation or samadhi, greater rejuvenation is possible. Longevity depends upon strengthening our prana, which implies slowing down and deepening the breath. We should not overtly try to suppress our breath or stop breathing, but should allow our breath to return to a deeper flow, which it naturally does when we turn our awareness within. We should let our individual breath, which normally flows like a stream, come to rest in the ocean of the Cosmic Prana.

Pranayama Practices

Below are a number of helpful pranayama methods for longevity, rejuvenation and opening to our inner Soma.

Tonifying and Reducing Forms of Pranayama

Pranayama can be developed either for tonification or reduction therapies, for either rejuvenation or detoxification. This depends upon how we use the breath, which itself is a vehicle or a carrier.

- Take in a deep breath and draw in the healing prana of nature from the plants, land and sky. On exhalation spread this prana of nature throughout the body to vitalize every cell and organ. This is a 'tonifying breath', which serves to build or create positive energy.

- Take in deep breath and draw in all the tension and toxins from the body and mind on inhalation. On exhalation, release and expel these toxins from the body. This is a 'purifying breath', which reduces negativity.

Tonifying breathing generally aims at prolonging inhalation, while purifying breathing aims more at extending exhalation. Inhalation brings in the Soma or nutritive power of the breath and has a magnetic or attractive energy. Exhalation has an expelling, reducing or releasing effect; an electrical or expressive energy connected more to Agni or fire. Inhalation as a drawing in of energy serves to feed the senses and the mind. Exhalation works to stimulate the motor organs, starting with speech that occurs on the outgoing breath.

Generally we should first use the breath in a purifying role in order to remove toxins and negative emotions as well as to release stress. Then we should develop a tonifying or rejuvenative breath to bring in higher healing energies and help these to circulate within us. However, the breath as a force of air tends to be more purifying and reducing to the body than it is nourishing and building. To make it more nourishing, we need not only to make the inhalation stronger but to make sure that we have proper fluids, oils and Ojas in the body to support the additional Prana – hence the importance of rejuvenative diet and herbs even for pranayama therapies. As we age the breath becomes shallower and drier. It is important to keep its flow deep and allied with greater moisture in the body and lymphatic system. Yet the breath can be better used to rejuvenate the mind, which like it is also connected to the air and ether elements.

There are many kinds of pranayama in the Yoga tradition. Generally speaking, rapid and strong forms like *bhastrika* and *kapalabhati* are purifying in nature and serve to remove toxins, impurities and mucus from the system. Such strong or rapid forms of pranayama can be of short-term help to stimulate rejuvenative processes in the brain, nervous system, circulatory system and lungs. Yet if we practice too much of them they can over stimulate and deplete the Prana and inner Soma. For this reason, we will not discuss them in detail here.

Tonifying forms of pranayama aim more at a deep slow breathing, with prolonged inhalation. Some require continuous breathing with no retention. Others develop retention naturally as a result of long-term deeper breathing. These are the main types of pranayama for rejuvenative practices. Alternate nostril breathing is probably the best of the rejuvenative pranayamas as it allows us to balance our energy and move into a unitary state of awareness and prana. It also allows us to hold or direct our pranic energy in an easier and more focused manner.

The Pranic key to well-being is simple:

- Be conscious of and observe your breath.

- Slow down the breath (and with it speech, mind and senses).

- Breathe more deeply on inhalation, taking the breath down to the navel.

- Balance the breath between both right and left nostrils.

- Breathe in the natural Prana around you.

- Relax the breath into a deeper state of observation and meditation.

Opening and Protecting the Sinuses

The sinuses are the place where Prana first gets absorbed into the brain, stimulating the senses and the higher chakras of the head. Unless the sinuses are clear, we cannot fully benefit from the Prana in the air. If the sinuses are congested or blocked, the brain's Soma cannot easily flow, whatever else we may do. An important aid to longevity is to keep our nostrils clear and the breath flowing evenly between them. Here the yogic use of the *neti pot* for cleansing the sinuses is very important, pouring a little salt water through the nostrils to clear them.[106]

Yet even more important are Ayurvedic *Nasya* or nasal oils. Those made with demulcent herbs like licorice in a sesame oil base (like *anu tail*) are best for lubricating the nostrils and so most useful for tonification and rejuvenation. Those made with spicy herbs like calamus and ginger are better for clearing the nostrils, for purification and detoxification. Keeping the nostrils properly lubricated aids in health and longevity. Strong forms of pranayama like bhastrika and kapalabhati, which involve forceful rapid breathing through the sinuses, help open the sinuses and can help revive the mind, but once this is accomplished, we should switch to deeper gentler breathing practices.

Taking the Breath Down to the Belly

Whatever form of pranayama we are doing, we should take our breath all the way down to the belly and the navel for its full revitalizing effect. In this way the breath can stimulate the digestive fire and invigorate the digestive system, massaging our internal organs from within.

1. Breathe in drawing the air down to the navel upon inhalation.

2. Hold the breath in the heart upon retention.

3. Breathe out through the head upon exhalation.

OM Pranayama

This is a simple but powerful pranayama method using the three letters of the *Om* (*Aum*) mantra along with the breath. It will allow your prana to move upward into a state of higher awareness.

*   Silently repeat the mantra A (aa) upon inhalation and the navel, drawing in the Brahma energy or creative forces of the universe.

*   Silently repeat the mantra U (oo) with retention in the heart, drawing in the Vishnu energy or sustaining forces of the universe.

*   Silently repeat the mantra M (mmm) with exhalation in the head, drawing in the Shiva energy or the transforming forces of the universe.

Continuous or Uninterrupted Breathing

A simple way to energize yourself with Prana, which can also open the lungs and sinuses, is through a continual breathing without any retention. One allows a deep inhalation to immediately follow with a deep exhalation.

For this practice, one can use the mantra *Om* on inhalation to draw in the cosmic Prana from the world around us, and the mantra *Haum* on exhalation to spread that energy through our entire being. After a few minutes of this practice, the Prana will naturally clear the head, nostrils and sinuses as well as give you more energy. This is often more calming and has the same results of stronger methods like Bhastrika or Kapalabhati.

So'ham Pranayama and Rejuvenation

So'ham is the natural sound of the breath, which is the sound of the Cosmic Spirit manifesting itself through us. Breathing naturally while silently repeating this mantra allows our breath to be linked with the cosmic breath. One silently repeats the mantra *So* on inhalation and *Ham* on exhalation drawing in the Divine energies on inhalation and expanding them through one's entire being on exhalation. *So'ham* increases the Soma of Prana within us. *So'ham* is the natural sound of the 'Soma of Prana'. You can do this practice at any time throughout the day.

Along with *So'ham* pranayama one can visualize the disc of the Moon (Chandra bindu), which represents the mind, ascending the spine on inhalation and coming to rest in its natural center in the thousand petal lotus at the top of the head, and then descending upon exhalation to renew the body with Soma.

As a general practice, it is good to visualize the breath going up and down the spine with inhalation and exhalation. Such spinal breathing will gradually stimulate the unitary flow of the breath through the Sushumna.

Alternate Nostril Breathing and Rejuvenation

Of the many helpful forms of pranayama, probably the best is alternate nostril breathing. This is also called *Nadi Shodhana* or 'purification of the channels', or 'solar and lunar breathing' because it helps balance the solar and lunar, right and left halves of the body, male and female, fire and water energies within us.

Throughout the day our breath gradually shifts from one nostril to another relative to our nature, actions and the environmental influences around us. Too much flow of the breath through the right or solar nostril causes us to overheat, become excessively active, agitated and aggressive. Too much flow of the breath through the left or lunar nostril causes us to become cold, heavy, slow, and unresponsive. In the process not only our longevity is reduced but also our awareness is fragmented into dualistic currents of attraction and repulsion, like and dislike, pleasure and pain, love and hate.

For health, rejuvenation and spirituality, we need to balance the breath between both nostrils. A balanced prana connects us with the immortal life force that is subtler than the breath and comes from within our own consciousness, not from the external air. It can help us enter into the breathless state that Yogis seek to reach.

However, the breath in the left nostril, owing to its lunar nature, connects more to Soma, and is moistening, calming and relaxing in nature. For rejuvenation purposes promoting the breath, particularly inhalation, through the left nostril can be an important consideration and helps stimulate Tarpak Kapha. It also depends somewhat on one's doshic type. Pitta and Vata types usually do better stimulating the breath in the left nostril, particularly for rejuvenation purposes. Kapha types do better stimulating the right or solar breath, which better counters their doshic tendencies.

Hamsa So'ham Solar Lunar Pranayama

We can balance the breath and awake the higher Prana through this simple pranayama that builds upon the *So'ham* approach, following a pattern of alternate nostril breathing. In this practice one inhales through the left nostril silently repeating the mantra *So*, and then exhales through the right nostril with the mantra *Ham*. This first phase of the pranayama is lunar in nature but connecting to the higher lunar forces of bliss, devotion, peace, cooling the mind.

Then one inhales through the right nostril with the mantra *Ham* and exhales through the left nostril with the mantra *Sah*. This second phase of the pranayama is solar in nature but connecting with the higher solar powers of awareness, discrimination, perception and consciousness.

This method of alternate nostril breathing is simple and easy, with both a balancing and a deepening effect upon the Prana. You can add yet more detail to the practice:

Shiva/Shakti, Solar/Lunar, Male/Female Energy Balancing

This practice extends the *Hamsa So'ham* pranayama along with bringing the energy up and down the spine.

- Breathe in through the left nostril with the mantra *So* and visualize the nourishing white lunar or Shakti (Divine Feminine energy) moving up the left side of the body.

- Breathe out through the right nostril with the mantra *Ham* and visualize the stimulating golden solar or Shiva (Divine Masculine energy) moving down the right side of the body.

- Breathe in through the right nostril with the mantra *Ham* and visualize the stimulating golden solar or Shiva (Divine Masculine energy) moving up the right side of the body.

- Breathe in through the left nostril with the mantra *Sa* and visualize the nourishing white lunar or Shakti (Divine Feminine energy) moving down the left side of the body.

If you perform this simple practice morning and evening for fifteen minutes, it can keep your Prana at its optimal condition throughout the day. It will also help balance the male and female, Shiva and Shakti energies within you.

Not only does our Prana tend to sink downward with the aging process, so does our Soma or sense of enjoyment, which causes us to feel tired, low in energy or depressed. Most of us hold our main Soma or enjoyment in our lower chakras which promotes the same entropy. Breathing in through the left nostril and drawing the Soma energy from the root chakra to the head can be a good way to counter this, breathing out through the right nostril and letting the energy descend.

Ayurvedic Pranayama Methods

Below are methods of using the breath to reduce the doshas of Vata, Pitta and Kapha and to promote Prana, Tejas and Ojas.

Dosha-Reducing Pranayama

In this practice we use the breath to help dispel the doshas from their primary sites of accumulation in the body. We place our right hand on the corresponding location of the body while performing this practice, using special mantras to draw the doshas back to their sites of accumulation. This is a kind of 'Pranayama Pancha Karma' involving pranayama, mantra and meditation. Yet done at the subtle level of Prana, it is milder in its effect, which also depends upon our power of concentration.

- **Vata** – Using the *Krīm Śrīm* in the large intestine.

Place your right hand on the region of the colon in the lower left of the abdomen. Then place the left hand over the right hand. Inhale gently, mentally repeating the electrical mantra *Krīm* (pronounced Kreem), drawing the energy of Vata dosha, the disturbed nervous energy of the entire body and mind into the colon. Then exhale using the lunar mantra *Śrīm* to disperse the energy of Vata out of the body and fill the lower abdomen with calm, strength and stability.

- **Pitta** – Using the mantras *Hrīm Śrīm* in small the intestine.

Place your right hand on the navel. Then place the left hand over the right hand. Inhale gently, repeating the solar mantra *Hrīm*, drawing the energy of Pitta dosha, the excess heat and fire from the entire body and mind into the navel. Then exhale using the lunar mantra *Śrīm* to disperse the energy of Pitta out of the body with a force of coolness, calm, nourishment and surrender into the navel.

- **Kapha** – Using the mantras *Śrīm Hrīm* in the stomach.

Place your right hand on the region of the stomach in the upper left abdomen above the navel. Then place the left hand over the right hand Inhale gently repeating the lunar mantra *Śrīm*, drawing in the energy of Kapha dosha, the excess energy of water, mucus, attachment and heaviness from the entire body, into the stomach. Then exhale using the mantra *Hrīm*, projecting a warm solar energy to disperse the accumulated Kapha out of the body and replace it with space, light, energy and strength.

Prana, Tejas and Ojas Pranayama

In this practice one uses the breath to increase the powers of Prana, Tejas and Ojas, the essences of the doshas, particularly that of Prana.

• Prana- promoting Pranayama

Draw in the energy of Prana from the world of nature around you, particularly from the plants, the trees and the atmosphere, silently repeating the electrical mantra *Krīm* on inhalation. Expand the energy of Prana with *Hrīm* on exhalation. In so doing fill your heart, entire body and mind with the energy of Prana.

• Tejas-promoting Pranayama

Draw in the energy of fire from the world of nature around you, particularly from the Sun, silently repeating the solar mantra *Hrīm* on inhalation. Expand the energy of fire with the fire mantra *Hūm* on exhalation. In so doing fill your heart, entire body and mind with the light of Tejas.

• Ojas-promoting Pranayama

Draw in the energy of Ojas from the world of nature around you, particularly from the earth, the waters and the Moon, silently repeating the watery mantra *Klīm* on inhalation. Expand the energy of Ojas with the mantra *Śrīm* on exhalation. In so doing fill your heart, entire body and mind with the strength of Ojas. Owing to the connection between Ojas and Soma, this practice is particularly important for rejuvenation.

Secrets of the Inner or Soma Prana

After we have developed the power of the breath, the inner Prana or Soma begins to flow.

Retention of the Breath

Once one connects with the inner Prana and feels a current flowing directly in the mind itself, one can gain a special rejuvenating energy through holding the breath. This is what is called *kevala kumbhaka* in Yoga.[107] The great Vedantic master Shankara called it the most important of all the pranayamas used in Hatha Yoga.[108] *This is an advanced stage and there should be no effort to forcefully bring it about.* If there is no inner flow of energy in the mind, which means directly through the Sushumna, one should be very careful not to try to hold the breath too long.

In this practice, one takes a deep breath followed by a relaxing exhalation and enters into the breathless state, drawing energy from the light of awareness within, and letting the outer breath flow gently, calmly or cease altogether. If one can enter into this state of drawing in the inner Prana while the outer breath is still, the rejuvenating effects are enormous.

As a preliminary practice you can begin by holding your breath until you feel the need to take a deep breath. Then allow yourselves to breathe deeply for a few moments (for this the *So'ham* mantra is very good). You can then hold the breath again, only for a little bit longer. You can gradually increase the length of retention over time.

Note that in this process no force should be used, just a gentle increase of effort. Holding the breath should be combined with deeper and longer breathing afterwards! In this way one will not only develop the power of the breath but that of attention and will power as well. In this process the prana flows inwardly through the Sushumna and the outer breath becomes peripheral or even ceases.

Khechari Mudra

Khechari mudra, explained in detail in Yoga texts like the *Hatha Yoga Pradipika*,[109] is a special Yoga practice placing the tongue back and up on the roof of the mouth.

When the Prana from the right and left nadis flows through the middle, in that state the Khechari mudra becomes perfect.

In the stream of nectar that flows from the Moon dwells the beloved of Shiva in visible form. The mouth of the unequalled, divine Sushumna must be filled at the back by the tongue turned upward into the roof of the palate.

Hatha Yoga Pradipika IV.43-47

This placement of the tongue allows the Soma or nectar from the head and crown chakra to flow down and for one to drink it with the tongue. Khechari mudra is a great aid to pratyahara and meditation. It an important practice to perform during pranayama, particularly on inhalation (one can lower the tongue to the base of the mouth on exhalation). It is also beneficial to practice it throughout the day and helps us control our appetite and need for stimulating beverages like coffee or alcohol.

In its more extreme forms, Khechari mudra involves cutting the base of the tongue bit by bit on a daily basis until the tongue can go all the way back to the throat. However, such a practice is very dangerous and should not be attempted individually without special guidance, if at all. It is enough to place tongue at the top of the mouth. If one curls the tongue back to the top of the mouth, the practice has yet more power. The use of certain mantras can also help.

Holding the tongue at the roof of the mouth aids in the control of speech, in the development of Mantra Shakti, sublimation of our desires, and the arousing of the Kundalini. It is helpful not only for pranayama, but for pratyahara (control of the senses) and concentration (dharana). It aids in longevity and keeps our Soma from dispersing through the emotions, mind and senses. Khechari mudra is usually accompanied with fixing the gaze at the third eye, though other sites can also be used, notably the top of the head.

Khechari mudra literally means 'moving in space'. Besides the outer method of moving the tongue, it also requires an upward orientation of our sense of taste and seeking of enjoyment in life, which implies devotion and inner search. We must be willing to give up outer enjoyments and search out the highest bliss, which ultimately dwells in space, not in any object, person or action. The space of consciousness itself is the highest form of happiness and freedom, as well as our true home. Khechari mudra is connected to kevala kumbhaka or the inner holding of the breath and the unitary flow of prana through the Sushumna and spine.

Yoni Mudra

Yoni mudra consists of using the fingers to block off the seven sensory openings in the head, the eyes, ears, nostrils and mouth. This allows us to focus on the inner light, sound and Soma in our deeper awareness. It usually occurs after deep pranayama and is accompanied by Kevala kumbhaka or prolonged retention of the breath.

Yoni mudra is meant to immerse us in our inner Prana and inner Soma, but we must get these to flow in order to really benefit from it. In this regard we must also learn to practice Yoni mudra at an inner level, which is to rest in the source of our own being, and not seek our happiness and support in the external world.

Developing the Soma of the Breath

It is important to develop the 'Soma of the breath', which occurs when we breathe with awareness, calm and contentment. Merely to do a lot of deep breathing while our minds or emotions are disturbed may not be helpful and can even be harmful.

The breath ordinarily has a rajasic or agitated nature owing to its connection with the senses, which causes us to lose our Soma through the breath and seek enjoyment in the external world. Deep breathing can give us more energy but that may not take us in a spiritual direction unless we develop an additional calm and contentment in the breath. We should make the breath sattvic or spiritual by allying it with a deeper awareness and aspiration.

Yoga requires a 'sattvic' or internalized prana, not a 'rajasic' or agitated prana, which implies following the life-style disciplines of the yamas and niyamas as a background for pranayama. Breathing should be a kind of meditation, not a mere exercise or effort. Otherwise pranayama can disturb the mind and increase the doshas, particularly Vata.

Once the power of Prana (Prana Shakti) and the Soma of Prana is developed, one can direct this force to any part of the body or to the body as a whole for healing purposes, making it a great tool for treating disease and promoting longevity. In this practice, one directs the inhalation to the part of the body intended, for example, the eyes. One holds the breath with one's attention on the eyes and then exhales as if breathing out through and energizing the eyes. In this way the Prana is made to move through the eyes.

You can make this practice more specific. If you draw in the breath through the left or lunar nostril, it will have a more nurturing or Soma like effect on the part of the body so energized. If you draw in the breath through the right nostril, it will have a more heating or Agni like affect on the part of the body so energized. In these practices it is best to breathe out through the opposite nostril in order to maintain balance. There are special mantras that can be used to make the practice yet more specific.[110]

The Need for Steady and Gentle Practices

Spiritual development in general and rejuvenation in particular is the result of a slow, steady, gentle organic growth, much like the cultivation of a garden. While certain outer practices can aid in this, inner attitude, devotion and calm are most important. There are no simple short cuts or rapid methods that can dispense with the need for steadiness and perseverance over time. If we try too quick or forceful methods, particularly of asana and pranayama, without a prior development of inner peace, we can disturb ourselves further or have a short period of inner growth that then comes to an end or causes us to abandon our efforts.

Whatever Yoga practices you take up here, please make sure not to look at them as short-term methods that you will expect quick results from, even without corresponding changes in your life-style or emotional condition. Do not use the ego to push your Yoga practice as some sort of personal achievement or power game. Let any techniques unfold naturally from your inner stillness. Let patience and contentment be your motivation, to return to the core of your being beyond all outer disturbances. Once that occurs you need not pursue any techniques but can rest in the highest action of non-doing, being one's true Self.

PRATYAHARA RASAYANA:
REJUVENATION AND THE
SENSE AND MOTOR ORGANS

With his tongue held at the roof of the mouth, steady in practice, drinking the Soma, within half a month without doubt, the knower of Yoga conquers death.

Hatha Yoga Pradipika III.44

Rejuvenation rests firmly upon the yogic science of *pratyahara*, without which it cannot go deeply. Pratyahara, which literally means 'withdrawal', is the fifth of the eight limbs of classical Yoga. It refers to the internalization of the prana, mind and senses necessary to take our awareness from the external world to the core of our being, the Divine presence within. That same internalization of energy is necessary for any deep rejuvenation or revitalization of body, mind or senses. Pratyahara is probably the key to rejuvenation, around which all the other Yoga practices should move.

Each one of us inherently possesses the capacity to access higher forms of energy and awareness within ourselves than what we normally access from the outer world of society. We also have the ability to access deeper and more transformative forces from the world of nature around us. However, to imbibe these higher energies, we must withdraw from the lower connections that currently preoccupy us, our attachments to the outer world and habitual responses that drag us down in life. Then we can experience the magic of the universe both within and around us as our daily life. This process requires pratyahara in various forms.

Pratyahara marks the dividing line between the outer aspect of Yoga as asana and pranayama, which mainly relate to the body, and the inner aspect as concentration, meditation and samadhi, which mainly relate to the mind. Pratyahara develops from and extends the yamas and niyamas or the self-discipline that is the basis of a true yogic life-style. Without pratyahara, Yoga remains asana little more than another form of exercise. Without pratyahara, pranayama remains only another means of giving energy to the ego. Yet following pranayama all Yoga leads to deep meditation.

Rejuvenation requires that we turn our vital energies within so that they can become increased and renewed. Normally our vital force flows outwardly through the sense and motor organs and exhausts itself in the external world and its attractions. This results in physical aging and in the loss of our awareness, even in the loss of control of our lives to external influences. It causes various addictions to external stimuli that leave us eventually depressed and devitalized.

Pratyahara takes us to a state of deep relaxation in which the nervous system can be revitalized, much like the refreshing effect of deep sleep. As long as a disturbed energy is flowing through our nervous system, it must create friction and wear out the body as a whole. Pratyahara allays this friction and soothes our nerves and emotions. *Pratyahara can be described as is the 'Yogic principle of conservation of energy'*, which is a conservation of our own Prana and a protection of our sense and motor organs from unnecessary or disturbing activity.

Traditional Ayurvedic rejuvenation therapies employ pratyahara as a primary strategy. They require that the patient enter into isolation in a special retreat hut in nature, cut off from all sensory impressions and human contact, much like a return to the darkness of the womb. This kind of 'isolation therapy' allows our energies to turn within and regenerate. But we must be adequately prepared for it or it can cause phobias within the mind, particularly if we approach it with unresolved emotions. We cannot simply impose isolation upon ourselves but must learn to embrace a greater aloneness in order to discover the wellsprings of vitality within us.

For ordinary rejuvenation practices, we need not enter into total isolation, but do need to retreat into nature and restrict our minds and senses to natural impressions, at least for the duration of the therapy. We must withdraw from non-pranic or non-organic sources of sensory impressions, like those from media or computer screens. Even in our daily lives, to maintain a positive energy of awareness, we should spend more time involved with natural impressions, solitude and silence than in social interaction or contact with the media.

Silence, stillness, rest, retreat, peace, equanimity and letting go are the foundation for rejuvenation. They are core values of pratyahara practice. Yet these values are opposite our current social norms of aggression, assertion, marketing and fighting on to the bitter end! This means that we must to some extent die to the world in order to be reborn within our own inner being.

For real rejuvenation to be possible, one should start with a rejuvenation retreat in nature or in an ashram for at least one week, preferably for an entire month or forty days. Outer rejuvenation practices like a rejuvenative diet, herbs and drinks should be combined with inner rejuvenation practices of pranayama, mantra and meditation. The mind should let go of stress and anxiety, and simply learn to be with life.

Generally during rejuvenation therapies, physical activity and exercise is reduced. However, gentle yoga asanas, particularly of a restorative nature can be helpful to slow down the body and mind. Asana aims at calming the motor organs, particularly the hands and feet, which is a kind of physical pratyahara. We need to employ a similar attitude and practices for calming all the sensory and motor organs. Below we will examine how to access a higher level of sensory impressions as well as how to turn our sense and motor organs within.

The Chakras and Rejuvenation

The five great elements of earth, water, fire, air and ether are not simply material forces or inert substances in the outer world. They represent the five root energies behind all existence, with pranic, mental, emotional and spiritual manifestations. The five sense organs, the five types of sensory impressions, and the five motor organs manifest from the influences of the five elements on different levels, which are reflected through the lower five of the seven chakras.

The seven chakras are the centers of the five cosmic elements, mind and consciousness, along with their corresponding sense organs, motor organs and sensory qualities. They grant us the energy and cosmic prana from these.

Location	Element	Dosha	Cognitive Sense	Sense Quality	Action/ Motor Organ
Root	Earth	Kapha	Smell	Aroma	Anus[111]
Sex	Water	Kapha	Tongue	Taste Sensations	Urogenital
Navel	Fire	Pitta	Eyes	Visual sensations	Feet
Heart	Air	Vata	Skin	Tactile sensations	Hands
Throat	Ether	Vata	Ears	Sound sensations	Vocal organs
Third eye	Mind space		Mind	Mind	Mental speech
Crown chakra	Space of Consciousness		Consciousness	Pure being	Divine Word

Well-being depends upon the proper balance of the five elements within us at both physical and psychological levels. Spirituality depends upon accessing the inner essences of the elements as the root powers of cosmic creation working through the chakras. Pratyahara aspects of rejuvenation consist of taking in the healing essence of the five elements through the outer and inner senses.

The chakras can function as powerful centers of rejuvenation. In the ordinary human state, the chakras work only at a diminished level, not taking in the cosmic energies in a way that can revitalize us or open us up to a higher awareness, but only reflecting our outward based sensory and emotional activity, the factors of our personal psychology.

We can renew our chakras through drawing in the respective cosmic elements through the natural sensory impressions that relate to them, by infusing them with prana and by energizing them with mantra. However to accomplish this, we must first unify our mind and prana, creating a steadiness and focus of both. Only a unitary awareness has the power to reach the Sushumna or central channel along which the chakras are located and can allow us access to their higher forces. Otherwise, we can only work on the chakras indirectly through their reflections at a physical or personal level. We must learn the art of using the chakras to draw in cosmic energy, which itself rests upon pratyahara or turning our focus within.

On this foundation, we will examine the rejuvenative powers of the five elements, five sense organs, and five motor organs, which should be looked at relative to their chakra correspondences as well.

The Five Elements and Rejuvenation
The Water Element and Rejuvenation

We begin our examination of the rejuvenative powers of the elements with water. Water is the primary element behind all rejuvenation therapies. This includes special healing waters, juices and herbal teas at a physical level, and bringing the cooling, nurturing energy of the cosmic waters at a psychological and spiritual level, some of which we have discussed already.

Water is the main element upon which life depends, from which it arises and which sustains it. Our body is dominated by the water element, which makes up its main fluids and tissues. Life depends both upon the proper type of fluid in the body and its right circulation. This is mainly reflected by the quality of plasma in the body, our dominant bodily fluid, what is called 'rasa dhatu' in Ayurvedic medicine. Water is a vehicle for Prana or the life-force, which moves through it. For health and longevity, it is important that the fluids we drink are richly imbued with prana. Prana is connected to the air and oxygen, but is also to the vital energy that we find in all of life.

Rejuvenation therapies are best performed in locations by water, lakes, rivers and streams. Mountain streams carry a powerful balance of water and prana. Natural lakes hold a calm and nurturing energy. Mineral springs carry special healing forms of water and also earth in the minerals that they contain. Bathing in special hot springs and mineral springs is an important aid in longevity. It brings in not only the healing power of water but that of earth as well.

Another important method is to bathe in special waters or simply take ones daily bath and shower along with reciting various mantras, especially rejuvenative mantras like *Aim*, *Śrīm*, and *Klīm*. We need to make our water sacred and empower the water in our lives with a healing prana for rejuvenation to occur. The waters of the heart, our inner ocean of consciousness, are most healing.

The Earth Element and Rejuvenation

The Earth is our foundation and support in all that we do. Rejuvenation depends upon being grounded and linked to the healing forces of the Earth, its rocks, minerals, woods, flowers, herbs and foods. We especially need the nurturing protection of the Earth for rejuvenation purposes. Traditional Ayurvedic rejuvenation therapy involved extensive periods of retreat and silence in a special hut (kutir), where one was not exposed to wind, cold, heat, dampness or dryness, but is protected by the Earth on all sides.

The forces of the mineral kingdom, particularly the rocks, have strong healing powers, holding an energy of existence that endures for millions of years. There are special healing forms of clay and the soil itself holds great healing energies. Mountains in particular hold the spiritual and regenerative power of the Earth. Crystals and gems carry subtle Earth energies as well.

One of the most important rejuvenative practices that we can do is to restore our personal connection to the Earth. This is to recognize the Divine Mother and Mother Nature working through Mother Earth. We all need our sacred earth, which is the ground of immortality. We need sacred earth in our homes as well, with special rocks and plants in the rooms where we spend most of our time.

It is important that we make the earth around us sacred, particularly the earth or place on which we sit. Yoga asana traditionally was a way of making sacred our connection to the Earth and linking us to the ground as our Yoga seat. To do this, however, we must look upon the asana as our connection to the Earth as a whole and consecrate it with mantras.

The Fire Element and Rejuvenation

Fire is more a purifying rather than rejuvenating force. Without previous work with the purifying power of fire, rejuvenation through the water and earth elements remains limited. Yet fire has its special rejuvenating effects as well. The energy of fire that we access outwardly can stimulate the inner fires of the mind, the eye and the body. Most of us have experienced how a campfire can stimulate our minds and senses.

There are special Vedic fire rituals or *Yajnas* for removing difficulties and diseases and extending the life, notably the *Mrityunjaya Homa* for Lord Shiva. Yajnas to planets like Saturn can also aid in health and longevity. In the ancient Hindu *Brahmana* texts gaining of the fullness of life is said to be one of the fruits of proper performance of fire rituals.

Honoring the sacred fire within and around us connects us with the cosmic forces of light and immortality. One can light candles (preferably aromatic) and ghee or other natural oil filled lamps. It is best to keep a flame burning in one's home in the evening. Gazing at such a flame is an important tool of concentration in Yoga practice (trataka). Contacting the flame of awareness in the spiritual heart and surrendering to it is an important means of Self-inquiry and accessing our inner immortality.

The Air Element and Rejuvenation

Air carries the prana or life-force on which our body depends and which stimulates the mind and senses to work. Special types of air hold more prana than others. For longevity and rejuvenation we need to breathe fresh natural air, filled with the energies of the earth, the waters and the Sun.

Air holds the best or special types of prana in mountain areas, by streams or by the ocean. We need to avoid the stagnant air of urban environments, offices and houses, in which chemical residues usually tinge the air. We should keep our air flowing, open and fresh. Above all we need healing air within our homes and work places. Even in the winter we should go outside and access fresh air on a regular basis. It will help prevent colds and flu and other respiratory ailments. However, we should avoid the wind, which can bring diseases into our bodies and disturb our minds.

The use of incense helps clear the air in our homes and buildings and turn it into a more rejuvenating force. Pranayama is the main method to work with the air element within ourselves.

The Ether Element and Rejuvenation

We need space in order to grow and to develop in consciousness, and also to rejuvenate ourselves, particularly space for the mind to release its narrowness and sorrow. Without first creating a sacred space, there can be no rejuvenation. Immortality is gained by taking our consciousness deep within our own inner space that extends beyond body and mind.

For rejuvenation, particularly of the mind, we need space around us, being in a natural setting that is open to a wide expansion of horizon and sky, like in the mountains, by a lake or by the sea. We also need a psychological space in which we are not caught in emotional conflicts or bound up in competition with others, in which our minds are not cluttered or burdened with disturbing thoughts or emotions.

There are many ways to connect to the space element. Looking at the sky and stars at night is important, particularly on dark nights. Even a good telescope can help in this regard. One can also gaze at the sky and clouds during the day (away from the bright Sun). Learning to observe the space between objects is another method. Above all, we need to create a space in the mind for meditation and a space in the heart for devotion. This requires letting go of any narrow opinions or judgments that restrict our awareness. Space is everywhere to heal and expand us, but we seldom look at it or open ourselves up to its energies. We must learn to live in space rather than in the world of form if we wish to discover our true nature.

Rejuvenation and the Five Sense Organs
Taking in of the Five Sensory Essences

The five senses form different means of accessing prana or the life-force. They bring us energy from the external world and stimulate the flow of vitality within us. They are the root of our activity and afford us the possibility of rejuvenation as well. One of the keys to longevity is to keep our senses active, engaged and sharp, not in media or technological pursuits but in contact with nature and with other people at the level of the heart. The more we are creatively engaged with our senses, particularly our eyes and ears, and relative to the world of nature, the more we are likely to live longer and be happier, the more we are accessing the cosmic prana. Do not neglect your senses or fail to develop their inner powers; as the *Vedas* say, they are the Gods or Devas within us.

Our five senses take in the five sensory qualities, which are regarded in Yoga philosophy as the five subtle elements (ether-sound, air-touch, fire-sight, water-taste, and earth-smell). These five sensory qualities constitute the main Somas for the mind. The five senses serve to bring in these subtle Somas.

Rejuvenation of the senses is closely related to the yogic practice of pratyahara, which refers to the withdrawal of the mind, senses and prana into the inner consciousness. In pratyahara practices, one usually first connects the senses with nature and then turns the senses within and draws them to key centers in the body like the third eye, the heart or other chakras for deeper meditation.

We can use our senses either in a way that increases our prana or in a way that depletes it. When we open up to wholesome natural impressions, our senses can nourish the mind and heart and touch the soul. When we pursue disturbed and artificial impressions, as in most of what we call entertainment, our senses cause us to lose energy from both body and mind and get us caught in a process of desire. One of the biggest health issues we have today, physical, psychological and spiritual, is the weight of negative impressions we take in daily through the mass media, which like toxic metals builds up in our tissues and cannot easily be dislodged. We must create our own positive impressions born of nature, art and meditation to counter these. This is a daily necessity and should be part of our every day routine.

Ayurvedic 'sensory therapies' are an important part of any rejuvenation therapy, particularly aromatherapy, color therapy and sound therapy. Rejuvenation requires sensory therapies to bring in a higher form of sensory nutrition for the mind and heart. These are very important not only in a clinic or spa but in your own home and meditation room. Make sure to bring in a higher quality of natural impressions every day for inner healing. This allows the Gods or divine powers to descend into our environment.

Ears – Sound – Space

The Soma of sound, though formless, is probably the most powerful of the sensory Somas, which we can observe in how easily song and music attract our attention and reverberate in our subconscious minds. Most of us spend a significant amount of our time pursuing audio sensations and some form of regular musical entertainment. It dominates our lives and defines our consciousness. It determines the nature of our mental space.

Sound connects to space and to the prana or vital force, the reservoir of potential energy, which permeates space. The ears connect us to the vast network of vibrations that underlies the universe, which are ultimately patterns of sound. The sound vibrations from space and the distant stars and galaxies are messages of cosmic intelligence that can draw us into a deeper awareness, if we open up to their energy. Subtle sound opens up many new inner dimensions to those who contemplate sound as sacred.

The ears reflect the deeper contemplative powers of the mind and allow it to expand. What we hear defines our space both inwardly and outwardly. How we listen similarly defines the type of space that exists both within and around us. If we open our inner ear then we can commune with all of life.

However, in order to deeply listen, one first must be silent within, not preoccupied with our own inner chatter. For most of us our inner space is cluttered with noise and memories, like a dust storm that blocks our deeper awareness. Yet silence is necessary to energize the ears, just as rest and relaxation energize the body. Silence helps rejuvenate our sense of sound. We should try to live more silent lives in natural settings where there are no irritating noises.

We need to reclaim the ears and our sense of hearing as a type of deep listening, honoring and worship of life, in which the voice of every creature and the sound of every object should be heeded with respect. We should strive to discover progressively more subtle sounds within and around us. This includes listening to the internal sounds of our own bodies and minds, and especially to the *nada* or the cosmic sound vibrations that flow in the silent mind.

A good practice for rejuvenating the ears is listening to the sounds of the five elements, particularly the sounds of water like the flowing of a creek, stream or river, waves on the sea, or the falling rain. The sounds of the wind are also very important but can be disturbing when very fast. We should try to listen to the sounds of nature, not simply human speech but to the birds, insects and other creatures. *Try to hear something new in nature every day.*

To rejuvenate the body, we must create our own revitalizing sounds through chanting and mantra. We must learn to listen to the sound of our own breathing and heartbeat and what they are reverberating. It is not enough just to listen to good music. We must discover a deep music inside ourselves, what is called *nada* in yogic thought. Our minds, down to the subconscious level, should reverberate with the universal presence.

Skin – Touch – Air

The Soma of touch is the most powerful and intimate of the sensory Somas. It is the basis of love, affection and sexuality. Touch triggers our emotions. Gentle touch awakens our sensitivities, while harsh touch can traumatize us. Touch carries prana or vital energy. Through the act of touching another, we link our pranas in a way that can be helpful or harmful, depending upon the intention and energy that we possess. We should be very careful about the type of energy we direct through our hands. We should also be very careful as to the energy that others touch us with, particularly those who may be doing some therapeutic work on us.

Our sense of touch is rejuvenated by healing and loving touch. This can be aided by applying oil to the skin, particularly warm sesame oil preparations such as found in Ayurveda. Sweating, steam baths and sauna therapies also help rejuvenate the skin. Bathing in special rivers or natural springs is also important. Touch is not just about human touch. We should learn to touch the subtle textures in nature, like that of leaves, flowers or the lichen on a rock. We should touch the soil with our own hands, and let the dirt flow between our fingers, noting also its fragrance. We are part of that Earth.

Eyes – Color – Fire

The Soma of light and color is extremely powerful, stimulating us and defining our vision of the world. It is the basis of all the visual arts and of the yogic practice of visualization.

Color helps revive and rejuvenate the eyes and our inner sense of vision, including the perceptual power of the mind. The bright artificial colors of computer and media screens serve to dull the eyes and narrow the range of our sensitivity to the colors of nature. Natural colors serve to awaken us to higher realities and subtler astral worlds. No screen, however high its power of resolution, can compare with the color variations that we find in nature, with its myriad earth tones as well as the blue of the sky, the colors of the setting sun amidst the clouds, or even the different colors of the stars.

Screens are two dimensional and make the mind superficial and two dimensional in nature. Out in nature we must develop depth perception, particularly looking at distant mountains, sky, clouds or stars. This serves to expand the mind and make it capable of holding more Prana.

Color therapy is an important sensory tool of rejuvenation. Generally cooling colors like white, green and blue are better for calming the mind and emotions. For soothing, nurturing and moistening the eyes, best is a creamy white, the blue of the sky or the green of grass or trees. For stimulating the acuity of the eyes warm and bright colors are best like orange, gold and red are best, particularly as found in flowers. Practicing night vision by looking at the night sky or stars helps rejuvenate our eyes. The natural colors of the ground, soil and rocks, the browns, grays and sandstone colors of the earth also help and make our perception subtler. We should avoid any bright shades, particularly of an artificial nature or colors reflected in too bright a sunlight.

Another important tool is eye exercises to open us up to new perspectives, like imagining a small rock as being a large mountain or vice versa. Examining the clouds or waves on the water to defocus the eyes from their fixation on solid or defined forms can also help. Such 'asanas for the eyes' can be very transformative and can help break up old emotional patterns and attachments as well. Many yogic Dharana practices are useful here as they relate to fixing the gaze in various ways. This includes the use of *yantras* or geometrical meditation designs, like the symbol below for opening the spiritual heart.

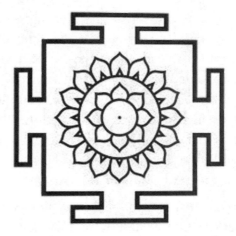

Tongue – Taste – Water

Taste connects directly to Soma, reflected in the tastes of our food and beverages at an outer level, and our inner sense of beauty and taste, both in art and spiritual practice, particularly devotion.

The tongue is the main sensory organ of taste but it is also connected to the motor organ of speech. Our ability to taste and our ability to speak are related. Poetic speech has a Soma quality to it and reflects this inner sense of taste that is also connected to sound. It is very important that we cultivate taste in life, so that we can eventually come to taste and imbibe the nectar of bliss that permeates all that we perceive. We need to develop a taste not only for foods and beverages but also for all the beauty and wonder of life.

The right spices help stimulate and revive our sense of taste. Loss of appetite is a common symptom and causative factor in many diseases and maladies like colds, congestion, allergies, asthma and depression. Best are sweet and stimulating aromatic spices like cardamom, ginger, basil, cinnamon, cloves, and mint. Right diet and right intake of beverages are important here as well, including good Soma beverages.

At an inner level, we need to learn to taste the nectar in our own brain and nervous system, which is also reflected in the breath and in our saliva. Normally we seek to please our palate with our taste in food. However, the palate also can be the place from which our own inner nectar flows. This requires that we make our brain and nervous system sensitive to the taste of bliss that lies behind all other sense qualities. Another helpful tool in right use of the tongue is Khechari mudra, holding the tongue at the roof of the mouth to connect our sense of taste with Divine grace and Soma.

Nose –Smell – Earth

It is curious that in the English language the word smell has basically a negative connotation. This reflects our lack of awareness of the beauty of fragrance and its transformational energy. The Soma of fragrance and aroma is the most immediate Soma for defining our own body, as well as our immediate environment and our interaction with it. Beautiful aromas help bring in celestial energies as well as clearing our pranic field. They are the foundation of all other sensory therapies.

Aromatherapy is an important method of working on the Soma of fragrance. Incense is another important aromatherapy that can be rejuvenating in nature. Regular burning of incense in the house is a way to keep a rejuvenative environment for body, mind and prana. That is why temples usually have incense burning all the time.

However, for aromatherapy to work, we need to keep our nostrils and sinuses clear. This is the importance of neti and nasya therapies in Ayurveda.[112]

As our inner awareness develops various inner fragrances can arise as well, particularly when the root chakra begins to open. Various aromas aid in the development of the subtle energies of the chakras, which are all nourished by the earth of the root chakra. In fact the fragrance emitted by our body reflects our consciousness. We need to cultivate our inner fragrance as it were. We should make sure that the perfume created by our thoughts and actions brings a higher awareness into the world.

To develop this higher sense of the cosmic aromas we should become familiar with the manifest fragrances of nature. This should begin with learning the fragrances of the Earth including those of different soils. Even rocks have a certain earthy aroma, particularly when they are wet. We should learn the fragrance not only of flowers, but also of grass, leaves and fruit, including pine needles and plant resins of all types. Morning and evening and the different seasons have their varying fragrances as well. We should learn to recognize the fragrances of the wind as it blows at different times or different directions.

Rejuvenation of the Five Motor Organs and Self-control

The five motor organs are the active counterparts of the five sense organs that are receptive in nature. Normally, we take in energy and information through the sense organs and express or release it through the motor organs. This means that there is a greater tendency to lose energy through the motor organs than there is through the sense organs. While the sense organs serve more to take in Soma, the motor organs are more a means of using or discharging it. We gain a certain pleasure or enjoyment in action and in our motor impulses, or we would not want to activate them.

Control of the motor organs is usually more difficult than control of the sense organs as there is a greater urgency in the impulses behind the motor organs. The senses organs owing to their perceptual functions have a more sattvic or receptive nature. The motor organs owing to their need to act and express have a more rajasic or potentially turbulent nature. To control them requires a certain discipline and effort maintained consistently over time.

Yet if we fail to control our motor organs, they will cause us to lose control of our lives on all levels. They will make us do things that we don't want to do and cause us regret. The problem is that our modern education, with its emphasis on entertainment, does not emphasize self-control or instill that into children. This means that as adults we lack that discipline and may find it hard to implement it. We are controlled by our impulses rather than consciously directing them.

Rejuvenation is more a matter of non-doing than it is of doing. It is a way of inaction more than action. As such, it requires calming the motor organs and bringing them back to a state of relaxation, checking their outgoing entropy through which vitality is lost, and using them only as really needed. Rejuvenation practices should rest upon a rejuvenation-promoting awareness, which is to conserve and transform, not to express and discharge our vitality. *This power of non-doing is the essence of rejuvenation.* It requires doing less, saying less, and being more decisive and clear when we are compelled to act.

Speech – Space

The organ of speech, including the vocal cords, mouth, lips and tongue is the most important, the most widely used, and the most widely abused of our motor organs. We lose the greatest amount of energy through the mouth, which is not only physical but also an emotional vitality. Many of us waste much of our time in useless talk, rumor or gossip, and do not know how to be silent and attentive. What we say gets us into trouble in many ways, but is even more so a loss of prana. Even random speech can cause us to lose energy, as well as to keep our minds confused. To control our motor organs we must first learn to control our speech. This begins with speaking only what is true and speaking it in a pleasant manner, with regard for the good of all.

The practice of silence and voluntarily not speaking (called mauna in Sanskrit) is the most important practice for rejuvenating our power of speech and for protecting our vitality overall. Many great sages were called munis for practicing this art of silence. Speaking less, speaking only when spoken to, or speaking only with a purpose are other considerations to help rejuvenate our faculty of speech. By not speaking, we learn to say more when we do speak, and gain a greater clarity in articulation in our speech.

Singing and chanting helps us control our speech, particularly when aligning it with the prana of devotion. Mantra is perhaps the key practice for developing the power of speech, performed vocally to strengthen the vocal organs and mentally to internalize and calm their energy. This does not mean that we should never talk freely but that we should always weigh our words carefully and speak only when there is a purpose or a need. It requires treating speech as sacred and speaking with courtesy, respect and kindness.

Excess use of the vocal organs or excess speech can cause many diseases starting with the common cold and sore throat, which can impair our immunity overall. It can result in insomnia or emotional unrest as the disturbed physical speech agitates our mind as well. Besides speech, we should control our mouths overall. This means controlling of eating and drinking and what we keep in the mouth. Try practicing keeping silence one day a week, particularly on Monday, the day of the Moon, or Wednesday, the day of Mercury. This will help you conserve the Soma of the mind.

Hands – Air

The hands are the most important part of the skin as a sense organ, where our sense of touch is strongest. Yet the hands are also a motor organ, through which we can do and make many things. Our special human hands provide us with the manual skills crucial for us to perform our actions in life. Like the voice, they can be used for communication.

The hands serve to hold, convey and direct prana, as well as to shape and make things. They are our conduits for vyana vayu, the expanding aspect of pranic energy, which is responsible for the outward movement and development of vitality and creativity. We must learn to become conscious of our Prana and direct it with our hands as a healing force.

The use of mudras is one of the best means of rejuvenating the prana of the hands, notably the Prana mudra.[113] Each finger has its own particular powers and qualities. Rubbing one's hands together also stimulates the prana and can be used to place a healing prana, as placing them over the eyes. One can also use one's hands to draw in positive prana from the atmosphere and draw it into the heart.

Feet – Fire

The feet are the motor organ counterpart of the eyes, which allow us to measure distance. They represent our outer connection to the Earth element and our inner connection to Fire. Keeping our feet grounded on the Earth helps us develop stability and calm and put us in contact with the rejuvenating power of nature. Foot massage is a way of relieving tension from the entire body.

Walking is perhaps the best exercise that we can do because it moves and massages the entire body, starting with the feet. Hiking is great because it connects us to Nature and to the earth, refreshing the nervous system as well. For every mile we hike, we add significant time to our lives and increase our overall longevity. In fact, if there is only one thing we could do for longevity, walking would be the best exercise. In Yoga, sitting poses like the lotus pose are very good for calming the energy of the feet and the navel chakra to which they are connected.

Staying in one place for a certain period of time is central to deeper Yoga practices and to rejuvenation. Cessation of outer movement allows inner rejuvenative energies to flow. When the body is naturally still, our inner Fire naturally rises.

Urogenital Organs – Water

The urinary system and sex organs represent our discharge of the water element from the body and also how we hold the internal water energy from which reproduction arises. Proper function of the kidneys is essential to life and longevity. Adequate and right intake of water and beverages is essential for this.

Taking spicy and diuretic (urination promoting) teas in the morning is very helpful for keeping the kidneys clear and well-functioning. Such herbs include ginger, cinnamon, basil, cloves, coriander, fennel, lemon grass and regular tea. The Ayurvedic herb punarnava is a common rasayana for the kidneys.

Right use of the reproductive system is another key factor of Yoga and pratyahara. We lose a lot of vitality in life through sexual indulgence, which depletes Ojas and weakens the immune system. We need to honor our internal water and not deplete it unnecessarily.

Organs of Elimination/ Colon – Earth

The colon represents the final product of our digestive process. It holds the earth element in the body. It allows us to absorb the deeper Prana from the food that serves to give strength to our deeper tissues of bone, nerve and reproductive.

Rejuvenation of the colon is essential to health and is different from merely stimulating the colon to be more active or to counter constipation. If the colon is weak, we tend to lose our energy downward, increasing Vata dosha and the aging process. Grounding the colon and the root chakra into the earth is an important means of protecting ourselves from gravity and the aging process.

Yet the organs of elimination reflect the principle of elimination, purification and letting go of the past in general. To create and renew, we must dissolve and let go of the past.

Other Pratyahara Practices

There are many helpful yogic pratyahara practices for longevity and rejuvenation. Relaxing and calming the body, prana, senses and mind is the main factor in all these practices. Asana, pranayama, mantra and meditation can be employed as a means of deep internal relaxation and letting go of stress and attachment from body and mind.[114]

Yoga Nidra

Yet more than a practice, pratyahara is the condition in which our energies and awareness is drawn within, which is what all of Yoga is about. Asana, properly speaking, should be a pratyahara of the motor organs. Pranayama is a pratyahara or internalization of the prana, particularly through retention of the breath. Asana practice often ends with savasana or the corpse pose, which helps hold the energies of asana practice and bring them to a deeper level.

Rejuvenation is much like the hibernation that animals undergo in the winter, reducing external activity, but combining this with developing internal sources of energy and awareness, which is a natural pratyahara. This means that probably the best practice for rejuvenation is *Yoga Nidra* or yogic sleep. It can be done in several ways. The main thing is to be able to enter into a state of internal rest without losing one's awareness, to be able to consciously, as it were, experience the state of deep sleep, to enter into the state of deep sleep while waking! Most of us suffer from a lack of deep sleep, which is a lack of deep peace and an inability to let go of all stress.

One can combine Yoga Nidra with savasana or make it one's preferred mode of sleep. But it is better to perform Yoga Nidra in a sitting pose, which keeps our energy moving up the spine. Yoga Nidra is a key to rejuvenation of the mind as well as the body. In Yoga Nidra, we also let the mind rest and return to silence. Yoga Nidra involves pratyahara of all the sense and motor organs, prana and mind. As such, it is the highest of all pratyahara practices and has powerful rejuvenative effects.

MANTRA RASAYANA,
THE REJUVENATING POWER OF COSMIC
SOUND AND THE DIVINE WORD

The golden one (Hari), putting forth his creative energies along the path of truth, directs his voice, like an oar a ship. Divine he reveals the secrets names of all the Gods, to declare them on the sacred grass.

Rigveda IX.95.2

Mantra has always been closely connected to Soma and is an important type of Soma itself. The chants or mantras of the *Rigveda* are said to give us Soma, particularly the Soma hymns. This 'Mantric Soma' is sometimes regarded as the most important of all Somas. Soma as the Moon gives inspiration to the mind that results in poetry and mantra. This association of poetry with the Moon and with intoxication, usually wine, is found in all poetic and mystical traditions of the world from the Sufis to the Chinese. A true poet must access that inner nectar, wine or Soma. So too, for mantras to really work they must be energized with that rasa, essence, Soma or immortal nectar.

Mantra is the main yogic tool for working on the mind on all of its levels and functions, from instinct, sensation, emotion and thought, to higher intuitive and inspirational energies. Mantras can serve to energize the mind, heal the mind, purify the mind, or calm the mind, depending upon the nature and application of the specific mantras involved. The magic of mantra on so many levels of life is perhaps unequalled by any practice![115]

Mantras are important medicines in themselves and have been lauded as such since Vedic times. The chanting of mantras can serve as a powerful rejuvenative therapy for the mind and heart. There are special rejuvenative or rasayana mantras that increase prana, feeling or perceptive powers. One creates a powerful flow of internal energy by repeating such rejuvenative mantras, bathing the entire psyche in its current, which can then electrify and revitalize us from within.

While mantras can be employed either along the Yoga of knowledge or the Yoga of devotion, mantras are primarily a tool of devotion and usually rest upon a relationship with the deity. We will explore the subject of devotional mantras more in the following chapter on Deity Rasayana.

Mantras are of three types by formulation: The first are single syllable seed or bija mantras like *Om* and *Hrīm*, which rest largely on the power of their sound vibrations. The second are Divine Name Mantras like *Namaḥ Śivāya!* or *Namo Narāyānāya!* which rest upon our connection to the Divine at a heart level. The third are longer prayers, propitiations and contemplations, which consist of specific verses to be meditated upon, like the Gayatri mantra or various Peace (Shanti) mantras. Yet all three types of mantras can be combined as well.

The first or bija mantras probably have the most powerful rejuvenative properties as they can alter the subtle sound and energy currents behind the mind and subtle body. Name mantras also have powerful rejuvenative effects, if we have a deep heart connection to the deity. There are special prayers for long life and immortality, as well as for warding off of death and disease like the famous *Mahamrityunjaya Mantra* to Lord Shiva.

Soft and Harsh Mantras

Mantras are usually divided into two main categories as soft or harsh. [116] Soft mantras are usually to benefic, watery or Soma forms of deities like Vishnu, Lakshmi, Sundari and Shiva. Harsh mantras relate to malefic, fiery and airy forms of deities like Rudra and Kali. Harsh mantras are used mainly for purification and detoxification purposes. Soft mantras aim more at tonification and rejuvenation purposes. Generally soft mantras reflect soft sounds and harsh mantras reflect harsh or strong sounds, but the intentionality with which the mantra is employed also comes into play here. Soft mantras imply a soft, gentle and nourishing intention. Harsh mantras are used to dissolve attachments and purify the mind. A few mantras are overall balanced and can be used either to purify or to revitalize.

STRONG OR HARSH, PURIFYING BIJA MANTRAS

Hūm	Energizes the Agni principle, including the digestive fire and the Kundalini fire in order to burn away impurities from body and mind
Krīm	Energizes the power of Prana, stimulating and opening the mind, senses and nervous system
Hsauḥ	Energizes a higher power of the breath and Kundalini Shakti
Kṣraum	Removes negativity from the navel chakra[117]
Ram	Seed syllable of the fire element, promotes purification through Agni or fire, strengthens the navel or fire chakra
Yam	Seed syllable of the air element, stimulates the heart or air chakra
Ham	Seed syllable of the ether element, creates space, Prana and movement

SOFT AND RASAYANA BIJA MANTRAS

Śrīm	Promotes the lunar force, rejuvenating the heart, lungs and emotions
Klīm	Power of attraction, for moistening, attracting, consolidating Ojas, love and bliss
Aim	Rejuvenates the mind and power of speech, developing the learning capacity, for Shakti overall
Sauḥ	Makes the Soma energy flow, gives poetic ability and creativity
Strīm	Awakens the inner Shakti and strengthening the female reproductive system
Lam	Seed syllable of the earth element and root chakra, but also reflects the higher energy of bliss and Divine speech

Vam	Seed syllable of the water element and sex center
Kṣam	Calms the mind, heart and emotions, allows the third eye to open
Śam	Seed syllable of peace or shanti, alleviates pain and calms emotions

BALANCED BIJA MANTRAS

Om	Energizes all processes, connecting to the Cosmic Prana, for the Shiva force
Hrīm	Purifies and rejuvenates the heart, drawing us into our inner being, Atman or Purusha
Rām	Calms the mind heart and mind and alleviating fear, particularly good for children

Of these bija mantras, *Klīm* is probably the best for drawing in and consolidating the Soma in the mind and heart. It not only helps us develop the Soma but also takes it into the spiritual heart. For this purpose, we can repeat the mantra by itself on a regular basis. But we also must have the proper intention and concentration.

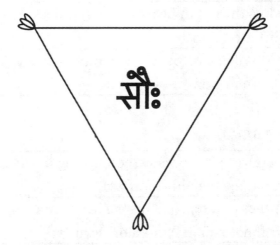

Sauḥ: the Shakti Bija Mantra for Soma to Flow

MANTRA RASAYANA PRACTICE

In this approach, one chants the mantra for one month, best from full Moon to full Moon, at least half an hour morning (before sunrise) and evening (before sleep). Best is to repeat the bija mantra 1000 times morning and evening. *Hrīm* is a good mantra to start with. Simple formulas like *Hrīm Śrīm Klīm* are very good, which is why we find them with such bliss-oriented deities as the Goddess Tripura Sundari. Her fivefold mantra as *Hrīm Śrīm Klīm Aim Sauḥ* stimulates the flow of Tarpak Kapha from the region of the Moon. One can also study the hymns of the great yogi and Vedantic guru Shankara, which include many chants to Tripura Sundari like his famous *Saundarya Lahiri*, the Wave of Bliss, perhaps the greatest of all Sanskrit and yogic poems.[118]

Another good mantra rasayana practice is to repeat mantras while bathing or standing in water (like that of a stream), which can include offering the mantras to the Sun or the Moon. We can even bathe ourselves with mantra, a *mantra snana*, letting the Soma of the mantra rain upon us. Another method is to use mantras to draw in the healing powers of nature from the Sun and Moon, from the wind and air, to the foods and herbs that we take. Using mantras to energize one's food and beverages is an important part of rejuvenation therapy as well. Yet any chanting of mantra can become a rasayana if done with devotion, love and surrender to the Divine within.

Types of Letters

Sanskrit recognizes three types of letters, as vowels, consonants and a third group of semivowels and 's' and 'h' sounds.[119]

- Vowels and vowel-based mantras, particularly *Om* and *Aim*, have primarily a Soma or lunar energy. They work on the higher chakras, particularly the throat chakra.

- Semivowel based mantras (*Lam, Vam, Ram, Yam*) and 's' and 'h' sound mantras (*Sam, Ham,* Śam, Ṣam, Kṣam) have a heat producing, Agni, fiery and purifying energy that stimulates the Kundalini. They work on the lower chakras, particularly the root chakra.

- Consonants have a solar energy and stand between the vowels and semivowels and their Soma and Agni energies. They work on the middle chakras, particularly the heart and navel.

- However, each letter of the Sanskrit alphabet has its own Soma, essence, meaning or beauty. Each serves to mark and energize one of the petals of the lotuses of the six chakras. Through the proper intonation of each letter of the Sanskrit alphabet, we can release the corresponding Soma of each chakra.

Another distinction relevant here is that short vowels in Sanskrit like the a-sound in the particle 'a' are more solar and masculine in nature, while the long vowels, like the a-sound in 'f*a*ther' are regarded as lunar and feminine in nature. Prolonging vowels brings out more of their Soma.

Ayurvedic Mantras

Bija mantras are very important in Ayurveda as well.[120] There are special mantras for the main marma points (energy centers in the body), including the different tissues and organs. Such mantras are

273

also connected to the chakras. Other mantras can help us balance the doshas of Vata, Pitta and Kapha or increase the subtle essences of Prana, Tejas and Ojas. Even chanting the Sanskrit alphabet can be an important tool for rejuvenating the body and mind. There are also chants to various deities like Shiva, Dhanvantari, or Shitali Devi (who protects us from fevers). Mantras for Vedic astrology or for Vastu are important as well.

Vedic Mantras

The Vedic language is the very language of Soma. Chanting Vedic hymns, particularly those to Soma, is a great way to increase our inner flow of Soma. Vedic Soma mantras trigger the subtle energies of the brain and mind in order to bring us into a deeper state of calm and contentment. There are also special Vedic mantras for health, happiness and longevity, many of which mention Soma and Agni. These include many *Shanti* or Peace mantras such as are commonly chanted at Yoga centers and ashrams. There are Vedic mantras for Prana, the doshas and for longevity (ayus) itself. Vedic mantras are perhaps the most powerful mantric medicines and have a wide range of application.

Such Vedic mantras are longer verses, not seed mantras, and require a special training to pronounce properly, though recordings of them can be found. In addition, there are several traditional and modern styles of Vedic chanting which have their variations.[121] Note our selection of Soma verses from the *Rigveda* in the appendix for some translations of these.

Vedantic Mantras

Along the Yoga of Knowledge are also many mantras, including special chants from the *Upanishads*. Usually these are not used for mundane purposes like longevity, but connecting with the higher reality help our karmas on all levels. Probably the most important Vedantic mantra for bliss, renewal and immortality is: *Sarvam Khalvidam Brahma* – Everything is Brahman (God or the Absolute).

We can use this mantra to discover the immortal essence of Being that is hidden in all of life and to draw into us all the healing forces of nature. We will discuss some additional mantras relative the next chapter on deities, particularly the use of Divine Names.[122]

Pronunciation of Sanskrit Mantras

Below are phonetic indications for pronouncing the main seed or bija mantras used in the book. I have included the indications for the long Sanskrit vowels in their transliteration for easier pronunciation. The same rules can be extended to other Sanskrit terms so indicated.[123]

Aim – Aym

Aum – au as in *ou*ch

Dham – 'a' as in '*a* book'

Ham – 'a' as in '*a* book'

Haum – au as in *ou*ch

Hrīm – Hreem

Hsauḥ – au as in *ou*ch

Hūm – Hoom

Īm – Eem

Jūm – Joom

Klīm – Kleem

Krīm – Kreem

Kṛṣṇa – Krishna

Kṣam – '*a' as in 'a* book', *ṣ* as in *sh*ip

Kṣraum – *au* as in *ou*ch, *ṣ* as in *sh*ip

Lam –'a' as in '*a* book'

Namaḥ –'a' as in '*a* book'

Om – Om

Ram, fire/navel mantra – 'a' as in '*a* book'

Rām, name of Rama – 'a' as in f*a*ther

Śakti – Shakti, 'a' as in '*a* book'

Saḥ –'a' as in '*a* book'

Śam – sham, 'a' as in '*a* book'

Sauḥ– au as in *ou*ch

Śiva – Shiva

Śrīm – Shreem

So – So

Som – long 'o' as in so

Strīm – Streem

Svāhā – Swaha, both 'a'-sounds as in f*a*ther

Vam – 'a' as in '*a* book'

Yam – 'a' as in '*a* book'

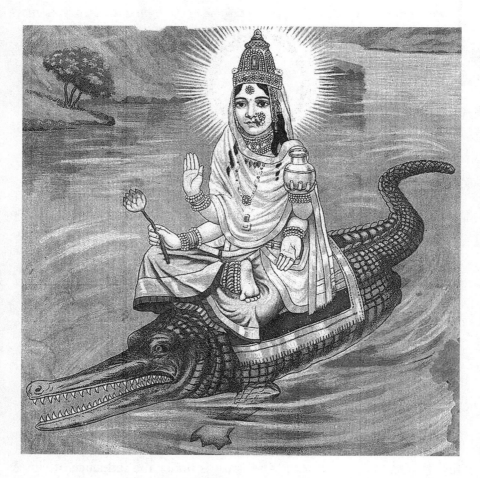

Ganga Devi, the Goddess of the Ganga River

Deity Rasayana: The Rejuvenating Power of Devotion

The seers meditated on the supreme Name of the light and discovered the three times seven supreme planes of the Mother.

Rigveda IV.1.16

The most powerful and enduring emotion for all creatures is love. True love is immortal and never dies. Love as the very power of eternity holds the secret of deathlessness. This is not just a romantic fantasy but also a Divine truth. Without love, no one wants to live, whatever else they may have gained in life. With love one can even accept death and will not fear it. It is only love that can take us beyond death. Only the love within us does not die, while all the other emotions must pass away.

Yet true love is not simply something physical or sexual, much less merely human. It is a love for life itself as eternal love in manifestation. It is a Divine love, not as an ethereal devotion but as a deep regard for the sacred essence in all beings. Such a supreme love is our true nature and is deeper than the names, identities and embodiments that the soul takes in its various lives. Death can only consume outer forms but not the inner spirit of love and devotion.

Death is allied with such negative emotions as desire, fear and anger, in which there is no love, trust, devotion, beauty or surrender. These fragmented emotions born of attraction and repulsion divide our energies and make us mortal. They put us under the influence of time and circumstance. Mortality is linked to the mind and its emotional reactions, which poison us, as it were, with energies of division and decay. Immortality is connected to the spiritual heart, which is the inner consciousness beyond the mind and its attempts to own, control, possess or dominate. This means that unless we move beyond such personal emotions to a higher force of love that happiness and immortality must elude us whatever else we may attempt.

Actually, it is negative emotions like fear, anger and desire that wear out the mind, not simply the aging process or physical disease. We accumulate negative emotions in our memory, which weigh us down and inhibit our inner growth. The key to well-being and happiness is an emotional rejuvenation, which includes a cleansing away of all negative emotions, fear, desire, anger, attachment and grief. Devotion, in which we connect with the immortal Divine love, is probably the best way to do this.

Love is probably the greatest of all rejuvenating forces. Love releases an inner flow of Soma into the body and mind. We have all experienced this in our ordinary human love and romance, which has its special exhilaration and fascination, and its hormonal stimulation. Bhakti or devotion provides an even deeper grace, rasa, delight and attraction.

Any contact with the Divine presence within our hearts opens us up to our inner immortality. The highest Soma is the flow of Divine grace within us. Yet it is the inner divinity of pure consciousness that grants this, not the outer deity of emotional belief, dogma or orthodoxy, which tends to stifle the mystical experience within us and itself is allied with mortality and ignorance.

The Soma of Relationship

Love is part of a broader 'Soma of relationship'. Our human contacts are a powerful source of either nectar or poison for our minds and hearts. We draw in the Soma or energy from the people we associate with or from the activities that we engage in along with others, from habitual activities to special events. When we have an audience in life to focus on us, we gain a certain Soma or delight from their attention. That is why public figures and celebrities can even forego other types of human enjoyment. They find that the Soma of adulation is enough.

How we form our associations and what types of people we most relate with at a heart level are very important to how our Soma develops in life. Yet our highest relationship is not with other people at an outer level; it is with the Divine in others, in ourselves and in the entire universe. To elevate our Soma in life we should always seek to relate to the highest. Developing a relationship with noble souls and teachers is what is called *Satsang* in Sanskrit or communion with reality. It extends into relationship with Divinity and human relationships that center around honoring or worshipping the Divine. Even in our ordinary relationship we should look to the good in others and try to support it, rather looking to the negative or imperfect in them.

The heart contains a magnetic energy to draw to it that which we are truly searching for in life. This is the magnetic power of the heart's Soma. It is the basis of devotion as a spiritual path. If we cultivate this 'Soma of relationship', which is the essence of Yoga as union, we will discover a network of Soma like gravity linking together everything in the universe and drawing the higher spiritual powers to us even without any overt effort on our parts.

Bhakti Yoga

Perhaps the most common, accessible and powerful form of Yoga is Bhakti Yoga, the Yoga of Devotion. Devotion has the power to heal the mind and heart, to remove negative emotions and to promote feelings that are positive, uplifting and unifying. Bhakti stimulates the inner sense of Divine love that is the supreme grace and most powerful Soma. In this regard, Bhakti is one of the most important tools of psychological healing. Those who have genuine devotion cannot fall into anger, depression, lust or greed. They remain even minded, content and concerned for others. The lack of devotion in our current culture is one of the main causes of psychological unhappiness as well as the wearing out of the mind among so many of us.

Even compassion for others should rest upon a higher devotion. Unless we share Divine love, which humbles us as well, our compassion may be little more than pity and can prove condescending and debilitating to others. Divine love has no boundaries of high and low but embraces all who are open to its energy. It does not look down upon anyone but looks to the light and strength within all.

There are two main yogic ways to reach the supreme reality, devotion and knowledge (Bhakti and Jnana). Both can be equally effective. The problem with knowledge-based approaches is that they easily become dry, conceptual or abstract, an encounter with emptiness, space or formlessness that can leave us ungrounded or unconnected. For knowledge-based approaches to be really effective, they require the background and support of devotion, whether to the deity, the guru or the higher Self within.

The beauty of devotion is that it takes our basic desire nature, our wanting to be loved – which is our biggest problem and greatest obstacle to the spiritual path – and turns it into a seeking of undying love. It uses form to take us beyond form to a pure all pervading love, beauty and delight.

The danger of devotion is that we can confuse personal emotions, including attachment to God or guru, with real devotion, and become bound to the names and forms of our devotional practices. To counter this we must not lose sight of the supreme beloved which is the inmost Self of all, not simply the deity of one religious tradition or another. We must ally devotion with a seeking to know God, not simply a worship of God on the outside. Blind devotion is not Yoga, nor can it take us to the supreme. Yogic devotion is linked to a deeper perception and realization.

The direct experience of the Divine and the eternal in all spiritual traditions is associated with bliss, grace, peace, contentment and delight – with we could calle Soma. Various spiritual traditions from the most primitive nature worship to the most sophisticated non-dualist philosophies recognize Soma or bliss in various forms, within and around us.

Surrender and Soma

We usually seek happiness in trying to gain things in life. However, a greater happiness can be found in letting things go. The main approach of Bhakti Yoga is surrender, what is called *Ishvara pranidhana* or 'surrender to God' in the *Yoga Sutras*, mentioned among the niyamas, though it also exists as an independent practice in the text.[124] Ishvara pranidhana is said to be the best means of entering into the state of samadhi, which means it is the best means of developing Soma or bliss.[125]

Yet this inward surrender is difficult, particularly today when we feel we must all be assertive in order to succeed in our competitive world. Most of us can surrender to an external influence, authority or even to a lover. But to surrender to the Divine within ourselves is difficult even to conceive. For this to occur, we must learn to surrender our personal will in life, which is to let go of our need to dominate, achieve or acquire and to accept instead the nature of reality, letting Divine grace guide us moment by moment without our resistance. This means letting go of our ego's need to be in control and let our inner consciousness come to the front. It means to accept the bliss and beneficence that is the true reality, and let go of all pettiness of thought and emotion within us that wants things to go our way.

It is only when we surrender that the inner Soma can really flow. We cannot make the Soma flow and the Soma will not flow for us based upon our desire, expectation or demand. But the Soma will flow and is always flowing if we accept the Divine grace that allows all things in the universe to function. It is Soma alone that allows all things to live and move. We are all seeking that Soma but must learn the laws of Soma or the *Soma Dharma*, which is the happiness of being in harmony with all.

Mantra and Chanting of Divine Names

The chanting of Divine names is probably the main practice for enabling the nectar of devotion flow in the heart. It draws our attention away from our ordinary preoccupations with other people and personal relationships to the Divine essence within all. The rejuvenating power of the Divine Name is well known to all mantric teachings. One can use whatever set of Divine names resonates most with one's own heart.

The 'nectar of chanting' is another term we encounter in yogic literature. Chanting, particularly in a musical form, opens the flow of grace through the vocal cords into our entire nervous system as well as into our Prana as a whole. Chanting may include Divine names but with bija mantras or with longer verses. This includes what is known as *kirtan*, which is a vocalized call and response chanting of a musical nature.

Inner and Outer Rituals

In order to access our inner Soma, we need to create the proper field or environment for it to manifest, which is a sacred space and sacred time. Rituals are ways of bringing the sacred into our lives and of expressing devotion in a formal manner. Yet for a ritual to enliven us it must be performed with attention, devotion and grace. Hindu pujas are important revitalizing rituals that express the Soma or nectar of devotion. They use flowers, fragrances, ghee lamps and incense to sanctify our environment and create a sacred space for divine energies to descend into our environment.

Rituals are usually done relative to a representational image like a statue or image. Special stones like Shiva lingas, or geometrical forms like yantras, can be used in the same manner. Bathing the linga or sacred stone with water, milk or other liquid substances is an important means of bringing more Soma into our environment. This process is called 'abhisheka'.

Most Hindu rituals include *Kalasha Puja* or worship of a pot of water, usually made of copper, which is decorated with mango leaves, a coconut and various mystic designs.[126] This also has a profound Soma symbolism. Soma is the water pot or pot of nectar. All Hindu rituals end with a distribution of *prasad* or food, generally sweets or sweet liquids. Prasad is another form of Soma and is meant to help awaken the flow of Soma in our minds and hearts. Indeed, the giving of prasad may well have developed from ancient Soma rituals.

Soma has a cleansing affect like water, in which case it is called *Pavamana* or the 'purifying flow'. In this regard, sacred bathing, such as is common in Vedic rituals or in Hindu rituals like bathing in the Ganga, is another important type of Soma ritual, which can be combined with Soma mantras for greater efficacy.

Inner rituals are Yoga practices in which the offerings are done within through visualization, without any actual substances being used, so they can be more elaborate. Yoga practices visualizing the flow of Soma from the head to the heart and throughout the entire being bring renewal to all that we do. Visualizing an inner *abhisheka* or pouring the Soma over the entire chakra system is a way of helping the Soma flow within.

FIVE FACTORS OF PUJA

Offering	Element	Sense Quality
Fragrant oil	Earth	Smell
Sweet liquid food	Water	Taste
Ghee lamp or candle	Fire	Sight
Incense	Air	Touch
Flower	Space	Hearing

In Vedic times there was a special *Soma Yajna* or Soma sacrifice. Soma was said to be the highest Vedic offering, given to all the deities to energize them, but particularly to Indra as the Supreme Lord or Vedic form of Shiva.[127] We must learn to ritually offer our Soma or the essence of our being to the Divine for transformation. Whatever we offer to the Divine within the heart becomes our Soma.

Deity Forms and Immortality

There are many Soma, love and bliss conceptions of the deity, in both male and female forms, and in naturalistic depictions, as well as relative to various attitudes to the Divine father and mother. The Yoga of Devotion has an entire set of practices involving rituals, chanting, worship and meditation.

The Divine, after all, is the immortal and eternal that we seek. There is a sense of Soma, bliss, delight, peace or grace in all sincere approaches to the Divine at an experiential level. This inner flow of grace produces great inspiration, poetry, music, and symbol. This flow of devotional grace is behind scripture, with its praise of the deity. It is there in great spiritual art, sculpture and painting as well.

The Yoga tradition has many forms that symbolize how to connect with the immortal essence or Being-Consciousness-Bliss, which is the universal reality beyond death and sorrow. Yet one can use whatever form or approach takes one in this direction. The form is a means of focusing the attention, not an end in itself. There are many options, as it is the way of the inner heart!

Importance of the Goddess, Shakti or Divine Mother

The mother represents the caring aspect of Divine energy. The father, on the other hand, represents more the purifying side. So the worship of the Divine Mother or Shakti is perhaps the most important devotional approach towards rejuvenation. The Goddess as the feminine form also represents beauty, delight and bliss, the Soma aspect.

There are many forms of the Mother Goddess in every traditional culture, particularly in all native and pagan traditions. She works through the Madonna or Mary in Christianity and Tara or Kwan Yin in Buddhism. The Mother is probably the prime form of devotion for everyone as she is the source of all. Worshipping the Great Universal Mother is our natural religion. The religion of nature, in which we feel the sacred presence all around us in our natural environment, is the basis of her worship. She seeks to emerge in whatever way she can through various religions, philosophies or artistic paths that honor the Divine Feminine. Whatever names or forms may be used or traditions developed honoring the feminine nature, it is really only Her in the end that is the real power of devotion and inspiration, encompassing and transcending all appearances.

The Goddess has a great diversity of forms and functions in the Hindu Yoga tradition in which she is honored as the great World Mother, who creates, preserves and destroys the universe, and is also the guiding power behind the development and evolution of the soul. She is *Sarasvati* as creative inspiration, *Lakshmi* as sustaining devotion, and *Kali* as transforming energy. She is *Durga* who protects and *Rajarajeshvari*, the Queen of the Universe. She is Mother Nature or Prakriti but also the Supreme Shakti of the Absolute beyond all manifestation. Every male deity has his feminine counterpart or consort. There are many ways to access the grace of the Goddess through ritual, pilgrimage, mantra and meditation, along with special sadhanas or practices of many types.

Soma forms of the Goddess reach their epitome in *Tripura Sundari*, the 'Beauty of the Three Worlds', who represents the flow of Soma from the thousand petal lotus of the head.[128] Her fivefold mantra: *Hrīm Śrīm Klīm Aim Sauḥ!* develops the Soma in the crown chakra and allows it to flow and fill the ocean of the spiritual heart. Her fifteenfold or *Panchadashi* mantra is yet more powerful.[129] She also has a very important Gayatri mantra of her own.[130] The Tantric cult of Soma is closely connected to her worship and part of a Shakti rasayana or rejuvenation through Shakti.

Forms of Shiva, the Conqueror of Death

Shiva is the great lord of immortality in Yoga. He is able to drink the poison of mortality and not be harmed by it. In this regard he is called *Nilakantha*, the 'blue throated deity', as he holds the poison at the level of the throat, meaning he does not allow it to enter into his heart.

Shiva as *Rudra* is the Divine doctor, the foremost of all physicians in the *Rigveda*.[131] Yet Shiva's energy is twofold as Agni and Soma. His Agni or fire aspect purifies. His Soma side heals and rejuvenates. Shiva is also the Vedic deity of healing touch and bringing the power of healing into one's hands.[132]

Shiva has a special form as *Mrityunjaya* or he who conquers death. This occurs through his connection to Soma. Like Soma, Shiva is connected to the Moon and worshipped on Mondays. For this is the famous Shiva Mrityunjaya Mantra. Shiva as the lord of bliss and Soma is also called *Sundareshvara*, the lord of beauty, and *Kameshvara*, the lord of love. Shiva is pure light of the Absolute (Prakasha), the essence of Om or sound vibration (Pranava), the great or immortal Prana and as the Primal Purusha or inner Self of all.

Shiva as the power behind all mantras has a tremendous healing power in his mantras, even in his very names. The rejuvenating power of Shiva is reflected more in his softer mantras, not so much in his harsher (Rudra and Bhairava forms).

Om Namaḥ Śivāya!
This simple five-syllable mantra calms the mind and heart and brings peace into the core of our being. Though it seems very simple, do not underestimate its power.

Śivo'ham
"I am Shiva", simple mantric affirmation of our identity with the supreme Shiva, can be used like *So'ham* along with the breath.

Om Haum Jūm Sah
This mantra awakens the immortal Prana (*Haum*), directs it with force and speed (*Jūm*) and holds it deep within our being (*Sah*). It is probably the best mantra for reviving a person, warding off death and stimulating rejuvenation within.

Mrityunjaya mantra

This is the longer *Tryambakam* mantra to Shiva. I have discussed it in my other books.[133]

The Rudram

The Rudram is a long chant to Shiva from the *Yajurveda*.

Dhanvantari

Dhanvantari is the Vedic deity governing healing and Ayurveda. He is a form of Vishnu, the Divine in the role of preserving and maintaining the universe. Dhanvantari holds all healing powers as the ideal or divine doctor. He arises from the churning of the cosmic ocean as a great gift to living beings. He carries both the powers of detoxification and rejuvenation. Rejuvenation is symbolized by the pot of immortal nectar (amrita kalasha) that he carries in one of his hands.

Whereas Shiva represents the supreme Prana and the power of healing touch, Dhanvantari represents the power of intelligence and compassion. There are a number of verses to Dhanvantari that are very good or the simple name mantra:

Om Dham Dhanvantaraye Namaḥ

Krishna

Krishna is the deity of Divine love, devotion, bliss and Soma. He is associated with the Moon and performs his dance of love at night. Krishna is a deity of beauty and bliss, much like Sundari among the Goddess, with whom he shares various mantras. Chants to Krishna enable the nectar of devotion, the Soma of Divine love, to flow within us. Curiously, Krishna is also famous for longevity as he was said to have lived 125 years.

Om Klīm Kṛṣṇāya Namaḥ

Hanuman and Rama

Hanuman is the son of the Wind God, the cosmic Vayu, and has the power of the immortal Prana. He has the immortal and indestructible diamond or vajra body. He is the great Yogi who can perform any asana, do any pranayama and who has all siddhis or magical powers through the power of his own devotion. Hanuman carries the higher energies of nature, represented by his ability to find and protect Sita, Rama's wife, who is also an Earth Goddess. Hanuman is one of the great long-lived sages in the Hindu tradition and so can grant longevity to his devotees, provided that they spend their time in service and devotion.

Om Haum Hanumate Namaḥ

The name of Rama itself is said to be a great rasayana. Repeating simply *Rāma Rāma Rāma Rāma* or *Om Rām* (initial 'a' pronounced long as in father) is one of the best ways of developing the power of devotion, particularly as allied with a higher spiritual aspiration and knowledge.

The Ashwins

The Ashwins are the divine twins, the miracle children, who carry all powers of healing, rejuvenation and going beyond death. They are portrayed as horseean, with the horse as a symbol of prana. They hold the secret knowledge of Soma in the *Vedas*. To them belongs the important *Madhu Vidya*, the knowledge of the honey-bliss that gives immortality even to the Gods and is the basis of many Upanishadic teachings.[134] There are several dozen hymns to them in the *Rigveda*. The Ashwins are also among the Divine progenitors of Ayurvedic knowledge as well and their constellation marks the rejuvenative powers at the beginning of the zodiac.

The Sun

As the source of prana, the Sun is a powerful source of healing and transformative energy. Mantras to the Sun, like the *Gayatri mantra* or *Aditya Hridaya Stotra*, are used as rejuvenative and revival practices for the heart as well as the mind,[135] though they can be over stimulating for the body or the feminine nature. The solar Soma complements the lunar Soma and should remain based upon it.

Serpents and Eagles

Soma is protected by the serpents or Nagas, which represent subtle pranic forces in which field the Soma is held in potential. The eagle, hawk or falcon (Shyena), on the other hand, is the bird of the Soma, who swoops down and can take the Soma away. One needs the blessings of both the serpent deities and the heavenly birds to gain the Soma. The Hamsa is not just a swan or bird of the Moon but also the Sun Bird that can take the Soma and draw it upwards. This requires a higher perception as well as a greater pranic force of aspiration and devotion.

SOMA

Soma is a Vedic deity that governs rejuvenation, longevity and immortality. Soma is honored in many forms from forces of nature like the Sun and Moon, to the sweetness derived from foods, herbs or honey. Soma is connected to mountains, rivers and to the ocean. Soma is sometimes regarded as a youth, other times as the father of all. He is lauded along with his sisters, who aid in his extraction and development.

Repeating Soma verses from the *Rigveda* can awaken that Soma power within us.[136] Even listing to the chanting of the ninth mandala of the *Rigveda* can aid in one's flow of Soma.[137] Learning to chant some of these mantras is yet stronger. Vedic Soma chants help develop the Soma within us and enable it to flow. Best is to learn a few of these verses, though even listening to these chants can help. They cool and calm the mind and nervous system and help develop samadhi or the state of yogic absorption. There is a simple Soma mantra that one can do.[138]

Om Īm Śrīm Somāya Namaḥ

The bija mantra *Īm* (pronounced eem) is also the seed sound of the eyes. It brings our awareness to the focused point of perception, the bindu through which the Soma of the mind can flow. *Śrīm* opens the lotus of the head or Soma, which is also the expanse of awareness. Soma connects us with the inner Soma to which we give our reverence.

Soma Gayatri

The Gayatri mantra to *Savitri*, the solar Godhead, is the most popular Gayatri and most important Vedic mantra, but Gayatris also exist for other deities. The Soma Gayatri is particularly important for healing purposes, including for preparing rejuvenative herbs and foods. It is included below along with a translation, though it is best to repeat that in the Sanskrit.[139]

Om Sudhākarāya vidmahe oshadhīshāya dhīmahi; Tan nah Soma pracodayāt!

May we know the creator of the nectar, may we meditate upon the lord of the healing plants. May Soma direct that towards us!

Deities and Pranayama

Deities are not merely powers of devotion; they also represent powers of knowledge and prana. As such, they are part of deeper Yoga practices of pranayama, mantra and meditation. This is particularly true of the *Dasha Mahavidya* or 'Ten Knowledge Forms of the Goddess'.[140]

We have already noted how Sundari, one of these ten great Goddesses, represents the Soma of the thousand-petal lotus of the head. Another, *Bhuvaneshvari*, who rules over cosmic space, grants us the Soma from the different directions. *Matangi*, who is green in color and holds both prana and Soma, helps us understand all the Somas of the healing plants, animals and other forces of nature.

Yet even fierce *Kali*, sometimes regarded as a Goddess of death or destruction, represents the kevala kumbhaka, the inner prana that flows through retention of the breath, as a power of immortality, and Yoni mudra, the closing off of the sensory openings in the head, to allow the prana to flow through the Sushumna. *Chinnamasta*, with her strange form as having cut off her own head, represents Shambhavi mudra, focusing the gaze within even while the eyes are open externally. *Bagalamukhi*, another strange form of the Goddess who grants control of speech, also helps us develop Khechari mudra, granting control of the tongue. Many other such examples could be given but these are matters of deeper and more detailed practices. Energizing yogic practices with the power of the deity grants a greater efficacy to all of them, particularly pranayama and mantra.

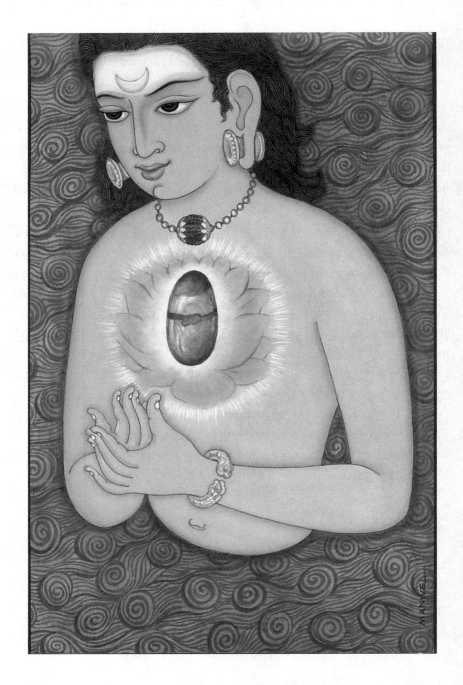

The Shiva or Soma Linga in the Spiritual Heart

MEDITATION, THE YOGA OF KNOWLEDGE AND REJUVENATION OF THE MIND

He made the Dawns into beautiful wives and placed the light within the Sun. Soma found the threefold immortal nectar hidden in the three luminous realms of Heaven.

He spread Heaven and Earth apart and yoked the chariot that has seven rays. By his secret power he placed the ripe milk within the souls; Soma upholds a fountain that has ten yantras (designs).

Rigveda VI.44.23-24

Most of us are unable to extract the Somas from our own minds. We are busy looking for Soma or happiness on the outside where it must always elude us. If we can learn this art of imbibing our own inner Soma, we will go beyond the need for any form of stimulation or entertainment. Yet we will also learn how to discover a lasting beauty and bliss beyond all that comes before our eyes.

Rejuvenation of the mind is the essence of the practice of meditation, which itself is a rasayana for the mind. 'Meditation therapy' is probably the most important of all healing therapies because it can remove suffering and ignorance completely from the whole of our lives. In fact, without meditation, all other wellness therapies are likely to be limited in their success. Only meditation provides us with the attention and clarity of mind to fully implement all other healing strategies.

To keep your mind young and healthy, it is best to meditate at least fifteen minutes in the morning and at least an hour in the evening. You can begin with whatever methods or approaches help prepare the meditative state, particularly mantra and pranayama. But always make sure to end your practice with meditative calm and silence, resting in the natural happiness and healing power of your own nature as pure consciousness, the Self of all.

Rejuvenation of the mind is most connected to *Jnana Yoga*, the

'Yoga of Knowledge' among the Yoga paths. This Yoga of knowledge is the path of *Advaita* or 'Non-dualistic Vedanta', such as taught in ancient times in the *Upanishads,* by later teachers like Shankara, and by modern teachers like Ramana Maharshi.[141] The Yoga of knowledge teaches us the way of inquiry, insight and meditative stillness to arrive at a direct perception of our true nature that is one with the universal being. Yet deep meditation leading to absorption or samadhi, the inner flow of Soma, is the pinnacle and essence of all Yoga practices.

Rejuvenation of the mind through meditation, by accessing the immortal powers of consciousness is the highest rejuvenation practice. Rejuvenation of the mind is possible without rejuvenation of the body, focusing on spiritual development alone. However, rejuvenation of the mind is usually made easier if we rejuvenate the body as well, because toxins and debility in the body naturally take their toll on the mind. Certain foods, herbs, exercises, and breathing practices can bring about major changes in how we think and feel. Working with subtle sensory energies can help in a major way as well as clarity of mind and senses always goes together.

However, the most important changes to revitalize the mind occur on the level of the mind itself, particularly in our deep-seated mental patterns down to a subconscious and instinctual level. We cannot rejuvenate the mind merely through reading books, listening to CDs or taking a few seminars, however helpful these may be. Rejuvenation of the mind requires major changes in our beliefs, attitudes, and values, including changing how we see ourselves and how we look at the world. It cannot be done mechanically or by another person but requires our own inner practices performed with regularity and consistency. The main practice for rejuvenation of the mind is meditation, not as the practice of a meditation technique, but as resting in the natural meditative stillness of the calm mind turned within to the sacred nature of all reality.

The Aging Effects of Memory

Just as excess weight and toxins at a physical level cause the body to age, decay and become susceptible to disease, in the same way accumulated weight and toxins at a psychological level make the mind old, heavy, and disturbed. Our mental and emotional overweight and toxicity, as it were, can be measured by the burden of memory, trauma and unfulfilled desires that causes our mental energy to decline.

We can easily weigh our bodies on a scale and see how much excess weight we carry for our height, sex and age. Similarly, we can easily determine the weight of our psychological burdens by the inertia, compulsiveness and shadows of our memories. Just as we need to reduce toxins and excess weight from the body, so too, we need to reduce the entropy of memory from the mind and heart. This does not mean that we should try to forget everything or lose our sense of facts and information. It means that we must let go of the burden of emotional memory, our personal history of guilt, regret and expectation.

This is not a matter of complex psychological analysis but of a simple understanding how the mind works. We are weighed down psychologically in life by the mind's burden of the known and the familiar. The shadow born of our habitual way of looking at life removes us from the newness and magic of existence and gets us caught in routine, compulsion, habit and addiction. Our mind's become old in the sense of becoming caught up in their past, looking through old and conditioned perspectives and responses. We can compare this old mind with the mind of a child, just as we can compare the old and the youthful bodies. The child experiences everything as if for the first time, living in the present moment with a certain innocence, curiosity and joy. The old mind experiences life through the veil of the past, seeking to repeat the glory of the past or rectify its sorrow.

We think we know ourselves and know the world in which we live. The fact is that we are only familiar with life at a superficial level. If we look deeply, we can find ever new and more beautiful potentials within ourselves, in others and in the world of nature around us. But to recognize these, we must first give up the arrogance that we truly know and instead embrace the vastness of the unknown that our minds can never circumscribe, that is beyond all thought, formulas, beliefs or expectations.

Rejuvenation of the mind requires first of all letting go of the past, which ties us to the energy of death. It means surrendering our opinions, likes and dislikes, and mental judgments in life. It requires being able to observe rather than to react, to be receptive to reality rather than proudly holding to what we think we know as real.

One need not totally forget one's past, of course, but one needs to let go of the mind's holding on to past experiences, ideas, emotions, attachments and traumas, which occupy it throughout most of the day and night. In fact, a good factual memory is only possible when the mind is not burdened by its emotional memories. Part of senility is not only forgetting things, but also living in the past and not seeing the present.

Actually every day is a new life for all of us and every night is a new opportunity to go beyond time. We can freely let go of our personal memories, our records of likes and dislikes, flattery and insult, success and failure, without losing who we really are. In fact, if we hold to these dualistic emotions, we only taint the purity of our inner being that is beyond limitation.

Our true being is not the self of our memories, which is but the shadow of the past, it is our capacity to see in the present with an open mind and heart. We cannot remember our true being, except by acknowledging its abidance in the present moment. Our true being resides in the light of consciousness beyond time and space. It is not our ego or self-image which is the weight of other peoples' ideas about us, but the imageless light of seeing within us.

We can rejuvenate our minds and hearts at any moment we are willing to let go of the past. Yet not only is it hard to let go of our positive experiences in life, we often find it more difficult to let go of our negative experiences. Many of us cling to our sorrow, oppression, unhappiness and even disease as a means gaining attention or importance for ourselves. In the modern world, in which we have made psychology so important, many of us are caught up in our personal psychodramas and try to draw everyone else into their net. We don't want to let our emotions go, but use them to get others drawn into our reactions. Psychodrama is a toxic reaction of the old mind, which is the mind not able to digest its experiences in life and move on. Without letting go of our psychodrama and embracing our inner being, our mind will remain trapped in its compulsions and fixations born of time.

Letting go of the past means dying to who we were, so that a new being can be reborn within us. We are ever new. We never die. We never enter into the past but remain behind the present as the power of all time. The past is our shadow self which turns our life into a shadow. We are not our past, which is but our shadow. We are the being who experienced the past but can experience life in a new way at every moment.

Beyond Information to a Direct Experience of Life

A related problem that causes our minds to age is the weight of information that we carry. We are caught up in names, numbers, personalities, packages, poses and external appearances. The result is that the mind becomes worn out by the burden of information. We no longer see the world directly but impose our ideas upon. Such factual based data is memory of a less emotional nature, but still a kind of matter, density or compulsion in the mind.

Rejuvenation occurs by attuning the mind to the nameless, the unknown, what is beyond quantification. It does not occur by any additional calculations, mechanical routines, names or numbers. We need to take a quantum leap, as it were, from the realm of quantity into that of the sacred that is beyond all measurement. This affords the mind the unbounded space in which it can be renewed and transformed.

What renews the mind is direct experience in the present, which has no limitations. Once we introduce name and measurement, we fall out of that direct experience into something quantifiable. The universe is a magical realm of mysteries in which the new, the immeasurable, the dynamic, the unpredictable and the eternal prevail. The problem is that we confuse our sense of the familiar with a true knowledge of the world and of ourselves.

Information is not direct knowledge. It does not reveal the nature of reality to us or serve to increase our own direct contact with reality. It is an indirect knowledge about things in terms of names, forms and numbers, which are but surface measurements. Such mediated knowledge can inhibit direct perception or substitute for it. To rejuvenate the mind we must give up our attachment to information and our belief that our information is true knowledge. Then we can once more directly live our own lives, seeing things as they are, rather than judging them according to a mental pattern, starting with our own thoughts and our own breath. This requires not only living in the present moment but also living in the presence of the light of awareness.

Rejuvenating the mind requires developing the higher mind, moving from an information based outer awareness to a perception based inner mind or true intelligence. When we awaken that intelligence within, we see everything as a sacred dance, feeling the light of consciousness pervading all things. Names and forms appear as but symbols or veils of a greater nameless and formless all-pervasive presence.

Restructuring our Perceptual Patterns

We have learned to structure our perception into meaningful patterns since we first opened our eyes to the world as a child and contacted its shifting chaos of forms, colors, sounds and movements. We learned to identify objects, people and actions, as well as how to function in the world ourselves. The result is that in our adult years, we automatically and often uncritically look at the world through the grid of our minds condition. These mental grids not only include objective factors of name, number, size, shape and distance, necessary for us to maneuver in the world around us, but also subjective factors of like and dislike, attraction and repulsion, fear and desire towards various objects that prevent us from seeing things as they are.

Our minds carry a certain pattern of perception reflecting how we have learned to interpret our experience through our education and conditioning, as well as our own inclinations. This way we look at the world could perhaps more rightly be called 'a pattern of misperception' as it usually reflects various personal and social biases, not merely a direct or view of reality. Over time our perception gets further covered over by the increasing weight of memory and habitual actions. We get so used to people and places, for example, that we may stop seeing them at all. This hardening of our perceptual apparatus results in a rigid, heavy or confused pattern of reactions that causes the mind to age and to become rigid.

Even such apparently objective factors as size or distance represent how our perception is structured, not necessarily the nature of reality. In a Japanese garden, for example, one learns to see the large in the small, like beauty of a small bonsai tree. We must remember that size and distance are relative. A tree is not the same size for an ant as for a person. The distance to the next city is very different if you are walking rather than driving. Time and space are fluid constructs of our perception and can be altered, lengthened or shortened by the nature of our attitudes and actions. Meditation seeks to liberate the mind from these limiting perceptual patterns, as the English poet William Blake so eloquently stated:

To see a world in a grain of sand, and a heaven in a wild flower,

Hold infinity in the palm of your hand, and eternity in an hour.[142]

There are special techniques of meditative gazing (Dharana in Yoga), in which we learn to look at things directly, giving up the interpretative filters of the mind and memory. This liberation of our perception from the sense of size opens us up to the magic of existence and the great beauty that is hidden everywhere.

To rejuvenate the body, senses and mind, we must clear and rejuvenate our perception. This requires learning to go beyond our mind's patterns of both practical information and emotional responses. We learn to see the light of consciousness behind the forms of the world, including behind space itself. This helps us let go of our limiting concepts about who we are and discover new ways of action that can improve our lives on all levels.

Developing our Higher Memory

Soma or our sense of happiness is strongly connected to our power of memory. The lower Somas create a memory that attaches us to past enjoyments. The higher Somas create a memory or recognition of eternal bliss that is the very ground of our being. Developing our power of memory (*Smriti shakti* in Sanskrit) is an important aid not only to meditation but also for longevity and rejuvenation of the mind. This higher memory is not the lower psychological memory or ego memory that causes the mind to become heavy or to age. This higher memory does allow us to factually remember the events of our lives, particularly experiences in which we have touched Soma, true love, beauty, creativity, inspiration, devotion or spirituality.

Yet more than this, our higher memory power is able to remember our deeper soul and Self and its immortal journey in consciousness from life to life. Sometimes it may involve memories from past lives, but more often it involves remembering the Divine powers and essences that pervade the universe. Mantra and meditation are important ways to develop this higher memory in which we can remember the eternal. To remember our eternal essence and home is to be able to transcend time and its limitations.

Creativity, Creation and Production

Soma can be defined as a flow of pure creative energy in the mind. That is why the Soma bearing mind so easily lends itself to mantra, poetry and art, and to all true genius and invention. All true creativity, starting with the creation of the universe through the forces of nature, is a manifestation of Soma or bliss. Yet at the highest level, Soma is pure creativity without expression. This is the Absolute or formless Brahman beyond time, space and manifestation. The highest art seems as simple as nature. The highest creativity does not need to express itself at all. Even if it does express itself, its reality is far greater than any of its expressions.

In the modern world and in western culture in general we value production, creating something that others can see and use. Sometimes it seems that we value production more than creation with all our artificially mass produced items that reflect little true creativity. Soma is not a product or a production. Soma can be expressed but its reality is always more than its expression.

To taste the inner Soma through meditation one must dive into the stream of pure creativity that is allied with silence - a dynamic current so strong that it does not create any form and develops a deep stillness in its steady flow. In meditation, we should learn to enter into the stream of creation, starting with the creative forces of nature, but moving into the unmanifest creativity of pure consciousness, which holds all potential energies in a singularity, without needing to say anything.

Cooling and Slowing Down the Mind

The mind ages as a result of overstimulation, which overheats it and causes it to burn up its Soma or power of peace, contentment, and delight. What overly stimulates the mind is too fast or powerful sensory impulses, such as our modern media abounds in. We speed up the mind through external stimulation through the senses and the media. In fact, the media is one of the main things that cause our minds to age, to get caught up in a net of memories, reactions, opinions and aggression, which also means to become heavy and emotionally toxic.

To counter overstimulation we need to cool down the mind, which is to detach it from its external fixations. Cooling down the mind also requires slowing it down. This does not mean that we should become slow minded, but should make the mind steady, attentive and aware, in a non-reactive state of passive observation. Such a state easily occurs when we align ourselves in the rhythms of nature. Disengaging the mind from media influences, particularly the visual media, is a great aid in its rejuvenation.

Yet as we slow down the outer mind, we learn to speed up the inner mind, which is to increase the flow of light and perception in the mind, including unfolding new creative powers. We no longer need to seek any stimulation or entertainment outwardly because our own current of awareness itself is a continual movement of transformation and delight.

Meditative stillness, however, is not an enforced stillness, lack of movement or blankness. It is not based upon resistance, an attempt to control, or trying to achieve a preconceived goal. It does not require an overt personal effort to stop thinking or suppress one's thoughts. Meditative stillness means moving to a deeper level of awareness, like diving deep within the sea, in which the surface waves, though they may continue to rise and fall, cannot disturb us or cause us to lose our composure. Thoughts like the breath come and go, but one no longer identifies with them, viewing them like passing clouds in the sky, not anything real or lasting.

Silence and stillness rejuvenates the mind, while activity and distraction wears it away. The foundation of any real Yoga sadhana is establishing a deep silence and peace in one's mind and heart as the basis of all else. This requires a surrender of our outer being to the inner Divine presence that is everywhere.

The meditative mind is the mountain lake in which Soma plants naturally grow. When the mind becomes still like a placid lake then Soma plants will spontaneously arise within it. These are astral growths, inner lotuses and flowers. The seven chakras or lotuses are such Soma plants and each reveals its own characteristic Soma essence.

Bringing Space into the Mind

To rejuvenate your mind you must first create space in the mind. Then the rejuvenating energy or Shakti will arise of its own accord. It does not require any other effort or action. The mind needs space in order to rejuvenate itself. This is not an empty space arising from boredom, frustration or loneliness. It is the space of clear awareness, not caught in any reactions of like and dislike, love and hate, attraction and repulsion. Soma can also be described as a 'flower of space'. Whenever we create space within, such flowers of light naturally arise within it.

The mind that is burdened by time, place, person and desire cannot experience space. The mind that is filled with memories, opinions, beliefs and preconceptions remains caught in their limited boundaries. To experience the space of pure awareness the mind must empty itself out, letting go of its attachments, fixations and assertions.

One way to create space in the mind is to go outdoors and embrace the space in nature, to deeply look at the clouds, the sky, the stars, the space of the mountains, the forests, the plains or the ocean – whatever natural space is available to your vision. Another way is to look at the space between objects rather than the objects themselves, seeing objects as but designs in space. Ultimately one needs to dive deep within and discover the mystic space within the heart, the space of consciousness that is subtler than the mind itself. In that small space within the heart, the entire universe dwells, along with all time and space, all creatures and all worlds. Learn to be aware of the boundlessness of space as the reality, not the forms or creatures that happen to move within it.

The Power of Solitude

The mind is best renewed in solitude, in a state of deep aloneness where one can commune both with the whole of nature and with one's inner Self beyond time and space. The mind needs solitude in order to heal itself. But this is not a state of loneliness, a feeling of lack, emptiness, isolation, or alienation. It is placing the mind in direct contact with one's inner being in which one needs nothing from the external world, in which the entire world can be forgotten and merged into a greater reality.

Such deep solitude is necessary for rejuvenation and immortality. There is no en masse way of entering the doorway into eternity. It is not a social event, class, party or political rally! Each soul must take that journey alone, letting go of all things and all associations along the way, ultimately surrendering one's own body, mind and human identity.

Old age is often associated with loneliness, in which we are removed from the vitalizing contact of other people. This loneliness occurs because we have not learned to access our inner aloneness that links us with all things. We cover over this inner isolation by keeping our minds distracted by people and events. This only causes us to avoid our inevitable contact with our own emptiness. Instead, we should learn the benefits of solitude, which allows us to connect to life at a deeper level, and loneliness will never be a problem for us. In fact, we are never truly alone because consciousness is everywhere if one knows how to look! Soma or bliss is not about being around other people but about finding our true Self both in the animate and inanimate realms.

The Positive Attitude of Eternity

Life is never perfect, which would mean to be fixed and final. Life is a work in process with birth and death, creation and destruction, formation and disintegration going on simultaneously all the time. Nature

303

itself shows us not only the beauty of the flower but that of the falling leaf as well. The outer world always presents challenges and difficulties for us to constantly deal with. These often increase with age as we have more health, work, family or social problems to attend to, which is why worry increases with age. However, the inner world and its stream of immortality is always open to those who sincerely seek it – and all of nature reflects it. If we let the world become greater than ourselves and defeat us with its obstacles and sorrows, we can have no real peace and happiness. We must learn to accept every outer challenge as a means of inner growth, and then nothing can ever defeat us

We need to cultivate a positive attitude in life. This does not mean affirming that all our personal desires will be fulfilled, which is not possible or even helpful. It means affirming that consciousness, bliss and immortality is the true nature of all – that nothing of any true value can be lost whatever we or anyone else may do or attempt to do. Only what is negative can be negated or lost. That which is positive, full of beauty, love and truth will always endure. Our work of healing or our Yoga practice should be conducted like cultivating a garden, not like fighting a war. It should arise from an inner contentment and inspiration not ambition or desperation. It should be part of embracing life as a whole, not trying to avoid what calls us into question.

We must keep ourselves light and full of light at a mental and emotional level. This means not to accumulate heaviness in the mind. Meditation requires a certain lightness of being. An ancient Vedantic text says that we should "Look at the world like a magic show lasting only a few days."[143] We should take neither the world nor ourselves too seriously. Humor is important because it is part of the positive attitude we need for meditation. This is not a superficial humor born of ridiculing others but a sense of Divine joy that our sufferings are but a play.

We are all immortal beings and in our essence we never die. Our body is but a garb we wear for a time. We can learn to make it last longer but if we need to, we can also feel free to move on to a new and better vesture if it better serves our karma. We should not turn the pursuit of longevity or rejuvenation into a burden on our souls. The outer world in any case is but a dream. We need not become desperate about gaining any outer goals or happiness, even a long life. We should live our lives with contentment, thankfulness and grace, knowing that a higher will and blessing exists behind everywhere. There may not be perfection in the outer world, but it always remains in the inner world of the spiritual heart.

The Practice of Meditation

There are many methods of meditation taught in various spiritual traditions. All are but expedient methods of entering into an abiding in the meditative state that is the natural equipoise of consciousness itself.

First, it is necessary to prepare the mind for meditation with the right life-style. Meditation is not simply something special that we do at a certain time, but the fruit of all else that we are engaged in during the day. It requires following dharmic principles and practices in our life as a whole (yamas and niyamas) and benefits from such support practices as asana (sustaining a sitting pose), pranayama (deepening and calming the breath), pratyahara (turning the senses within) and mantra (focusing speech and thought), as well as having self-control and an observant mind during our daily activities.

Soma Dharana, Concentration on Soma

Dharana, the yogic practice of concentration, is often left out of modern approaches to meditation. People are asked to be still, to be aware, to observe or to witness, though they usually lack the power of attention or concentration to accomplish it. The mind's power or Shakti is its power of attention, just as that of the muscles is the ability to lift weights, we could say. To cultivate concentration is not just a matter of effort or will-power, it means developing a higher motivation in life, a will to know the truth, which alone can enable us to sustain an enduring power of attention.

The stronger our power of attention, the greater is our capacity to rejuvenate the mind. The power of attention itself can rejuvenate the mind. The power of attention is the mind's ability to revitalize both itself and the senses. A key to physical and mental longevity is to have a strong power of attention, to be in control of your own power of attention by rooting it in a greater spiritual aspiration and the regular practice of meditation. Most of what we call entertainment is a giving over of our mind's power of attention to the external world. It promotes entropy and causes the mind to deteriorate or prevents it from developing in the first place. Dharana or cultivation of attention is the foundation for meditation.

Soma in Vedic thought is an essence that comes forth from a certain pressure or concentration. The more we are able to concentrate the mind, the more its essence of delight can come forth. Yet concentration also distills that essence of delight and makes it fuller and stronger. We must learn to continually press out and concentrate the Soma of the mind through yogic concentration and meditation.

Dhara in Sanskrit also means 'flow'. The 'flow of Soma' or *Soma Dhara* is also the steady flow of attention or concentration in the mind, *Soma Dharana*. The mind naturally gives its attention to whatever provides it happiness. We are always concentrating or refining our Soma or pursuit of happiness. Yogic concentration is about developing our inner Soma or inner happiness. True yogic concentration or Dharana is letting our Soma or inner inspiration of the mind flow freely, which is back to its source within our own deeper awareness. What we are concentrating on in Dharana should be our own Soma, which is our inner search for the Divine and eternal.

The secret of meditation is that if we let our Soma flow, we can find happiness directly in that flow itself. We need not look for Soma on the outside. That free flow of Soma will become strong, steady and full, leading us into deep meditation and samadhi. We must cultivate a flow of Soma to the Cosmic Being, which is the flow of Soma of the Cosmic Being itself.

Prana Dharana

Prana Dharana means sustaining a focus on the life-force through a continual awareness of the breath. Perhaps the simplest way to do this is to hold one's gaze and attention at the navel, and to draw the breath from there.

Another way is just to maintain awareness of the breath throughout the day. Whatever else is going on during the day, strive to continually redirect your awareness back to the breath. Then you will not lose your focus or become disturbed by anything. Our power of prana and power of attention are linked together. When our prana is deep and full our attention is more likely to be complete and sustained as well. By this practice we can hold the Soma of our Prana within us.

Dharana of the Five Elements and Five Chakras

In this practice, one focuses one's gaze and attention at the sites and energies of the chakras in order to stabilize their energies.[144] It can be accompanied by using the seed mantras for the chakras, which can be repeated along with the breath. Additionally, one can meditate upon the qualities of the elements in the respective chakras or their respective deities, particularly their respective Somas.

1. Hold to the calm grounding energy of the Earth element, the Soma of the root chakra – *Om Lam Som Somāya Namaḥ*

2. Hold to the fluid invigorating energy of the Water element, the Soma of the sex chakra. – *Om Vam Som Somāya Namaḥ*

3. Hold to the radiant illuminating energy of the Fire element, the Soma of the navel chakra. – *Om Ram Som Somāya Namaḥ*

4. Hold to the dynamic, transformative energy of the Air element, the Soma of the heart chakra. – *Om Yam Som Somāya Namaḥ*

5. Hold to the still, receptive energy of the Ether element, the Soma of the throat chakra. – *Om Ham Som Somāya Namaḥ*

6. Hold to the perceptive and probing energy of the cosmic Mind, the Soma of the third eye. – *Om Kṣam Som Somāya Namaḥ*

7. Hold to the infinite, unmanifest energy of Pure Consciousness and Bliss, the Soma the crown chakra. – *Om Om Som Somāya Namaḥ*

Shambhavi Mudra

It is important never to place your center of awareness or attention outside yourself, but to hold it within. *Shambhavi Mudra* is the practice of holding one's awareness within even while looking or acting externally.[145] It is related to the practice of *Bhairavi Mudra* in Kashmiri Shaivism. Its foundation practice is to hold the gaze within, while keeping the eyes open and not blinking. Its expanded practice includes holding one's point of awareness at certain places in the body like the heart, third eye, top of the head or navel. It can be performed during meditation, as a kind of dharana or concentration or *Drishti Yoga* or 'Yoga of Seeing'. Yet it can also be performed while acting throughout the day to sustain our spiritual focus in life.

Shambhavi Mudra can be combined with Khechari Mudra (holding the tongue at the roof of the mouth), which maintains the upward movement of our senses. This makes its practice yet stronger.

- Holding the awareness at the top of the head connects us with the higher light and unbounded awareness.

- Holding the awareness at the third eye sustains our higher judgment, discrimination and insight.

- Holding the awareness at the navel gives us greater Prana and Agni, vitality and digestive power and also helps arouse the Kundalini.

- Holding the awareness in the heart connects us with the source of Divine love.

- Holding the awareness at the soft palate of the mouth grants control of the mind, senses, detachment and inner delight.

Soma Dhyana or Soma Meditation

Most forms of meditation serve to develop Soma, which can also be described as the energy of silence, peace and contentment that true meditation must unfold. True meditation consists of accessing the mind's natural flow of meditative well-being, which is its natural Soma. Meditation is the unfoldment of our inner Soma, like a lotus in the lake of the mind. We must learn to dwell upon the Soma of the mind, which is its deeper core of stillness and contentment, and let go of its poison, which is its addiction to the outer world and its conflicts. Being itself is Soma or bliss; no action is required to create it and no action can bring it about. Dwelling in the presence of Pure Being, which is all pervasive, the Soma or Ananda of Brahman is the highest form of meditation.

- The first stage of Soma Dhyana is to allow the mind to flow like a river. One learns to follow the current and let go of the thoughts that arise within it.

- The second stage is to let the mind become still like a mountain lake, not through overt effort but through the full release and freedom of the mind's flow.

- The third stage is for the mind to be like a mirror, still and fully reflective of the reality. One merges into the ocean of consciousness-bliss.

Soma meditation requires developing a receptive awareness beyond the reactivity of the mind. We must learn to observe and to contemplate, rather than to react and judge. We must bring a greater space and time into the mind. Our minds must become like a placid lake or Soma vessel. We should learn to let our mind's reflect reality like the Moon, rather than project their conditioning upon it. For this we must bring the mind and heart into alignment, uniting the deepest feeling, knowing and seeing.

Meditation on the Spiritual Heart: Self-Inquiry

Perhaps the simplest and most direct method of meditation is to merge the mind into the heart, which is to dive deep within to one's inner home or heavenly origin before birth and beyond death. This is the main Soma approach or approach to immortality followed in Jnana Yoga, the Yoga of Knowledge. It can be stimulated by asking the question, "Who am I?" – seeking not just our personal or psychological self but the essence of our being and consciousness which is universal.

This process is called 'Self-inquiry' or *Atma-vichara* and goes back to the *Upanishads*,[146] the prime scriptures behind the Yoga tradition.[147] Its main modern teacher is the great sage Ramana Maharshi, who emphasized this path in all of his writings and transcribed talks.[148]

Other primary questions of life can be brought into the inquiry such as: "Why am I alive? What is the purpose of my existence?" "From what has this world arisen? How has it come into being?" "What is the eternal truth behind this transient world?" "What was I before I was born and what will I become after I die?" The inquiry can be aided by repeating the bija mantra *Hrīm*, which is the seed sound of the spiritual heart and source of awareness. We can also inquire through the breath, tracing back the root of our life-force in the spiritual heart. In short, it is not a mental inquiry but an inquiry, search and prayer with our entire being, life and consciousness.

The fact is that we do not know who we really are. We are lost in the outer world where we constantly have to deny our inner being, happiness and freedom for our ego identity and self-image. Similarly, we do not really know what the world truly is. What we call the world is but a shifting set of appearances, shadows of a greater reality that we judge wrongly. Once we take up this inner search, our outer desire based seeking begins to fall away. We begin to discover the happiness and bliss of our own nature, which is the nature of all.

For Self-inquiry, we must learn to use our thinking process in a positive way to root out wrong ideas about reality. We do not just try to stop the mind directly, but rather trace it back to its origin in our deepest aspirations. We can begin this practice with deep study, especially of Vedantic texts that teach this approach.[149] We continue with deep thought of our own, questioning our mental processes down to the subconscious mind. We then can move into a steady deep meditation on the ultimate questions of life.

Our normal thought pattern based upon the ego is mechanical, reactive and rooted in the past, a kind of half daydreaming mentality. We need to replace it with a current of thought that is creative, observant and based upon the present. This is the awakening of our higher intelligence and perception, which we can then use to connect with our deeper Self.

We must learn to question our every thought, why it is there, where it arises from, and what are its consequences. Most of us in life are breeding illusion with our thoughts. We are mulling over and digging deeper into our minds with thoughts of desire, fear, anger, worry or hatred that cloud our perception and create a wrong motivation within us. This mechanical stream of thoughts causes the mind to age and the heart to become heavy. Its concern is with the transient and the mortal, not the eternal and the immortal and so increases our own transience as well. It is a kind of pathology, as it were, breeding conflict, disease and sorrow through our emotions.

Conscious inquiry is a means of countering this inertia of thought, which will take us into a deeper silence as these questions gradually become resolved. To begin to question oneself at a deep level is also to awaken a transformative energy that can renew the mind, freeing us of the past and its limitations. Without this churning of inner inquiry or vichara, it is difficult to really awaken the higher mind or clear out the karmic patterns in the subconscious mind. It is essential to getting the mind's inner Soma to flow.

We must question the very nature and origin of happiness. We wrongly ascribe the source of our happiness to the various external people, objects or circumstances that seem to make us feel happy (though sometimes the same things cause us sorrow). The truth is that actual happiness arises from within. These external factors only serve to trigger our internal happiness mechanism, the flow of Soma in the mind and heart. If we can allow this Soma to flow directly through Yoga and meditation, then we can go beyond sorrow.

After all, whatever is dear to us is only so because we are there. Without our own presence, all that we hold dear has no meaning. Our self is what is most dear to all of us. In this regard there is an important Upanishadic teaching, which the great sage Yajnavalkya gave to his own wife Maitreyi:[150] "It is not for the sake of the husband that the husband is dear but for the sake of the Self. It is not for the sake of the wife that the wife is dear but for the sake of the self. It is not for the sake of all that all are dear but for the sake of the Self."

The Self is the dearest of all objects because it is the source of happiness. The question is "What is that Self?" because it is something more than the body and mind which are its instruments of experience. We all find happiness even in the state of deep sleep in which there are no external experiences or even movements of the mind. Deep sleep reflects the happiness that is inherent in our own nature, in consciousness itself. We must learn to go back to that original Ananda through deep meditation. Then we will discover that bliss is the nature of all. We can find bliss in all things as we find that all beings dwell within us:

He who sees the Self in all beings and all beings in the Self cannot be disturbed.

In the knower in whom the Self has become all beings, where can there be any delusion or any sorrow, for one who sees only unity?

Isha Upanishad 6-7.

While Soma reflects the crown chakra as its place of overflow in the subtle body, its origin, support and goal resides in the ocean of consciousness-bliss in the spiritual heart, which can also be regarded as the core of the crown chakra. This Soma of the heart has a magnetic quality to draw all things towards it. Besides the Sushumna that rises from the root to the crown chakras is another channel called the Amrita nadi, which consolidates the cool Soma energy in the head and draws it back to the spiritual heart. This is the current one follows in the return to the spiritual heart. We need to return to that ocean of the heart, which is the ocean of Soma.[151] *The entire universe dwells within your own nature, in the heart, in the ocean, in all life. May we realize that wave of bliss!*

Rigveda IV.58.11

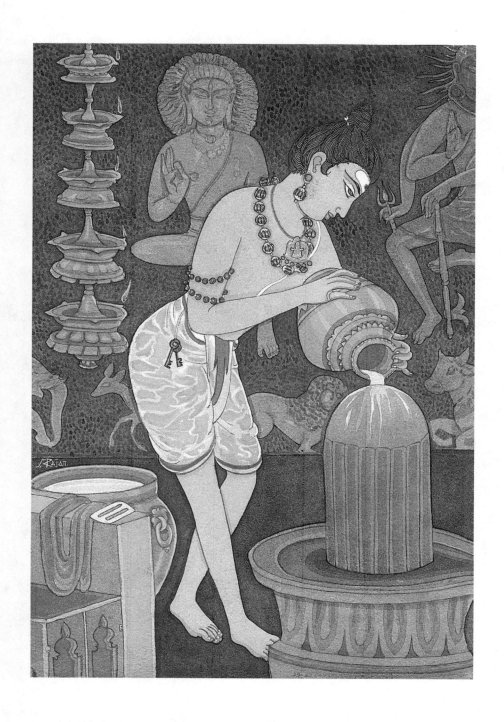

Abhisheka or Water pouring over the Shiva Linga

PART IV

Esoteric Soma Teachings

The golden one, moving on the path of truth, energizes his voice, like an oar a ship. Divine, he reveals the secret names of the Gods, to declare them on the sacred grass.

Rigveda IX.95.2

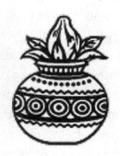

Vedic Astrology and Longevity: The Influence of Time and Karma

Soma as a light form in the outer world is represented by the Moon. The Moon is the Soma vessel that the Gods fill up during the waxing Moon, and then drink during the waning Moon. Vedic astrology gives tremendous importance to the Moon and has several special ways of measuring its influence, particularly through the Vedic calendar or Panchanga that uses lunar months. Through the Moon in the birth chart of a person we can read the nature of the mind and our happiness potential in life.

The factors of rejuvenation in the chart are also closely related to the Moon and to Soma, but pervade the entire chart. Soma and rejuvenation is not limited to the Moon but reflects all the planetary influences. In Vedic thought, there is an honoring of the Soma of the Sun or the forces of bliss, water and nourishment that come to us through the Sun. Each planet has its own Soma or power of delight. This is more obvious in the inner planets, those near the Sun, like Mercury and Venus, which like the Moon wax and wane or increase and decrease in light as they are moving away from or towards the Sun. But even the outer planets, those outside the Earth's orbit like Mars, Jupiter and Saturn, have their variations in light and are brightest, like the Moon, when opposite the Sun. Oppositions of these planets from the Sun are the best time to access their Soma.

Vedic astrology provides us with a wonderful system for understanding our karmas in life and their likely unfoldment through the course of time. Our birth chart shows the overall karmic potential that we are born with, which is reflected through the placement of planets in signs and houses, and the aspects and yogas (planetary combinations) that occur between them. The timing of our karmas is revealed through the dashas (planetary periods), transits (current movements of the planets relative to positions in the birth chart), and the annual chart or solar return.

Health and well-being is an important factor in the chart and is determined by the overall placements of planets within it. It is closely connected with vitality, as a strong vitality usually translates into good longevity. However, sometimes people live long but are not healthy. Other times healthy people may die prematurely from accidents, in battle, from calamities, or from contagious diseases, though their body is otherwise healthy. Yet while the issue of longevity has its complexity, a good astrologer can see ones health potential in life, the times at which our health may be in danger, including favorable times and periods for rejuvenation and other healing therapies.

Certain planets and their combinations tend to cause disease, injury and death as the negative rays they cast upon us can be disruptive to our life energy. Other planets and their combinations promote health, safety and longevity as their rays are healing and strengthening. Yet Vedic astrology teaches us that as we age, all the planets become stronger in their disease causing potentials and even good planets begin to cause us harm in our later years. This is part of the entropy inherent in the movement of time.

One may ask: "Why should we bother trying to prolong our lives, if the planets have the last say and our longevity is likely to be written in our birth chart?" In this regard, we should recognize that we can work with the influences of the planets to improve or transcend our karmas, or at least to project better karmas for future lives. Karma is a set of probabilities that we have set in motion and can be modified. We should not turn ourselves into victims of our karmas but rather learn to master them.

It is quite possible to extend one's longevity or to develop one's spirituality through special methods of propitiating the planets. In fact, working with planetary energies is one of the best ways to help us move beyond the limitations of time and karma. Our ignorance of planetary influences and resultant failure to adjust to them causes us a great deal of unnecessary suffering in life. We can compare this with the negative effects of not adjusting to the weather, for example, like not dressing up properly to deal with the cold of winter. No one looks at seasonal changes as a destiny that one must passively accept, but as environmental variations that require adaptation. The same is true of planetary influences. The difference is that while we can easily perceive and adjust to outer environmental changes, inner astrological forces are difficult for us to perceive and require special guidance in order to recognize them and adjust to their shifting influences. In addition, the planets wield cosmic forces that we can connect to in order to take our awareness to a higher plane of existence, if we can learn how to direct their energies with skill and wisdom.

Vedic astrology provides us with a number of tools to optimize our karma, including those for helping us live longer and wiser. Even if one has indications of a short life in the chart, it is possible to extend it. There are certain critical times astrologically, during which our health may be threatened. If we are careful and know how to protect ourselves during these difficult periods, we can continue on to safer periods in which our health may not be a problem.

Planets and Longevity

Certain planets cause disease or accidents and the onset of their periods tends to make these happen. The *Ascendant* or rising sign and its lord is the main factor in our physical well-being and outer happiness in life. Its strength must be examined first. The Moon governs our psychology and our emotional happiness and must be considered as well. If these are unafflicted then our well-being is likely to be steady through life.

Saturn is the main planet that governs Ayus or longevity, along with the eighth house, called the house of longevity (Ayur Bhava) and its lord. These factors must be considered as well. Generally, Saturn will promote disease and aging, unless we know how to work with its influence. Propitiation of Saturn is probably the key astrological factor for health and longevity.

Jupiter, on the other hand, is the planet that indicates life, positive health and the capacity for rejuvenation. It reflects the grace and vitality of the soul, the life principle at the core of our being. Jupiter also shows the influence of the guru or spiritual guidance in our lives, including the help of teachers, doctors and counselors. Honoring Jupiter is important for achieving our positive goals in life, including overall health and well-being.

Generally speaking, benefic planets, those that have soft, nurturing or expansive energies – which are the Moon, Jupiter, Venus and Mercury – promote life, longevity and rejuvenation. Malefic planets, those which hold harsh, depleting or contracting energies – which are the Sun, Saturn, Mars, Rahu and Ketu – promote decay, injury or disease.

Rahu and Ketu, the two lunar nodes that cause eclipses of the Sun and Moon, symbolically represent the two halves of the serpent who wrongly gained immortality. They represent the immortality that exists in the dualistic world, which is covered by death and rebirth. Going beyond the negative influence of Rahu and Ketu, which requires uniting their two rulers in the birth chart, is another important consideration in all higher spiritual development. Rahu, in particular, represents the outer Soma forces or power of Maya that can mislead us. Reuniting the influences of Rahu and Ketu in the chart, on the other hand, helps us regain our natural immortality.

Benefic planets protect our health, particularly if in the birth chart they are located in angular houses (houses one, four, seven and ten) or trines (houses five and nine), or if aspecting or conjunct the Ascendant and its lord. Meanwhile malefics located in these houses or influencing the Ascendant and its lord tend to weaken the health and longevity of a person. Yet malefic planets located in houses three, six and eleven usually protect the health and longevity of a person.[152]

The sixth house governs disease, the eighth house is that of death, and the twelfth house is that of loss. These are the three difficult houses or *duhsthanas*, particularly where benefic planets like the Moon suffer and cause health problems, if they are located in them. Yet even malefics can suffer in these houses.

However, the effects of all planets is altered by the houses in the birth chart that they rule over. The lords of the sixth, eighth and twelfth houses (the planets ruling the signs that mark these houses from the Ascendant) in particular are disease causing influences. The lords of the second and seventh house can cause disease or death, if the chart is otherwise weak or the person old in age.

There are several rules that Vedic astrology examines in this regard, of which those above are only a few key principles. Best is to have your chart done by a Vedic astrologer with insight and experience in the field of Ayurveda or medical astrology. A good Vedic astrologer can tell if your planetary periods are favorable for longevity, rejuvenation or spirituality, and how you can best propitiate their negative energies, when these exist. [153]

Gems, Protecting the Life and Longevity

Gems are probably the simplest astrological method, though an expensive means, to help promote the life and longevity of the person. Most important are the gemstones for benefic planets like Jupiter, Venus, Mercury and the Moon, the ascendant lord and the lord of the benefic ninth house and fifth house. These help bring in positive and life-giving energies into the chart.

Jupiter	Yellow sapphire, yellow topaz	Protects immunity, strengthens Ojas, aids in rejuvenation
Mercury	Emerald, aquamarine	Increases power of prana, protects nervous system, keeps the mind youthful
Venus	Diamond, clear sapphire	Strengthens sexual vitality and Ojas
Moon	Pearl	Calms mind and heart, protects bodily fluids, particularly good for women

Besides wearing the gem, the bhasma (Ayurvedically prepared ash) or tincture of the gem can be taken internally for similar rejuvenative effects. We have already mentioned pearl ash or moti/mukta bhasma for this effect, as the pearl is the gem of the Moon. Diamond ash (hira bhasma) is also very powerful, but such preparations can be very expensive as well.

Gemstones for malefic planets like the Sun, Mars, Saturn, Rahu and Ketu are only helpful for health and longevity if they rule good houses, are afflicted in the chart and do not themselves significantly afflict other benefic planets. If they rule the Ascendant for your chart they can be considered, but they should be used with caution, particularly blue sapphire and ruby. One should consult a good astrologer before wearing them, particularly gems for Saturn.

Sun	Ruby	Protects heart, digestive system, gives self-confidence
Mars	Red coral	Improves blood, muscles, liver, vital strength
Saturn	Blue sapphire	Strengthens bones, nerves, improves longevity, gives emotional calm
Rahu	Hessonite garnet	Improves physical and psychological immunity, counters poisons
Ketu	Chrysoberyl cat's eye	Improves immunity, counters infections, improves perception

Planetary Mantras and Rejuvenation

Our own efforts are usually more effective for improving our karma than simply using some outer aid like a gemstone. One cannot simply remove negative karma by putting on an expensive gem, if there is no change of attitude or life-style that goes along with it. Even for the gem to really work requires some empowerment through mantra. Below are listed some important planetary mantras that can aid in the rejuvenation of body and mind. Many others exist.[154]

• Mantra for the Moon – *Om Som Somāya Namaḥ*

Strengthens the influence of the Moon, particularly at an inner level. As the Moon is Soma, this is probably the best planetary rasayana mantra.

• Mantra for Jupiter – *Om Bṛm Bṛhaspataye Namaḥ*

Strengthens the influence of the planet Jupiter and increases Ojas. Promotes positive growth and expansion in life.

- Mantra for Venus – *Om Śūm Śūkrāya Namaḥ*

Strengthens the influence of the planet Venus, the reproductive system (shukra) and Ojas.

- Mantra for Mercury – *Om Bum Budhāya Namaḥ*

Promotes youthfulness and rejuvenation of the mind and intellect.

The gems and mantras of natural malefic planets like the Sun, Mars, Saturn, Rahu and Ketu can also be used at times, particularly when these planets govern the Ascendant. Saturn is most important as the indicator of longevity. The Sun helps bring a higher Prana into our lies.

- Mantra for Saturn – *Om Śam Śaṇaye Namaḥ*

Protects our longevity and immunity and brings peace of mind.

- Mantra for the Sun – *Om Sūm Sūryāya Namaḥ*

Helps bring the cosmic prana into our energy field, reviving the heart, senses and power of perception.

27 Nakshatras or Lunar Mansions

Besides the twelve signs of the zodiac, which follow largely a solar symbolism, Vedic astrology employs a zodiac of twenty-seven constellations or lunar mansions called *Nakshatras*. They mirror the movement of the Moon, which takes about twenty-seven days to go around the entire zodiac. Actions are best performed at a time in which the Moon is in a favorable Nakshatra.

Each of these twenty-seven Nakshatras, a bit like Sun signs, represents different soul or personality types and provides us a key as to our inner or spiritual nature.[155] They are very important in Vedic astrology, particularly relative to the unfoldment of our karma during the course of our lives.[156]

15 Tithis and 16 Kalās of the Moon

Vedic astrology divides the lunar month into two phases of the waxing and waning Moon. Each of these two phases is further divided up into fifteen phases called 'tithis' in Sanskrit, making thirty in total. During each of these fifteen phases, the Moon moves twelve degrees

322

relative to the Sun.

Besides the fifteen tithis, the Moon possesses an additional inner aspect that neither waxes nor wanes, which allows the Moon to wax again after having become new. These sixteen aspects of the Moon are called 'kalās', which literally meaning sixteenths. The sixteenth Kalā that neither waxes nor wanes is the immortal or amrita Kalā. Each of these Kalaas represents energies that one can access. For rejuvenation and immortality one should imbibe the energies of the immortal sixteenth kalā or portion of the moon. These sixteen kalās also exist inside of us. The essence of our own mind is its immortal portion or kalā. The aspects of the mind involved with the sense organs, motor organs and sense objects, of which there are five each, reflect the fifteen mortal factors or kalās.

To reach that immortal essence of the Mind like that of the Moon requires going beyond all waxing and waning, all the dualities of thought and emotion, to the unitary immortal essence. It is one of the main goals of inner Yoga practices.

Astrological Timing of Longevity Practices through the Moon

Healing practices work best if timed with consideration to the position and condition of the planets, particularly the Moon that is the lord of plants and healing energies. Rejuvenation practices are best performed, or at least started, during the waxing Moon, while the waning Moon is better for purification. Our bodily fluids increase during the waxing Moon and dry out as the Moon wanes.[157] Of the fifteen tithis or lunar phases, the best are the tenth and eleventh of the waxing moon (dashami, ekadashi). The mind's virtue is strongest at these times.

The signs and constellations that the Moon is located in also make a difference. Rejuvenative practices do best if commenced during an auspicious *Nakshatra* or lunar constellation. Among the best are Ashwini (00 – 13 20 Aries), Rohini (10 00 – 23 00 Taurus), Mrigashira (23 20 Taurus – 06 40 Gemini), Punarvasu (20 00 Gemini – 03 20 Cancer), Pushya (03 20 – 16 40 Cancer), Uttara Phalguni (26 40 Leo – 10 00 Virgo), Hasta (10 00 - 23 20 Virgo), Chitra (23 20 Virgo – 06 40 Libra),

Uttarashadha (26 40 Sagittarius – 10 00 Capricorn), Shravana (10 00 – 23 20 Capricorn), Dhanishta (23 20 Capricorn – 06 40 Aquarius) and Uttara Bhadra (03 20 – 16 40 Pisces). Note that these are the positions of Vedic astrology, not western tropical astrology.[158]

- Ashwini Nakshatra, which marks the beginning of the zodiac in Aries, rules over revitalizing Prana. It relates to the Ashwins, the twin horseman, who are the original teachers of Ayurvedic medicine and the healers of the Gods who hold the secret knowledge of Soma.

- Rohini Nakshatra, said to be the favorite of the Moon and also the Nakshatra of Lord Krishna, is also very good for Soma, beauty and delight.

- Mrigashira Nakshatra, which includes the Orion nebula where many stars are born, rules over Soma and is connected to Lord Shiva. It is the doorway beyond death to immortality in the sky.

- Pushya Nakshatra ruled by Brihaspati, the priest of the Gods, where the planet Jupiter is exalted, is said to be good for all rituals and healing practices.

- Shravana Nakshatra, ruled by Vishnu, is very good as Vishnu governs over the highest light and wisdom.

The sixteen kalaas and the twenty seven Nakshatras make the total of forty three, which is the number of triangles in the Sri Yantra, the Yantra of the subtle body and the thousand petal lotus or crown chakra, the domain of Soma. This mystic side of the Moon should not be forgotten.

Vastu, Directional Influences and Rejuvenation

Vastu is the Vedic sciences of directional influences, which is employed primarily in building and architecture. Directional influences affect our health and well-being and are considered relative to rituals. Rejuvenation is connected to the north, northeast and eastern directions, where spiritual, nurturing and watery energies prevail. Meditation while facing these directions is important. Placing one's altar or images of deities and gurus in these directions is particularly helpful.

DIRECTIONAL DEITIES AND COSMIC PRINCIPLES

NW	N	NE
Vayu - Air	*Soma* - Mind	*Ishana* - Ether
W	C	E
Varuna -Water		*Indra* - Earth
SW	S	SE
Nirriti - Intelligence	*Yama* - Ego	*Agni* -Fire

North specifically is the direction of Soma from which rejuvenative influences can flow into the mind and heart. The northeast in particular is the direction of positive health, well-being, Ojas and divine guidance. The center also has a supportive and nurturing energy. The east relates to prana and light, new birth and growth. Southeast and South directions have energies of fire and purification.

Meanwhile the influences of the northwest, west and southwest tend to be inimical to health as they promote airy (Vata disturbing) forces. The northwest in particular is the direction of disease and Vata dosha overall. One should particularly avoid sleeping in the northwest, which tends to promote the energy of disease and decay. By honoring the influences of the directions, we can bring positive forces into our lives and avoid the negative.[159] There are also Vedic mantras, rituals and yantras for this purpose.

THE SEARCH FOR THE
ORIGINAL SOMA PLANT

There has been a long search for the identity of the original Soma plant and several plants have been proposed as representing it. The view we will propose here is that Soma was never simply a single plant, though there may have been one primary Soma plant for certain times and locations. Soma referred to several plants, sometimes a plant mixture or preparation, and more generally to the sacred usage of plants overall, to the extent that it is a plant metaphor. Beyond its botanical side, Soma referred to an entire cosmic duality of Agni and Soma forces from the Sun and Moon to fire and water and all aspects of life.

Vedic Soma is mentioned as existing in all plants and many different types of Soma are indicated, some requiring elaborate procedures and preparations.[160] Water itself, particularly that of the Himalayan rivers like the Ganga, is said to be a kind of Soma.[161] In Vedic thought, for every form of Agni or Fire, there is a corresponding form of Soma as water, fuel or food. In this regard, there are Somas throughout the universe. There is quite a bit of mythology about Soma in Vedic, Ayurvedic and yogic thought. This, however, is not because the nature of the original Soma plant was forgotten but because Soma was always part of an extensive mystical view of the universe. The same mysticism pervades the Vedic view of Agni or fire or the Sun.

The great ancient Ayurvedic doctor, Sushrut, mentions twenty four types of Soma plants found in the mountain ranges of India, with the majority growing on Himalayan lakes and many named after Vedic meters. Soma, therefore, was part of an entire science of sacred plants and not just one plant in particular.

"The one and the same Divine Soma plant may be classified into twenty-four species according to the difference of their habitats, structures, epithets, and potencies. They are as follows: Amshumat, Munjavat, Chandramah, Rajataprabha, Durvasoma, Kaniyan, Svetaksha, Kanakaprabha, Pratanavan, Talavrinta, Karavira, Amshavan, Svayamprabha, Mahasoma, Garudahrita, Gayatrya, Traishtubha, Pankta, Jagata, Shankara, Agnishtoma, Raivata, Yathokta, and Udupati. All these kinds of Somas secure for the user a mastery of the Vedic chant and are known by the above auspicious names mentioned in the *Vedas*."[162]

"In the Himalayas, Arbudas, Sahyas, Mahendras, Malayas, Sriparvatas, Devagiris, Giris, Devasahas, Pariyatras, Vindhyas, Devasundas and Hladas are the inhabitants of the Soma plants. Somas of the best kind, the Chandramah species, are often found to be floating here and there on the mighty stream of the river Sindhu), which flows down at the foot of five large mountains beyond the north bank of the Vitasta. The Munjavat and the Amshumat species may also be found in the same region, while those known as the Gayatri, Traishtubha, Pankta, Jagata, Shankara, and others looking as beautiful as the Moon are found to float on the surface of the divine lake known as the little Manasa in Kashmir."[163]

Soma is said to grow in all the different mountain ranges of India, north and south. Soma is a plant of all the mountain ranges of India but specifically the higher ones, the Himalayas. The Chandramah (lunar) Soma, called the best Soma, appears to come from the upper Indus region, in the direction of Ladakh and Leh, as Vitasta is the ancient name for the main river of Kashmir. The greatest diversity of Somas, however, comes from Kashmir and its famous Manasa Lake.

In other verses in the *Rigveda*, there is an association of Sushoma, Arjika, and Sharyanavat [164] as lands of the Soma, though Somas can be found everywhere. The lands of the Soma are described:

Which Somas are in the superior region, which are in the inferior region, or which are in Sharyanavat, which are in the well-made Arjikas, which are in the middle of the Pastyas (home regions), or which are among the five peoples. [165]

Sharyanavat is said by the medieval commentator Sayana to be a lake in the Sarasvati region near Kurukshetra, reflecting a statement in certain *Brahmana* texts.[166] The implication of all these statements is that there were many types of Somas in many different regions around India and among all its different peoples.

Modern Proposed Soma Plants – Ephedra and Amanita

Some modern scholars emphasize the plant ephedra as the main Soma plant and connect it with Afghanistan and Iran, where ephedra is common, though ephedra is also not uncommon in India. They note that ephedra was the main Soma plant of the Persians, which they called 'Haoma'. Ephedra commonly grows in different places in India even today, and is sometimes even called Somalata or 'Soma creeper'. Yet that only means that ephedra is one of the Soma like plants, particularly those of a stimulating rather than nutritive nature, but does not prove that ephedra was the only Soma plant, nor does ephedra resemble the characteristics of the primary Soma plants described in the *Rigveda*.

Soma is part of a vast watery and oceanic symbolism of Soma in the *Rigveda*. The *Rigveda* describes Soma as growing near water[167] and as flowing with a milky juice gained by crushing the plant. Ephedra, on the other hand, is a dry plant with very little juice.

Other scholars propose that the original Soma was the Amanita muscari mushroom, which is used by many shamans, particularly in Siberia. While I cannot say for certain that this mushroom was not one of many kinds of Soma, the Vedic Somas are described in different ways and mushrooms are rarely used medicinally in traditional Ayurvedic medicine or known to be a common food of Yogis or of Indians overall. On the contrary, mushrooms are usually not recommended for pure yogic diets. The Vedic Soma plant is described with leaves, which mushrooms do not have, and said to be fibrous (amshuman), with filaments. It is often said to grow in water like a lotus or lily.

More Specific Possible Ancient Somas

Sharyanavat, probably the main *Rigveda* Soma land,[168] refers to a lake and means 'abounding with reeds', with shara (Saccharum sara) the name a type of reed related to sugarcane. Shara was mainly used to make arrows and was sacred to both Agni and Soma. Another later great Soma land of Munjavat[169] also means 'abounding with reeds' with munja being a type of reed related to the same plant as shara and considered to be the best of the Somas. This again shows Soma growing in marshy or aquatic areas and being some sort of reed grass, perhaps even a type of bamboo, some of which are rejuvenative agents in Ayurvedic medicine.[170]

Some scholars have gone so far as to identify Soma with the sugarcane,[171] another Saccharum species cultivated in ancient India, as after all, sugarcane is sweet like Soma, is fibrous, has a sweet juice that can be pressed out, and is the basis of various beverages, including those that can be intoxicating. Sugarcane was probably used in certain Soma preparations, if not another type of Soma, though I am not certain if it was the prime Vedic Soma. In any case, the main Vedic Somas probably included certain reed grasses, some of which do have significant nervine and nutritive properties.

The *Atharva Veda* specifically mentions five great plants of which Soma is the best, including marijuana, barley and darbha (kusha or munja), showing that many plants had Soma-like qualities.[172] Here Soma is again connected with another type of grass, darbha or kusha, which is an essential component in Vedic rituals down to the present day. Soma is also connected with marijuana, suggesting that mind-altering plants were regarded as different types of Soma.

Soma is sometimes called a tree[173] and is connected with the Ashwattha or sacred fig tree, which also grows in the Himalayan foothills as mentioned in the *Atharva Veda*.[174] The Ashwattha tree, like many fig trees, has a white resinous juice and very strong healing properties that can extend to rejuvenation.[175] Other plants connected with Soma, which was often said to grow on mountain lakes, are the lotus and water lily. Like these plants, Soma is described as having leaves that come out in a circular pattern like the Moon. In this regard, Soma is connected to the lotus of the head or the crown chakra on an inner level.

Additional potential Soma like plants include other members of the orchid and lily families. A number of these plants are nervines. Like Soma, they have milky juices, unusual leaves, and filaments. Their juice can be pressed out between rocks. The Ayurvedic tonic shatavari, a kind of asparagus root, that is commonly used as a rejuvenative agent, particularly for women, is such a lily family plant. Some milkweed family plants, like certain Sarcostemma species, are sometimes regarded as Soma plants, but this seems to be a later interpretation than the Vedic period.

The Mysterious Himalayan Saussurea Plants

The Vedic Soma is mainly described as a mountain plant and connected to the Himalayas. A number of unusual plants grow in high altitudes, particularly above tree line, throughout the world. The difficulties of survival at such high altitudes, dealing with cold, wind and unusual atmospheric conditions has brought about special adaptations in the plants, including an ability to resist the elements and bringing in cosmic energies from the higher altitudes. Such high altitude plants can promote higher awareness and rejuvenation, stimulating our primary vitality and our higher awareness.

The *Vedas* say that the Somas or rejuvenative plants grow particularly near mountain lakes. In the Himalayas, there are many such unusual plants, but perhaps most important are the plants of the Saussurea species. Soma is in other places connected with kushta (Saussurea lappa), a kind of spicy nervine. This is one of the herbs that Soma is said to grow along with, a type of Soma, or perhaps the main Soma itself.[176] This plant also called costus (from the Sanskrit kushta) has entered into herbal pharmacies all over the world. It is noted as a blood purifier and has its value in promoting longevity.

Though Saussureas are part of the sunflower family, they grow in quite unusual shapes for such plants. They have adapted to the above tree line environment in a way that affords them special forms, properties and powers. There are several important exotic plants of the Saussurea species that grow in the high Himalayas often by lakes. They are renowned for their herbal powers and some look like lotuses.

Most famous is the Brahma Kamal (Saussurea obvallata), the lotus of Brahma, which is the state flower of Uttar Khand, one of the Himalayan states of India from which the headwaters of the Ganga and Yamuna rivers arise. The plant looks a bit like candle or a flame coming out of a lotus. It blooms only at night and usually lasts only one night. Like the ancient Soma, it grows in the high mountains often near lakes. Hem Kamal is another Saussurea that looks like a lotus. Clearly these

330

were ancient Soma plants as well. The Snow Lotus (Saussurea invo-lucrata) is another related plant also used in Tibetan medicine. Such Saussurea plants may be the closest to the ancient Soma plants used in the *Vedas*.

Along with these Himalayan Saussureas is the famous sanjivani herb brought by Hanuman back from the Himalayas to revive Rama and Lakshman who had been wounded in battle by Ravana in the story of the *Ramayana*. Sanjivani appears to be a kind of Soma for the mind, stimulating awareness.

The Rare Ashtavarga Rejuvenative Plants

Ashtavarga is a group of eight Soma plants that were the main active ingredients for Chyavan prash in ancient times. The Amalaki fruit was simply the base used for holding their energies. These herbs are said to be cool and moist in nature and to increase Kapha, Ojas and Soma. A number of the rejuvenative herbs we have discussed are likely types of Soma used in Vedic times. Shatavari in particular, which like Soma is a vine with cool and moistening properties falls into this category.

Today this ancient group of eight Soma plants is usually represent-ed by the following plants: 1) Ashwagandha, 2) Shatavari, 3) Vidari Kand, 4) Fritillary, 5) Lily, 6) Bala, 7) Nagbala or Mahabala or Ati-bala, 8) Dioscorea. We have mentioned most of these plants under Ayurvedic rejuvenative herbs. This modern Ashtavarga group clearly contains a number of substitutes and does not claim to represent the original plants.

B.D. Sharma and Acharya Bal Krishan have identified what they be-lieve may be the ancient eight plants of this group. They are predomi-nately sweet in taste, cooling in energy, reduce Vata and Pitta, increase Ojas, strengthen immunity and strengthen the nervous and reproduc-tive systems. They are mainly members of the lily and orchid families, though some ginger family members may also belong.[177]

1. Vridhi – Habenaria acuinta or Habenaria edgeworthii – Orchid family

2. Ridhi – Habenaria intermedia – Orchid family

3. Jeevak – Malaxis acuminate or Microstylis wallichii – Orchid family

4. Rishabhak –Malaxis muscifera or Microstylis muscifera – Orchid family

5. Kakoli – Roscoea alpina or Roscoea procera – Ginger family

6. Kshirakakoli – Lilium polyphyllum – Lily family

7. Meda – Polygonatum verticillatum – Lily family

8. Mahameda – Polygonatum cirrifolium – Lily family

Relatives of these plants grow in the Himalayas and may be effective substitutes. The ancient doctors were not always botanically precise in identifying individual plants and often had to use related plants as substitutes when the primary plants were not available.

Soma Preparations

The Vedic Soma is commonly referred to as a preparation, cleaned, ground, extracted and cooked in various ways and in different mediums. In general, Soma was prepared in three forms, as cooked with grain or barley (yava), milk (go), or curds (dadhi).[178] While some Somas had their fresh juice used, it seems the majority were part of elaborate preparations.

Soma was often used along with ghee (ghrita) and honey (madhu), which are sometimes synonyms for Soma. In fact, Soma is often called madhu (honey or mead) and sweet (svadhu). Special herbal honey preparations and herbal ghee preparations were additional types of Somas. As connected to honey and flowers, Soma is connected to lotuses and other flowering aquatic plants. Soma, however, was discriminated from Sura or wine and alcohol, though fermentation may have been used in preparing some types of Somas.

As a plant extract, Soma can be linked to an entire herbal science, including extractions of heavy oils, aromatic oils and other essences. Soma was even connected to minerals and with the practice of alchemy and as early as the *Rigveda,* it was prepared with gold and possibly lapis lazuli, perhaps even with seashells or pearls.

General Types of Soma Plants

We see, therefore, that there were a number of Soma plants in ancient India. The first group includes several lily and orchid plants like the Ashtavarga group, as well as various lotuses and water lilies. A second group consists of the various Saussurea plants and others growing near tree line. A third group is various grasses and reeds, perhaps extending to sugar cane. A fourth group consists of various nervine stimulants like ephedra and calamus. A fifth group consists of narcotics like cannabis, perhaps even opium. Yet other possible Soma plants are there. More research needs to be done but clearly Somas were a variety of plants and different types existed, with the nutritive and calmative Somas being the majority. On top of all these types of Soma plants are different types of Soma preparations, which also probably involved using a number of Soma herbs. To look for a single Soma plant therefore makes as much sense as to look for one type of fire recognized in Vedic thought.

The Somas in India were mainly special powerful plants growing in mountain lakes and river regions, along with a special art of extracting them. With the shifting of the rivers, this cult appears to have changed or became lost, but reverence for Himalayan plants and rivers remained a characteristic feature of the Hindu religion and the people of India. It is curious to note that along with the drying up and shifting of the waters of the Sarasvati River the Soma cult largely disappeared as well. This may be no mere coincidence.

However, we must remember that the real Soma is a secretion in the brain from spiritual practices of Yoga, pranayama, mantra and meditation. Soma at a yogic level refers to the crown chakra, which is opened by Indra (yogic insight) and releases a flood of bliss throughout the body. This inner Soma is the main subject of the Vedic hymns, though outer Somas did have their place. It is only through the inner Soma that lasting bliss and immortality is gained, not through any mere plant extract.

It is wrong to look for a single Soma plant. Rather, Soma is part of the ancient, yogic and shamanic usage of sacred plants, including tonics, nervines and mind-altering plants of various types as well as special preparations of a number of them used together. Each group, community or geographical region in India probably had its own Somas or sacred plants, as does each ecosystem today. Soma is a transformative substance that can be found in many plants and reflects corresponding mind-altering substances that can be produced by the brain itself. We can never exhaust all such Soma plants, though we can reduce some Soma species to extinction.

What we need to do therefore to solve the mystery of Soma is not to find the original Soma plant botanically but to discover the original nature of Soma inside ourselves, the original yogic Soma, which is the flow of bliss or Ananda within our deeper mind and heart. Once that Soma flows, we will forget about all other plants and all other intoxicants or enjoyments. In your inner being you are the original Soma plant!

Shiva as Nilakantha:
Turning Life's Poison into Soma

Shiva is the great ecstatic deity of Yoga, the supreme Lord of the highest inner energy and transformation. He has the deepest experience of bliss (ananda) as his constant state of being and consciousness. He is the foremost drinker of the Soma, the amrita or mystic nectar that is the delight inherent in all existence. For him everything is bliss or grants bliss. He knows how to extract the Soma everywhere.

Shiva is also *Nilakantha*, the Deva whose throat is blue from being able to drink poison and not be harmed by it. He is not only the foremost drinker of the Soma but also the best drinker of poison. He can drink any poison and survive, in fact flourish from it. There is an important connection between these two aspects of Shiva and several lessons to be drawn from them in our own experience.

Actually everything in life can be poison. Even our most blissful and happy experiences of love, prosperity or vitality as limited by time and death can become a poison to the soul, if we attach ourselves to them. Brooding over the joys of the past can become as painful as going over past sorrows. The end of our success or fulfillment in life itself can cause a greater pain than failure and loss in the first place.

At the same time, everything in life is nectar or Soma. Even our most painful experiences of death, sorrow and parting contain an immortal nectar that we can draw from them. There is in these painful events the rasa (essential feeling) of being able to connect to what transcends this mortal realm, if we look at them as pointing out a greater eternal peace. There is the ecstasy of the witness and of knowing a Divine grace is always with us to save us and take us beyond, if we but take refuge in it during life's difficulties.

Shiva is also the great lord of time (Mahakala). He is Eternity, and he is also the present moment. As the eternal, he extracts the enduring essence from the fleeting dance of time. He holds eternity as he dances through every moment, never losing his equipoise or missing a step.

In dynamic stillness, he holds both being and becoming. He is both the nectar of eternity and the poison of time. Time turns eternity into poison. Eternity turns time into nectar.

Shiva's most famous chant is the *Rudram* from the *Yajurveda*. This long set of ancient, cryptic and melodic Vedic mantras honors Rudra, the fierce form of Lord Shiva, in all the terrible, dangerous and challenging aspects of life like sorrow, pain and conflict, in the snakes and the wild beasts, in the butcher and the thief, in natural calamities, in sickness, separation and death – in all that life can use to take us down.

It is only after one has gone through the trial and tribulation that one can find real peace. It is only after one has taken in the poison and transformed it that one can find the inner nectar. Yet this is not a matter of stoically enduring sorrow, having a stiff upper lip or being thick skinned so as not to be hurt by anything. It is a matter of positive joy in which one rests in the poignancy of all experience, in the delight of being, and the beautiful light of consciousness that pervades everything. Doing this in the happy side of life is one thing. Finding it even in the unhappy side is another. One must be able to feel the pain without becoming pained by it. One must touch happiness in sorrow, delight in pain and love even in rejection.

Life presents us with various rasas (essences) and *bhavas* (feelings and emotions) through which our experiences are colored. It is the rasa and the bhava that matters, not simply the form. The rasa is the nectar hidden in the flower of our experience. Do we imbibe that nectar or simply pick the flower and watch it fade? How we handle our experience is more important than what that experience is in its own right.

Great Tantric teachers like Abhinavagupta have taught us the secret of all the rasas. In this regard, all emotions are rasas. The nine emotional rasas are love, anger, disgust, courage, joy, fright, compassion, wonder and peace. Like a great artist or performer one must come to understand and be able to express all these rasas in their full scope. Then emotion becomes a tool of divine feeling and eternal joy, which raises us up, not a poison that brings us down. These emotions belong to the Divine artist. When we expropriate them at an ego level, they become poisons. We must not be incapable even of negative emotions like anger or fear, but should touch the energy behind them, not contract in the circumstances that create them.

In Tantra, emotion is the main area in which our life energy, our prana or Shakti is held. Suppressing emotion is like suppressing life. It causes death. But expressing raw emotion at an ego level is also destructive and disintegrating. The key is to go to the rasa of the emotion in the dance of Shiva, in which the Shakti will naturally be released.

Of course, the nature of the experience we seek is important. We should seek out the higher rasas or immortal influences in life: the beauty of nature, the sacred energy of temples, the company of spiritually exalted souls, meditating on great teachings or contemplating great works of art. We should not waste our time running after what is vulgar, petty, trivial or superficial. Yet we should not become fixated upon the lesser side of life negatively either by opposing it, by being judgmental, moralistic or hypersensitive. We must look for the higher rasa and pursue it, not worry about the lower rasas, which many will always pursue.

The Importance of Rasa

Today most of our lives in this commercial world contain little of any real rasa in them. They lack the inner juice, vitality or substance as it were. We are caught in a mundane world of personal assertion and acquisition that leaves us overextended, if not exhausted. We have little free time to experience much less enjoy life. We are constantly on the run working, going to and from work, keeping our lives in order, avoiding disease and in our little free time, we pursue pleasure outwardly as a distraction to give us some space from our hectic routines. The rasas that we pursue are either financial or media based, measured in money or social recognition. These rasas do not engage the soul, leave out our real heart and so we end up empty in the end in spite of all the apparent abundance around us.

The most we get is the comfort of good entertainment for which we are usually little more than a passive spectator. We may count our gains in wealth but our time is bleeding away and with it any possibility of a deeper existence drains off as well. We have forgotten to nourish our inner being for which the rasa is the food.

We cannot avoid some poison in life, whatever we do. Even if we pursue the inner life, we have to deal with the poison of negative emotions from family or friends who feel that we are leaving them behind. If we cannot handle this poison, then our spiritual search comes to an end and we fall back into the confines of ordinary emotions, becoming merely puppets of the needs and desires of others. If we endure this negative force, like the devotional poet Mirabai confined in her room for her love of Krishna, we will find that Krishna will come to us wherever we are. But that requires a special courage that few are able to find. It is easier to conform then to chart out new inner worlds.

Yet even if we only pursue the outer life, there is the jealousy and enmity of others that we run into in the business, academic or media worlds; wherever it is that we are stationed. If we try to avoid facing the poison of life, we must hide from everything and the poison will seep in from somewhere anyway.

We have many poisons to contend with in our ordinary life struggles. For this we have doctors, lawyers, accountants, public relation firms, bodyguards or even armies to help us. Yet these only entrench both ourselves and our opposition in the struggle. Often what we thought was nectar turns into poison with failed relationships, failed businesses or friends that become enemies. We end up projecting our own poison on the world as well. We usually find more pleasure and comfort in the pain and failures of others than in their successes. We find more entertainment in destruction than creation, which our modern movies so clearly reflect.

Our entire culture is hurling poison on our environment with a callous insensitivity. This takes many forms as the pollution of the air, water or soils from toxic chemicals of all kinds, as agitated radio waves from our mass media and communication networks crowding the atmosphere, or as the noise, junk, debris and garbage that we mindlessly use to lay waste to nature. Do we really think that this poison will not affect us or that we can achieve the nectar of health or happiness while we are spreading it?

Our bodies are often swimming in poison from the many pharmaceutical or recreational drugs that we take, from our fast food that is devoid of prana, or from the air or noise from the polluted world around us. We pursue detoxification at the level of health, not realizing that this is just the tip of a greater problem.

So we must ask: What is the secret of how to handle the poison and find the nectar? Shiva's throat is blue from having drunk the poison. The poison never reaches his heart. He holds it at the level of the throat. The inner heart or hridaya, the heart of Shiva, the seat of the soul or Atman is ever free of this poison. It is untouched by whatever happens in the realm of time, space and action. Yet it is their essence as well.

This pure awareness is the rasa of rasas. It is the illuminating power of light, the life-giving power of water, the warmth and radiance of fire and the unpredictable impetuous power of the wind. It is the love that embraces life and death, joy and sorrow. It is the prana of prana, the eye of the eye, the mind of the mind as the *Upanishads* say.[179] It is the beauty of the young woman, the strength of the young man, the fearlessness of the lion, the shade of a vast tree, the stability of a high mountain. Whatever rasa or essence that makes anything into the unique object that it is, the pure awareness or Shiva consciousness is the supreme rasa behind all of these.

But unless we reach that center of the heart of Shiva, the poison will affect us. We must learn to hold the poison at the level of the throat and not let it reach the heart. This is to turn the poison to nectar at the level of the throat. The throat is the seat of the buddhi or discriminating mind in yogic thought.

Discriminating the Nectar from the Poison

We must learn to discriminate the nectar from the poison in our experience. Both factors are always there in whatever happens to us. Will we embrace the immortal nectar or the poison of transience? This is the basic choice we have in life, the basic action of our inner intelligence that determines the real value of all that we attempt.

The problem for us is that we think that what is poison is actually nectar. And what is nectar for us is actually poison. When the bearer of the Divine wine cup offers us the ecstatic drink, we turn away from it as poison. Instead, we imbibe our mundane poisons as nectar, going after food that makes us sick, or experiences that land us up in sorrow. We first need discrimination in order to know what is truly nectar and what is truly poison. This requires already having developed a taste for the immortal nectar, which means that our cravings for the mortal nectars, the hidden poisons, has waned. It requires aspiring for something beyond ordinary humanity and our mundane affairs.

Actually nothing is really poison and nothing is really nectar. Whether anything is poison or nectar depends upon how we see and use it. The inner vision in going to the essence pursues the nectar. The outer vision in holding to the form ends up with poison. True discrimination is not a matter of analysis but a change of vision.

Shiva is the mountain God and Soma grows in the high mountains. The mountain in one sense is the meditative mind. The mountain is the mind in its state of stillness that allows the Soma to flow. This is the mind merged into the heart, not the intellectual mind caught up in its own concepts. The state of inner stillness allows the Soma to come forth.

Whatever we respond to with a deep silence and peace must become Soma for us. In Vedic thought, Soma is extracted by being crushed between two rocks. The rock is the mind like a mountain, which is also the philosopher's stone that can transmute base metal into gold, which is another metaphor like turning poison to nectar or darkness into light.

How do we reach that inner heart of Shiva? It is first by embracing death and sorrow. Let the poison put an end to that which must die. Let the poison poison itself as it were. If one becomes the death of death, then there is nothing left over that can die.

This means being able to withdraw from our senses, vital urges and mental impulses into that aspect of our nature which is eternal, into the presence of Shiva within us. However, this is not to deny the senses, emotions or mind. It is to hold to the rasas or essences that they reveal. This using the rasas to withdraw within in is another Tantric secret.

340

It also uses the rasas to expand our awareness to the entire universe around us. It makes Yoga not into a dry asceticism but an alchemical search for cosmic delight.

The real poison is that of the ego itself, the outer self born of desire, time and karma. Whatever the ego becomes fixated on becomes a kind of poison. This ego is not our true Self or real individuality, the real person within us. It is the poisoned or toxic self that reflects the influence of the forces of time and disintegration around us. We must learn to let that ego-self go along with its poisons and hold to the deeper longings of the soul behind its outer actions.

This means that we must learn to accept our share of poisons in life. It is not that life has some special vendetta against us. Enmity, opposition and resistance pervade this world that is built on duality. One cannot be in this world and not encounter such forces. And we must understand that the poison is most likely to come from those close to us, whether those working in the same field who feel competition with us, or our friends and family members with whom we are connected to at personal emotional levels that can easily agitate us. It is not only our enemies, whom we are already cautious with, who can poison us but also our friends that we trust, if that trust is not rooted in a spiritual bond.

Should others be critical and hurl insults against us, why should it matter? We all share the same human weaknesses. There is not one of us who cannot be criticized and who is free of blame. But we should not take these poisons personally. They are part of the rasas of life. Even the venom of a snake has great healing powers if taken in small dosages. Poison can activate Prana and get us to make changes. Yet whatever poison is projected upon us, we must first wish the other person well for it. We must assume the attitude of Shiva, the giver of peace and happiness, when dealing with the negative attitudes of others. We must not embrace the poison or even try to fight against it.

When life's poisons come to us, let us remember Nilakantha, Lord Shiva's ability to turn poison into bliss. Let us remember that whatever poison we do not react to, but rather look for the nectar hidden behind it, becomes neutralized. The ocean can take in even muddy waters

341

without becoming tainted itself. As we learn to discover this Soma essence, we may find that the ordinary actions of life lose their attraction or we may find them to reflect a greater cosmic passion and delight of which they are but a reflection.

It is only the Soma that endures. If we find and hold to our Soma, the poisons of life may continue to challenge us but cannot enter into us. Shiva in the heart remains our Soma. We must learn how to work with both Nilakantha and Soma, Shiva's protective and bliss aspects. Nilakantha takes us to Soma.

Selected Soma Verses from the *Rigveda*

The Vedic hymns to Agni or the sacred fire form the root of the Vedic teachings. Yet the hymns to Soma form its fruit. The Vedic Yajna or sacrifice, which reflects the entire cosmic order, involves enkindling the sacred fire in order to prepare the Soma, which itself is the highest offering to the fire. The outer aspect of the sacrifice consists of offering various substances like wood, cow dung or ghee into the sacred fire along with special mantras to gain the blessings of the Gods, starting with the rain from heaven above. The inner aspect of the sacrifice consists of offering speech, mind and prana into the inner sacred fire of meditation, with yogic practices of mantra, meditation and pranayama, in order to gain Divine grace, the flow of Soma or bliss from the heavens of higher consciousness.

Soma is associated with the Vedic hymns themselves, which are said to impart Soma to those who recite them. Soma is specifically connected to the Vedic meters (chandas), and the Vedic language itself is called the metrical language or chandas. We could say that the Vedic hymns are the very language of Soma. Ancient Soma plants were named after the Vedic meters like gayatri, trishtub and jagati.[180] The Vedic meters reflect the rhythm and intonation of the Vedic mantras, including their essence or Soma.

Soma and the Moon are said to bring about an increase in poetic and mantric power in a person, inspiring the brain and the crown chakra. This means that to understand the Vedic Soma hymns one must have a sense of their vibratory power and flow of inspiration, which is best revealed in the original Sanskrit. The Soma hymns reflect the language of the crown chakra, which holds a thousand syllables, or all the variations of sound and meaning that can arise from seed mantras like *Om*.

The ninth book or mandala of the *Rigveda* consists entirely of Soma hymns, 114 in number. There are only a few other Soma hymns elsewhere in the text, mainly the first and eighth books, though Soma is frequently mentioned relative to other Vedic deities, particularly to Indra, Agni, the Maruts, the Ashwins, and as among the hymns to the Universal or All Gods (Visvedeva).

Below are a few important Soma verses from the *Rigveda*, not any complete hymns, according to my translation and commentary. I have included these to show the vast symbolism associated with Soma in the Vedic period.[181] This includes the connection of Soma with meditation, samadhi, the crown chakra and the spiritual heart. All the secrets of Tantric and Kundalini Yoga can be found in this Vedic Agni-Soma approach, which is their ancient origin. You will also see how little botanical symbolism is there in most Soma hymns, which are cosmic in nature.

Kavi Ushanas

Relative to his universal form, Krishna in the *Bhagavad Gita* states that he is the Ushanas among the seer-poets or kavis.[182] Ushanas is the foremost of the Bhrigus, one of the two most ancient families of Vedic seers famous for their spiritual and occult knowledge, including the power of rejuvenation. Ushanas in the *Rigveda* has several Soma hymns and his family the Bhrigus is closely connected to Soma; note a few verses below.[183]

The Most Secret Light - *Rigveda IX.87.3*

The father and generator of the Gods, the pillar of Heaven and support of the Earth, the seer, the sage, the guide of men, skillful, wise, Ushanas by his poetic power: he found that which hidden, the mysterious secret name of the light.

That which is most hidden is the secret light of truth in the spiritual heart which contains the entire universe and makes us one with all beings. It resides deep in the small space or cavity of the heart, beyond the three states of waking, dream and deep sleep. Searching that out is the process of meditation and Self-inquiry. This verse plays on the sounds of related words *Go* for cow but also light and soul and *Guha* for secret but also the cave of the heart.

Soma or bliss is the ultimate magnetic energy that sustains everything in the universe. Once we open to its power, our entire being will be upheld both in time and space and beyond. The pillar of heaven is the Shiva linga, the ascending cosmic masculine force, which originally was a Soma pillar.

Soma Gayatris

Gayatri is the name of the most famous of the Vedic verses by the Rishi Vishvamitra to the Deity Savitri, who represents the transformational aspect of the Divine light through the Sun. Gayatri is also the name of a meter and many Vedic hymns are composed in it, including a number of Soma hymns. There are three special Gayatri mantras in the hymns of Vishvamitra, which follow immediately after his Savitri Gayatris.

Soma Gayatris - *Rigveda III.62.13-15*

Soma goes forth as the finder of the path. He moves to the special place of the Gods to sit at the origin of truth.

May Soma grant freedom from disease and give vitality to us, and to all two-footed and four-footed creatures.

Increasing our longevity, self-powerful and strong, Soma sits at the seat of truth.

Soma is regarded as the guide, guru and finder of the path. One always follows one's bliss or inspiration, and one's deepest inspiration is usually one's best guide. That deeper inspiration takes us to the origin of truth itself, the supreme reality. Soma grants us health, longevity (ayus), well-being and immortality, bringing grace and happiness to our entire being by connecting us to our inner joy.

The First Verse of the Soma Mandala – *Rigveda IX.1, 6, 7*

With the sweetest and most intoxicating current, O Soma, flow extracted for Indra to drink. The daughter of Heaven purifies the poured out Soma by the eternal and extended moment.

The ten maidens, who are subtle (atomic) in form, grasp the Soma in the encounter, the sisters on the other side of Heaven.

Soma flows for Indra who represents the Seer or Purusha, the higher Self. Our Indra consciousness can be defined as the prime focus of our life energy, our seeking of transcendence and going beyond all limitations. The daughter of Heaven is the Dawn Goddess, the muse who directs our inspiration. The ten maidens or sisters are the five sense organs and five motor organs, which when purified, reveal the Divine Soma in all that we experience. When the mind is concentrated on the moment of bliss it can move beyond all time.

The Single Eye – *Rigveda IX.9.3-4*

The pure bright son at birth made his two Mothers shine reborn, the great God, the two great Goddesses who flourish in truth.

By seven insights held, Soma invigorates the guileless currents that have magnified a single eye.

Through the currents of the seven chakras, Soma energizes the single vision of the third eye. That flow of bliss is required to open our inner vision, which is the vision of Soma or Ananda in all. His two mothers are Heaven and Earth or mind and body, which he fills with light and delight.

The Lord of the Mind – *Rigveda IX.11.8-9*

Who destroys the unfriendly, wide in power, O Soma, flow as peace for the light, as you grant all wishes for the Gods.

Soma is poured for Indra to drink for his ecstasy, the mind and the lord of the mind. Flowing Soma, grant us strength and abundance, as the drop (Indu) united with Indra.

Soma is the mind and Indra as the Self is the lord of the mind. When our inner Self absorbs the mind, then our memories are transformed into bliss. The mind as Soma becomes the purified drop or point, the *bindu*, which is united with Indra or the consciousness of the Supreme Self.

The Lord of the Word – *Rigveda IX.12.5-6*

Indu directs the Word over the summit of the ocean, energizing the sheath that drips honey. Soma is the eternal chant, the great forest tree, and the wish-yielding cow within our inspirations, directing all the ages of mankind.

Indu is Soma as a drop or point focus, much like the bindu of Tantric thought. The ocean is the ocean of the heart into which the Soma flows from the crown chakra once awakened. The Word is the Divine Word, *Pranava* or the original seed mantra that creates all other sounds. The sheath that drips honey is the bliss sheath or Anandamaya kosha. Soma as in many places is said to be a great forest tree (vanaspati), which is symbolic of the cosmic tree that arises from the mantra and the Divine Word. This Soma is the power guiding and inspiring mankind throughout all history, all the yugas or world ages.

The Supreme Light – *Rigveda IX.17.5-6*

Transcending the three luminous celestial realms, you illuminate heaven; directing your energy, you expand like the Sun. You the sages and poets have called at the head of the sacrifice, holding what is delightful in the eye.

Soma as the supreme light of consciousness pervades even the highest heavens, here the three luminous realms of Being-Consciousness-Bliss. Soma is the Sun of truth, the original eternal light. That Soma the sages invoke with their mantras, at the head of the sacrifice, which is also the crown chakra, as the bliss of higher perception.

Soma and Indra – *Rigveda IX.19.1-2*

O Soma, what is the bright, laudable heavenly or earthly treasure, bring that to us as you flow. Soma, you and Indra are both the lords of the sun world, the lords of light. As co-rulers overflow our intelligence.

Soma as bliss and Indra as consciousness are the supreme ruling principles that can invigorate our higher intelligence. They are the interrelated powers of light and delight. Soma or bliss flows for Indra or our higher awareness to drink, imbibe or absorb. That Soma or power of perception brings us the abundance and beauty of all that we see.

The Original Powers of Life – *Rigveda IX.23.1-2, 4-5*

The swift Somas have poured in the flow of the honey ecstasy, over all seer powers. As the original powers of life, they have reached the place that is ever new. For light they generate the Sun.

The Somas as the life powers have poured the ecstatic honey wine over the sheath that drips with bliss. Strong Soma flows holding the juice (rasa) of the power of perception (indriyam), heroic, the remover of all negativity.

The Somas are the original powers of life and longevity (ayus) that arise from the Divine creative vision. Though eternal, they bring into being that which is ever new. They generate the Sun of truth. As the Soma flows it opens up the *madhu-kosha*, the sheath of the honey wine, which is also the sheath of bliss or Anandamaya kosha. Soma is the essence of all that is revealed to the power of perception, the power of Indra, the seer.[184]

The Mothers of Truth – *Rigveda IX.33.4-6*

Three voices are elevated. The mother cows bellow. The Golden one continues to roar.

The Priestesses, the mighty Mother streams of truth have sung. They cleanse the child of heaven.

Soma, pour for us from every side four infinite oceans of splendor.

The forces of the Divine Word as the great Goddesses prepare the Soma or bliss consciousness as their Divine child. This Soma is articulated as the Divine speech. Soma's sisters are said to be ten, which scholars have tended to look at as the ten fingers of the hands. However, they represent the five sense organs and five motor organs along with Soma as the mind. The four oceans are the four directions of space, which under the bliss of Soma become unbounded.

Generating the Luminous Realms of Heaven – *Rigveda IX. 42.1-2*

Generating the luminous realms of Heaven, generating the Sun in the waters, the Golden one, wearing the light and the waters, Divine Soma flows pressed out in a stream by the original intuition.

Bliss is the creative power that creates the visible universe outwardly and inwardly creates the higher Heavens of consciousness. The Sun is the Divine Self hidden in the waters or the ocean of the deeper mind. The original intuition is that of our true nature beyond time and space.

The Divine Poet – *Rigveda IX.44.2-3*

Welcomed by the thought, placed by insight, Soma speeds in the beyond, the poet by the flow of the sage.

The one wakeful among the Gods, extracted he passes through the purification filter; Soma moves with the power of vision.

Soma relates here to poetic and rishi inspiration that moves by mind and intelligence according to the flow of bliss. He is the wakeful power within us that is always seeking a deeper experience of life and dwells even in deep sleep. The true Soma of bliss arises only through enhanced wakefulness, not through any mere drunkenness, inebriation or stupor.

Soma as the Supreme Creator – *Rigveda IX.64.7-9*

Of you the purifier, the knower of all, your creations have streamed forth like the rays of the Sun.

Creating the illumining light from Heaven, you generate all forms, O Soma, as the ocean you overflow.

Directing the Word, you flow, the purifier in the wide Dharma; you stride Divine like the Sun.

Soma is the supreme creative force, generating both the lower and the higher worlds. This Divine creativity overflows like the ocean. It is not the product of any lack or want. Soma is the power of the Divine Word and the Divine Light, the supreme ocean and the Sun of suns.

The Original Void – *Rigveda IX.70.1*

Three times seven milch cows have yielded for him the elixir of truth in the original ether. Four other beautiful realms he made as an adornment, when by the truth he flourished.

Desiring to partake of the beauty of immortality, he opened up both the Heavens by his seer power. By greatness he encompassed the most radiant waters, when by inspiration they knew the place of God.

Soma holds the three times seven or twenty-one mantric powers of the Goddess or cosmic Mother through all the seven chakras. Through these he fashions higher realms of truth beyond this mortal world. That Soma pervades space and is present even in the void, particularly the original ether in the heart. Soma reveals all the beauties of the immortal realms and the very place of God or the seat of our own higher Self.

A Thousand Currents – *Rigveda IX.73.7*

A thousand currents are extended in the purification filter as the wise seers purify the Word. The powers of Rudra are the most invigorating, free of illusion, as seeing powers that move in harmony, beautiful and with the vision of the soul.

The guardian of truth who has good will cannot be deceived. He has created three purification filters in the heart. The knower he perceives all the worlds; the unwelcomed falsehoods he places in constriction.

Soma opens up the thousand currents of the crown chakra or thousand-petal lotus. The Rudras are the powers of Shiva, the powers of the higher Prana. The three purification filters, or means of perception, are the powers of Fire, Air and Sun as the ruling forces of the three worlds of the Earth (body), Atmosphere (Prana) and Heaven (mind). These dwell in the spiritual heart.

The Tongue of Truth – *Rigveda IX.75.2-3*

The tongue of truth pours the delightful honey wine, the speaker, the Lord inviolable of this insight. The son holds the secret Name of the two parents, in the third of the luminous realms of heaven.

Flashing forth, he roars into the chalices, led by men into the golden sheath. The milkings of truth have resounded over him; in the third summit he illuminates the dawns.

The Divine Word arises from bliss or Ananda. It enters into creation as the immanent consciousness that is able to realize the supreme truth and take us to the highest heaven. The tongue here may reflect the yogic practice of Khechari mudra. The golden sheath or *hiranmaya kosha* is the same as the Anandamaya kosha or sheath of bliss. The third summit is the non-dualistic realm.

The All-knowing Ocean – *Rigveda IX.86.29*

Yours are the progeny of the heavenly seed. You rule over the entire universe. Thus the entire world is in your control. You, Indu, are the first giver of the law.

You are the all-knowing ocean, O Seer; yours are the five directions in the wide dharma: You extend beyond heaven and earth. Yours are the lights, flowing Soma, who are the Sun.

The heavenly seed is the soul's immortal nature within us, which reflects our deepest Soma. The all-knowing ocean is the ocean of consciousness that encompasses the entire universe. The bliss-consciousness of Soma embraces all manifestation but extends to the Absolute beyond all time and space.

The Divine Father – *Rigveda IX.96.5-6*

Soma flows as the generator of our thoughts, as the generator of Heaven and the generator of the Earth; the generator of Agni and the generator of the Sun, the generator of Indra and the generator of Vishnu.

The priest among the Gods, the guide of the Seers, the rishi among the sages, the water buffalo among the animals, the falcon among birds, the axe in the forests, Soma flows through the purification filter singing.

Soma is the generator, father and mother of all. He creates all mortal creatures but also manifests all the Divine powers through Ananda. Soma is the essence of all things, the best or highest form or archetype or prototype. The artist and the mystic are able to grasp this essence. Whatever we place our Soma in; we will excel in that as well.

The Rishi Mind – *Rigveda IX.96.18-19*

The rishi mind, the maker of the rishis, who conquers the world of light, who has a thousandfold guidance, the guide of the seers: The great one displays his third nature. Soma as the singer illumines the original splendor.

The falcon in the chalices, the bird of omens who moves widely, the drop, the point of the light, carrying his weapons, the wave of the waters merging into the ocean, the buffalo reveals his fourth nature.

Soma as the power of bliss is the supreme awareness of the rishis who manifest through his power and for whom Soma is the original teacher or guru. Soma takes us to the higher reality beyond duality. Our own Soma or bliss can merge into the supreme ocean of Consciousness-Bliss, as the drop returns to the sea. The buffalo symbolizes the power of the Divine Word. The fourth nature or *Turiya* is the state of pure awareness beyond the three lower states of waking, dream and deep sleep.

The Vedic Soma Yoga – *Rigveda IX.100.3*

Soma, the insight yogically linked to the mind (dhiyam manoyujam), you release like thunder does the rain. You nurture all earthly and heavenly treasures.

Soma unites the insight or inner intelligence (dhī or buddhi) with the mind, bringing about the unfoldment of our higher consciousness. This is part of the ancient Vedic 'Soma Yoga', which is harnessing the power of bliss to yogically control the mind. It is only Soma that can truly control the mind or bring us to the yogic state of samadhi, which is the mind resting in its core Soma.

The Vast Truth – *Rigveda IX.107.14-15*

The Somas that carry the power of life pour the ecstatic juice over the crest of the ocean, as the exulting sages who have the knowledge of the world of light.

The Divine King, the Vast Truth (Ritam Brihat), flowing Soma crosses the ocean by the wave. Pouring the Dharma of the Divine Lord and Friend, giving energy to the Vast Truth.

Soma is the Vast Truth, *Ritam Brihat*, the supreme Brahman or Being-Consciousness-Bliss. The wave of the Sushumna or central channel of the subtle body takes us across the ocean, merging everything into bliss. Soma has the power of ayus, which is not just longevity but the immortal life of the spirit.

The Bull with a Thousand Flows – *Rigveda IX.108.8*

The bull with a thousand flows, who increases the juice, the King, the deity, the Vast Truth: Who by the truth is born of truth.

Soma is *Ritam Brihat*, the Vast Truth, meaning the truth beyond all time, space and action. That is Being-Consciousness-Bliss or Sat-chit-ananda (Sacchidananda). We should never forget the importance of truthfulness in allowing the highest Soma to flow.

Soma and Indra, the Immortal Life-spirit – *Rigveda III.32.8-10*

Indra's actions are manifold and perfect. All the Gods cannot diminish his laws. He upholds Heaven and Earth, and with his magic power generates the Sun and the dawn.

Your truth is without illusion, O Indra, when by greatness, instantly born you drank the Soma. The heavens cannot limit your power and strength (Ojas). Nor can the months or years obstruct you.

At the instant of your birth, O Indra, you drank the Soma for ecstasy in the supreme ether. Then you entered into both Heaven and Earth, and became the primal power that sustains the chant.

Indra is the inner Self and immortal life spirit that drinks the Soma through its power of perception and awareness. We must awaken that Indra spirit within us in order to be able to imbibe the eternal nectar. Then we too will enter into the entire universe as our own Self.

PART V

Appendices:
Glossary, Index, Resources

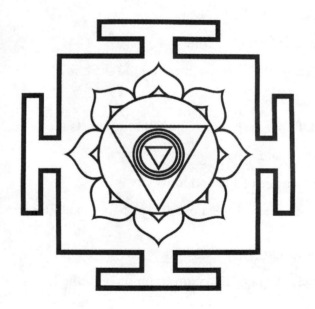

SANSKRIT TERMS

Agni – fire as a cosmic principle, digestive fire

Ahimsa – yogic principle of non-violence or non-harming

Apana Vayu – downward moving Prana governing elimination and reproduction

Ama – toxins born of wrong digestion

Amrita – nectar or Soma

Amrita nadi – channel from the crown chakra to the spiritual heart

Arishta – Ayurvedic herbal wine

Asava – Ayurvedic herbal wine

Ashwins – twin Vedic horsemen who hold the knowledge of Soma

Atman – higher Self

Avalambak Kapha – type of Kapha that supports the heart

Ayus – Life or longevity

Ayurveda – science of life and longevity

Bandha – lock, special Yoga practice as Mula, Jalandhara and Uddiyana

Bhakti – devotion

Bhakti Yoga – Yoga of devotion or union with the Divine at a heart level

Bija mantra – single syllable or seed mantras

Bindu – point focus of energy and awareness

Bodhak Kapha – type of Kapha governing taste and salivation

Brahma – deity governing creation or manifestation

Brahman – the Absolute or Godhead

Brihmana – tonification or building therapy

Buddhi – higher mind

Chakra – energy center of subtle body

Chandra – Moon

Dasha – planetary periods of Vedic astrology governing one's life and karma

Devi – Goddess or Divine Mother

Dhanvantari – Ayurvedic deity of healing and rejuvenation; form of Vishnu

Dhara – flow of liquid, oil or Soma

Dharana – concentration

Dharma – natural laws, principles of consciousness

Dhatu – tissue-element, seven in number in the body (rasa/plasma, rakta/blood, mamsa/muscle, meda/fat, majja/nerve/ shukra/ reproductive)

Dhi – higher mind

Dhyana – meditation

Dosha – biological humor

Gayatri – special Vedic verses for invoking the higher powers

Ghee/Ghrita – clarified butter, symbolizes the clarified state of the mind

Gunas – qualities of nature or Prakriti

Hanuman – Deity of the cosmic Prana, with the form of a monkey

Hatha Yoga – Yoga of balancing solar and lunar forces

Hridaya – spiritual heart

Ida nadi – lunar channel running to left nostril, has Soma nature

Indra – Vedic deity of Purusha and Prana, drinker of the Soma

Indu – Soma as a drop

Ishvara – God as the cosmic lord

Jatharagni – digestive fire

Jnana – spiritual knowledge

Jnana Yoga – Yoga of knowledge

Jyotish – science of light or Vedic astrology

Kala/Kalaa – 16 digits of the Moon

Kali – Goddess governing death and immortality

Kapha – biological water humor

Ketu – south node of the Moon

Khechari mudra – holding the tongue at the top of the mouth and related practices

Kicharee – Ayurvedic food of equal parts basmati rice and split yellow mung beans

Kirtan – chanting, singing or praising

Kledak Kapha – type of Kapha that moistens food and protects digestion

Kosha – sheath or layer around the soul or inner Self, usually five in number (anna/food, prana/breath, manas/mind, vijnana/intelligence, ananda/bliss)

Krishna – Vishnu as the avatar of Yoga and devotion

Kundalini – electrical power behind consciousness, energizes the chakras and subtle body

Lakshmi – Goddess of preservation, devotion and abundance

Langhana – reduction therapy, allied with detoxification

Madhu – honey, symbolic of Soma or bliss

Manas – mind

Mandala – book of the *Rigveda*

Mantra – sacred sounds, syllables and chants

Marmas – Ayurvedic pressure points

Mudra – hand gesture, yogic action

Muladhara – root chakra

Nada – cosmic sound vibration

Nadi – channels or currents of the subtle body

Nadi shodhana – alternate nostril breathing for balancing solar and lunar energies

Nakshatras – twenty-seven lunar mansions

Nama – offering of devotion, reverence or surrender

Nidra – sleep

Nilakantha – name for Shiva relative to his blue throat

Niyamas – yogic practices of self-discipline

Ojas – vital essence of Kapha dosha

Pancha Karma – five main purification practices of Ayurveda

Pavamana – Soma as the purifier or self-purifying in its flow

Pingala nadi – solar channel running to right nostril

Pitta – biological fire humor

Prakriti – nature and one's Ayurvedic constitution

Prana – vital energy, breath

Pranagni – fire of the breath

Pranayama – control, development and transformation of Prana

Prakriti – nature or natural condition

Pratyahara – inward turning of mind, prana, sense and motor organs

Puja – devotional or flower based worship, helps generate inner Soma

Purusha – higher Self or soul

Rahu – north node of the Moon

Raja Yoga – eight-limbed Yoga

Rajas – quality of action, agitation, disturbance

Rama – Vishnu as the avatar of dharma and knowledge

Rasa – plasma, essence, juice

Rasayana – rejuvenation

Rigveda – oldest Vedic text, bases of Vedic chants

Rishi – Vedic seer

Rudra – Vedic form of Shiva, Divine doctor

Sadhak Pitta – type of Pitta governing the nervous system

Sadhana – Yoga practice towards Self-realization

Sahasrara – thousand petal lotus

Samadhi – absorption into inner awareness

Samana Vayu – balancing or centering prana

Samyama – deep yogic concentration rooted in Samadhi

Santosha – yogic principle of contentment

Sarasvati – Goddess of wisdom

Sattva – quality of purity, clarity and spirituality

Savitri – transformational aspect of solar energy and deity

Shakti – Goddess as the cosmic power

Shamana – Ayurvedic palliation or digestion promoting therapy

Shambhavi mudra – holding the gaze within even while looking to the outside

Shani – Saturn

Shiva – deity in role of destruction and transformation of the universe

Shodhana – Ayurvedic radical purification therapy like Pancha Karma

Snehana – oil application

Sleshak Kapha – type of Kapha that lubricates the joints and provides ease of movement

Soma – water as a cosmic principle, power of rejuvenation and immortality

Sri Chakra – meditative worship of the Sri Yantra

Sri Yantra – main yantra of Soma and the subtle body

Sundari – Goddess of bliss and Soma

Surya – Sun and solar deity

Sushumna nadi – central channel or Soma nadi

Svaha – mantra for energizing other mantras with fire or Agni

Svedana – sweating therapies

Tamas – quality of darkness and inertia

Tantra – Yogic teachings on Shiva and Shakti as the universal powers

Tantric Yoga – Yoga of Shiva and Shakti, Agni and Soma

Tapas – yogic purification practices

Tarpak Kapha – type of Kapha governing the nervous system

Tejas – vital essence of fire

Tithi – 15 phases of the Moon

Udana Vayu – upward moving prana, draws our awareness upwards

Vajikarana – aphrodisiac, reproductive system tonic

Vastu – Vedic architecture and directional science, related to Sthapatya Veda

Vata – biological air humor

Vayu – air as a cosmic principle

Vedic Yoga – Vedic Mantra Yoga of balancing Agni and Soma

Vidya – way of knowledge

Vikriti – disease

Vishnu – deity in the role of preserving, maintaining the universe

Vyana Vayu – outward moving prana

Yamas – yogic attitudes

Yantra – energetic concentration devices for meditation

Yoni mudra – closing off the sensory openings of the head with the fingers and related practices

BIBLIOGRAPHY

Aurobindo, Sri.
The Life Divine. Twin Lakes WI: Lotus Press, 2001.

Aurobindo, Sri.
Secret of the Veda. Twin Lakes WI: Lotus Press, 2001.

Balkrishna, Acharya.
Secrets of Indian Herbs for Good Health. Divya Publishers: Haridwar, India, 2008.

Chopra, Shambhavi.
Yogini: Unfolding the Goddess Within. Delhi, India: Wisdom Tree, 2006.

Chopra, Shambhavi.
Yogic Secrets of the Dark Goddess. Delhi, India: Wisdom Tree, 2007.

Dikshit, Rajesh.
The Dasa Mahavidya (Sanskrit and Hindi). Agra, India: Deep Publications, 2003.

Dikshit, Rajesh.
Sri Vidya (Sanskrit and Hindi). Agra, India: Deep Publications, 2003.

Joshi, Sunil.
Ayurveda and Pancha Karma. Twin Lakes WI: Lotus Press, 1995.

Pandey, Dr. Gyanendra.
Dravya Guna Vijnana (three volumes). Varanasi, India: Krishnadas Academy, 1998.

Rao, S.K. Ramachandra.
The Tantrik Practices in Sri Vidya (with Shri Sarada Chatussati, English and Sanskrit). Bangalore, India: Kalpatharu Research Academy, 1990.

Shankaracharya.
Saundarya Lahari (V.K. Subramanian trans.). Delhi, India: Motilal

Banarsidass, 1986.

Sharma, B.D. and **Acharya Balkrishna.**
Vitality Strengthening Astavarga Plants. Divya Publishers 2008:
Haridwar, India, 2008.

Satguru Sivaya Subramuniyaswami.
Dancing With Siva. India and USA: Himalayan Academy, 1993.

Woodroofe, Sir John/ Avalon, Arthur.
The Serpent Power. Minneola, NY: Dover Books, 1974.

Yogananda, Paramahansa.
Autobiography of a Yogi. Los Angeles CA: Self-Realization Fellow-
ship, 2007.

SANSKRIT TEXTS

Atharva Veda Samhita
several versions available.

Bhagavad Gita
several versions available.

Bhavamishra
Bhava Prakasa
Prof. K.R. Srikantha Murthy translation. Varanasi, India: Krishnadas Academy, 2000.

Caraka Samhita
several versions available.

Complete Works Of Sankaracarya
Sanskrit only. Chennai, India: Samata Books.

Vasistha Ganapati Muni.
Collected Works Of Vasistha Kavyakantha Ganapati Muni (Sanskrit only),
eleven volumes, edited by K. Natesan. Tiruvannamalai, India:
Sri Ramanasramam 2003-2007.

Hatha Yoga Pradipika
of Svatmarama, several versions available.

Rigveda Samhita (Sanskrit, with some English).
Bangalore, India: Sir Aurobindo Kapali Sastry Institute of Vedic Culture,
1998.

Susruta Samhita
several versions available.

Upanishads, One Hundred And Eighty Eight
(Sanskrit only). Delhi, India: Motilal Banarsidass, 1980.

Patañjali, **Yoga Sutras** (Sanskrit only)
Varanasi, India: Bharatiya Vidya Prakashana, 1983, with commentaries of
Vachaspati Mishra and Vijnana Bhikshu. Note also the modern commentaries
of Swami Veda Bharati for a deep study of the text.

RELEVANT BOOKS BY THE AUTHOR

Frawley, David.
Ayurvedic Astrology: Self-Healing Through the Stars.
Twin Lakes WI: Lotus Press, 2005.

Frawley, David.
Ayurvedic Healing: a Comprehensive Guide, second edition.
Twin Lakes WI: Lotus Press, 2001.

Frawley, David.
Inner Tantric Yoga: Working With the Universal Shakti.
Twin Lakes WI: Lotus Press, 2008.

Frawley, David.
Mantra Yoga and Primal Sound: Secrets of Bija (Seed) Mantras.
Twin Lakes WI: Lotus Press, 2010.

Frawley, David.
Tantric Yoga and the Wisdom Goddesses: Spiritual Secrets of Ayurveda. Twin Lakes WI: Lotus Press, 2000.

Frawley, David.
Wisdom of the Ancient Seers: Selected Mantras from the Rig Veda.
Twin Lakes WI: Lotus Press, 2000.

Frawley, David.
Yoga and Ayurveda: Self-Healing and Self-Realization.
Twin Lakes WI: Lotus Press, 1999.

Frawley, David.
Yoga and the Sacred Fire.
Twin Lakes WI: Lotus Press, 2004.

Frawley, David and Vasant Lad.
The Yoga of Herbs.
Twin Lakes WI: Lotus Press, 1986.

RESOURCES

Acharya David Frawley (Pandit Vamadeva Shastri)

Acharya David Frawley is the author of more than thirty books and several distance learning courses written over the past thirty years. His books are available in twenty languages and include important publications in the fields of Ayurvedic medicine, Vedic astrology, Raja Yoga, Veda, Vedanta and Tantra. His works are noted for their depth and specificity and often serve as textbooks in their respective fields.

Vamadeva is one of the most respected *Vedacharyas* or teachers of the ancient Vedic wisdom in recent decades, East and West. He is honored in traditional circles in India, where his writings are well known and often discussed. He is also regarded as a teacher or acharya of Yoga, Ayurveda and Vedic astrology, reflecting his rare ability to link different Vedic disciplines and teach them in an integral manner.

American Institute of Vedic Studies, www.vedanet.com

The American Institute of Vedic Studies is an internationally recognized center for Vedic learning, with affiliated organizations worldwide. Directed by Dr. David Frawley (Pandit Vamadeva Shastri) and Yogini Shambhavi Chopra, the Vedic institute serves as a vehicle for their work, their books, CDs and activities. Located near Santa Fe, New Mexico, USA, the institute offers in depth training, including distance learning programs, each of which offers over a thousand pages of original material. Our courses are available in a number of different languages as well.

- Ayurvedic Healing course (Ayurvedic Life-Style Consultant certification). Probably the most widely used distance learning program in Ayurveda in recent decades with over five thousand students worldwide since 1988. The course covers the philosophical background of Ayurveda, the Ayurvedic view of anatomy and physiology, physical and mental constitution, the disease process and stages of disease, diagnosis through pulse, tongue and abdomen, an introduction to Ayurveda and Yoga, and treatment through diet, herbs, colors, counseling, mantra and meditation among other topics.

- Yoga, Ayurveda, and Meditation course, (Yoga and Ayurveda Health Educator certification). A comprehensive integral approach to Raja Yoga, Vedanta and Ayurveda, covering all eight limbs of Yoga according to an Ayurvedic view. Includes a complete and original translation and study of the *Yoga Sutras* from an Ayurvedic perspective, with sections on Bhakti Yoga, Jnana Yoga, Karma, Yoga, Mantra Yoga, Asana and Pranayama.

- Ayurvedic Astrology course (Ayurvedic Astrologer certification). One of the first and most popular English language course in Vedic astrology, since 1985, and one of the few to include traditional Ayurveda and its healing aspects from an astrological perspective. Explains the fundamentals of Vedic astrology, planets, signs, houses, aspects, yogas, dashas, Nakshatras, ashtakavarga, and muhurta, and the foundations of Ayurvedic medical astrology for body, mind and spirit. Includes remedial measures of mantras, yantras, rituals, deities and gems.

- Mantra Yoga course (Mantra Yoga Consultant certification). New course based upon Dr. Frawley's books, *Inner Tantric Yoga* and *Tantric Yoga and the Wisdom Goddesses*, as well as the current Soma book, and Yogini Shambhavi's books and CDs. Examines the place of Mantra Yoga in Veda, Vedanta and Tantra, with special reference to the role of Shakti and the role of deities, with usage in Yoga, Ayurveda, Vedic astrology and Vastu.

- The institute conducts regular tours and retreats, including in India, notably an annual March "Ma Ganga Yoga

Shakti Retreat," that brings students from all over the world for a deeper level of instruction with Vamadeva and Shambhavi. We also participate in various international programs and events.

The institute website features extensive on-line articles, on-line books and a full range of Vedic resources for the serious student, including a regular newsletter and on-going newsgroup.

Yogini Shambhavi

Yogini Shambhavi Chopra, co-director of the American Institute of Vedic Studies, is one of the foremost women teachers coming out of India today, and the author of several important books on the Goddess (*Yogini: Unfolding the Goddess Within* and *Yogic Secrets of the Dark Goddess*), noted for their experiential approach to higher consciousness. Her *Yogini Bhava* and *Jyotish Bhava* CDs provide guides for traditional chanting and mantra sadhana. Shambhavi also offers consultations in Vedic astrology and spiritual guidance, including initiation into Shakti Sadhana, for students from all over the world. She is a great inspiration for all who come into contact with her.

Sources for Ayurvedic Herbs and Supplements

There are a number of good Ayurvedic companies in India and in the West, which keeps growing. Among our favorites are: Divya Pharmacy (Patanjali Yog Peeth of Swami Ramdev and Acharya Balakrishna), Sri Sri Ayurveda (Sri Sri Ravishankar), BAPS Swaminarayan Herbal Care and their many temples (Akshardham) in North America and India, Banyan Herbs (USA), Trihealth Ayurveda (Hawaii), and Kerala Ayurveda. A number of western herbal companies now offer Ayurvedic herbs, including several like ashwagandha, shatavari and amla mentioned in this book.

COMMENTS ON BOOK

Soma in Yoga and Ayurveda weaves together with remarkable clarity rejuvenation of the body, revitalization of the mind, and awakening to the inherent immortality of the Spirit. The book reveals special healing secrets of Soma from the ancient Vedic rishis and yogis reflecting a profound vision and wide range of application that can transform both our individual lives and our collective culture. Vamadeva Shastri has provided one of the most important and original books on Yoga and Ayurveda in recent times that is bound to be studied for decades to come.

Deepak Chopra, author *Reinventing the Body,*
Resurrecting the Soul: How to Create a New Self

Vamadeva's tour of well-being, incisive and empirical, always comes back to us, to the goodness in our life. His understanding of the doshas and what each of us needs to find balance within and ward off disease is uncanny. This book's fundamental message reminded me of Abraham Lincoln's maxim: "In the end, it's not the years in your life that count. It's the life in your years." The difference is, Vamadeva teaches us how to put the Divine life into all our days and years.

Paramacharya Sadasivanatha Palaniswami, *Hinduism Today,*
Editor-in-Chief

Once again, David Frawley has produced a book of unparalleled depth and insight.

Soma in Yoga and Ayurveda synthesizes profound teachings and practices from Yoga, Tantra, Ayurveda, and Jyotish for rejuvenating the body, elevating emotions, awakening the intellect, and realizing the true meaning of immortality. Vamadeva is one of the few authentic voices sharing this transformational knowledge, making it available and accessible to the modern reader. I am continually grateful for his work.

Gary Kraftsow, American Viniyoga Institute,
author *Yoga for Wellness* **and** *Yoga for Transformation*

Soma in Yoga & Ayurveda cracks the secret code of "Soma" and demystifies the myth and logic about its practical application. Dr. Frawley has clearly outlined that the real fountain of Soma is well within you and tapping into that nourishment will make your life enlightened and blissful.

Dr. Suhas Kshirsagar BAMS, MD (Ayu), Director, *Ayurvedic Healing*

Soma is another classic from the master translator of Vedic knowledge and wisdom of our time and culture. Vamadeva once again takes a profound subject, previously obscured by barriers of esoteric language and concepts, and offers it in a way that preserves, respects and elucidates its mysteries while rendering them accessible and practical to all.

David Crow, author *In Search of the Medicine Buddha*

Soma is the mystic nectar of the ancient Vedic rishis and the Tantric Yogis, the inner Shakti of rejuvenation, immortality and bliss, which is the supreme creative force. Vamadeva has revealed the hidden secrets of Soma and special powerful Yoga practices, rarely taught even in India, particularly how Soma is necessary to facilitate the proper unfoldment of Kundalini and the opening of the chakras. A profound guidebook for all higher Yoga practices.

Yogini Shambhavi, author *Yogic Secrets of the Dark Goddess*

Uniting ancient wisdom and penetrating insight, David Frawley has written a jewel that explores the inner alchemy of physical and emotional rejuvenation while illuminating the spiritual quest for enlightenment. The book provides the student with the yogic and Ayurvedic tools necessary to achieve optimal health, peace of mind, and the eternal happiness that can only be found through spiritual awakening.

Dr. Marc Halpern, author,
Healing Your Life; Lessons on the Path of Ayurveda

This multifaceted book combines Yoga, Ayurveda, Tantra, Vedanta, and the Vedic sciences in a natural and transformative manner around the central concept of Soma or the science of immortal bliss. Such a vast capacity of synthesis in a profound and authoritative way of approaching the higher knowledge is most rare and shows a special connection with the higher forces of cosmic intelligence that govern the planet.

Narayananda (Dr. Jose Rugue) *Suddha Sabha Yoga Ashram Brazil*

In *Soma in Yoga and Ayurveda,* Dr. David Frawley successfully brings out the true significance of Soma, 'the immortal delight of existence', as envisioned by the ancient Indian Rishis. Here we find a comprehensive description of the Vedic idea of Soma, which insightfully reveals Soma's secret of Immortality and bliss. Dr. Frawley shows here how to apply the principle of Soma to our lives through useful techniques, for the rejuvenation of the body and mind and most importantly, for the resurrection of the immortal spirit within us."

Dr. Sampadananda Mishra, *Sri Aurobindo Society India*

ENDNOTES

1 *Enā soma stavena te pra viśema guhā dhiyām*

Yā te tejāṁsi pārthivā yā divyā tāny āviṣkṛdhi Enā te kratunā soma pra carema guhyā matīḥ

Ye te vahnayaḥ pārthivā ye divyās tān samindha na*ḥ*

Original Soma verses by Swami Veda Bharati, among the many Vedic verses he has envisioned in his different writings, including his *Chandasi*, his own special collection of Vedic verses he has composed.

2 *Yajurveda* mantra.

3 *Rigveda VIII.48.12, hrtsu pītāḥ.*

4 *Madacyut...Somo gaurī adhi-śritaḥ. Rigveda IX.12.3.*

5 *Eṣa...viśva-vin manasas-patiḥ. Rigveda IX.28.1.*

6 *Manaścin manasas-patiḥ. Rigveda IX.11.9.*

7 Note the following references for this paragraph's statements: *Dhiyā yāty aṇvyā. Rigveda IX.15.1.*

Pra vācham indur iṣyati. Rigveda IX.12.6.

Pratnam nipāti kāvyam. Rigveda IX.6.8.

*Eṣa pratnena manman*ā*. Rigveda IX.42.2.*

*Eṣa divam vi dh*ā*vati. Rigveda IX.3.7.*

8 This famous Vedic chant is said in the *Upanishad*, which presents it to be a chant to Pavamana Soma, to the immortal nectar.

9 Paramahansa Yogananda, *Autobiography of a Yoga*, note index for many references to Babaji.

10 Notably Sri Aurobindo's the *Life Divine*.

11 Such a new humanity beyond the divisive ego-mind and its conflicts is the real need of the world in any case.

12 *Bhagavad Gita II.16.*

13 Note the teachings of Ramana Maharshi that center on abiding in the spiritual Self within the heart.

14 Note books of Sir John Woodroofe (Arthur Avalon), like the *Serpent Power,* which reflect traditional Kundalini Yoga and are free of the many distortions that have come up in recent years.

15 Note *Autobiography of a Yogi,* story of Sri Yukteswar's resurrection, pages 466ff.

16 Gaudapada, *Mandukya Upanishad Karika.*

17 Note the life and teachings of Ramana Maharshi. Most of his books are available at the ashram website.

18 In *Katha Upanishad*, Yama, the God of Death, teaches the youth Nachiketa.

19 Note the teachings of the *Bhagavad Gita II.22.*

20 Like Agnihotra, the daily fire offerings at sunrise, noon and sunset, which constitutes the main practice of the Brahmins and other twice born and initiates.

21 The fifth of the eight limbs of Raja Yoga in the *Yoga Sutras II.54,* which internalizes the mind and senses to allow meditation to proceed.

22 Note *Gods, Sages and Kings* (Frawley) and *In Search of the Cradle of Civilization* (Feuerstein, Kak, Frawley) for such a different view of world history and the ancient history of India.

23 The *Zend Avesta*, the scripture of the ancient Persian Zoroastrians, provides much emphasis to Soma or Homa, which was part of many of their rituals.

24 Note Dr. Suhas Kshirsagar: Soma is nothing but Nature's Intelligence at every level of existence. It is the subtle link connecting Matter, Energy and Consciousness. Soma is understood as the purest and subtlest form of material expression, which connects mortality with immortality.

25 Note the author's translation of various Soma hymns of the *Rigveda* in *Wisdom of the Ancient Seers.*

26 *Taittiriya Upanishad II.7. Raso vai saḥ.* "The Self is the rasa or essence," meaning the essence of delight or Ananda.

27 The Samkhya system of philosophy as explained in the *Samkhya Karika* of Ishvara Krishna, the main traditional text on the subject. Samkhya is also explained in detail in the *Mahabharata*.

28 My first writings on the *Vedas*, consisting mainly of translations of hymns from the *Rigveda*, began in April 1980, when M.P. Pandit, the then secretary of the Sri Aurobindo Ashram in India, began serializing my writings in various ashram publications like *World Union* and the *Advent,* extending to the publication of several dozen articles. Aurobindo himself was one of the greatest modern Vedic scholars, which was a mere sidelight to his greatness as a Yogi and Seer, being a rishi himself.

29 Note the *Katha Upanishad VI.1:* "With its root above and branches below, such is the eternal Ashwattha (banyan) tree. That is the luminous; that is Brahman; that indeed is the immortal."

30 *Rigveda* X.97.5-7.

31 Importance of vamsha or reed in the *Vedas*, notably in the *Aitareya Aranyaka*.

32 These are tamasic Somas, Somas in which the quality of tamas, which is ignorance, darkness and attachment prevails.

33 Note Dr. Suhas Kshirsagar: The lunar essence of Soma is adversely affected with our modern lifestyle. Inflammation, the "silent killer" is at the backdrop of many chronic diseases. Computers, Cell phones, WiFi, polluted air, food and water, will lead to cellular toxicity and dry out the cooling essence of Soma. It can create an under active or over active immune and nervous system.

34 *Charaka Samhita Chikitsa Sthana I.*

35 Amrita or Chandra in Sanskrit.

36 Indra is *Somapā* or the drinker of the Soma, which is extracted mainly for him. In this regard Indra is connected to Vayu, which is not just wind but the Spirit, which drinks or imbibes the Soma of bliss.

37 Soma in the *Rigveda* has a profound watery symbolism and is often referred to as *samudra* or ocean, *sindhu* or river, *nāḍi* or current, *dhārā* or flow, *saras* or lake, *vṛṣti* or rain, ūrmi or wave and *indu* or *drapsa* or drop, as well as called *Pavamāna* or flowing. In terms of liquids, Soma is called āpas or water, *rasa* or juice, go and *payas* or milk, *madhu* or honey, *ghṛta* or ghee, *pīyuṣa* and *amṛta* or nectar. Its flow is described in various ways and through different verbal roots as well. These reflect a cosmic water symbolism, not simply that of a particular plant. Yet water or āpas and light or *jyoti* are one in Vedic thought and so Soma has its light forms as well.

38 Bhutagnis of Ayurvedic thought.

39 Dhatvagnis of Ayurvedic thought.

40 The five forms or subtypes of Pitta dosha are also regarded as the five types of Agni.

41 Rasa, Rakta, mamsa, medas, asthi, majja and shukra in Ayurveda.

42 What is called *ambhuvaha srotas* or the channel system carrying water in Ayurvedic medicine, which also governs the sugar metabolism.

43 What is called annavaha srotas or the 'channel system carrying food' in Ayurvedic medicine.

44 That is why the *Upanishads* say that the essence of food is the mind; *Chandogya Upanishad VI.5.*

45 Purusha Sukta, *Rigveda X.90.13.*

46 The term Hatha is commonly divided as 'Ha' indicating the Sun and 'Tha' indicating the Moon. Ha and Tha are also used in Mantra Yoga as seed mantras for the Sun and the Moon.

47 *Hatha Yoga Pradipika, II.44,* commentary.

48 *Aitareya Upanishad III.*

49 This is part of the practice of Khechari Mudra that we will discuss later in the book.

50 *Hatha Yoga Pradipika III.44* and commentary of Brahmananda.

51 The Kapha subdoshas can be regarded as types of Soma and help sustain positive health. Yet too much Kapha in the body can also cause them to deteriorate.

52 What is called Shringataka marma in Ayurvedic marma therapy. Note *Ayurveda and Marma Therapy* (Frawley, Ranade, Lele).

53 What is called Sarasvati nadi, which flows from the throat chakra to the tip of the tongue.

54 When a higher Tarpak Kapha develops the saliva or Bodhak Kapha reflects it by becoming sweeter, a kind of internal nectar or Soma flow.

55 Generally we are most prone to the diseases of our own constitutional type, or if we are dual types, of one of the two dominant doshas within us.

56 Taken from author's book *Yoga and Ayurveda*.

57 Kapha dosha is most active in spring. Pitta dosha is most active in summer. Vata dosha is most active in the fall. Early winter is more Vata and later winter more Kapha. However, different ecosystems have their climate variations as well.

58 Note Dr. Suhas Kshirsagar: According to the Ayurvedic texts, Soma is the purest form of Kapha, Shukra and Ojas. This cooling essence further regulates Agni and Tejas. The cosmic dance of Prana, Tejas and Ojas, which pervades in the universe, is held together by Soma.

59 Dhatu does not just mean tissue but whatever supports or upholds the body. As such supportive factors, the doshas are also dhatus.

60 What is called vyadhi kshamatva in Ayurveda.

61 Note author's *Yoga and Ayurveda Chapter 7*.

62 *Hatha Yoga Pradipika I.57-63.*

63 Generally cool tastes, yet not too cold, promote rejuvenation, while heating tastes are more detoxifying. This also means that cooling foods and herbs are better overall for rejuvenation.

64 Including Ayurvedic salt based formulas to improve digestion like Hingashtak or Lavanbhaskar churnas.

65 Saag which is mainly spinach and mustard greens is famous in this regard.

66 *Suta* in Sanskrit.

67 *Pavitra* or purification filter.

68 *Ghṛta* and *madhu* in Sanskrit.

69 Please consult Ayurvedic herbals like the author's *Yoga of Herbs* or other books mentioned in the bibliography.

70 The role of mineral supplements and rejuvenation would come in this area as well.

71 But take some caution to get a reputable source for the herbs. Some of these are listed in the resource section of the book.

72 For this purpose it is important that the bees are treated well!

73 There are many other rejuvenative herbs for the mind in various herbal traditions throughout the world. Chinese medicine has a number of interesting herbs in this regard likely zizyphus and schizandra. In western herbal medicine, lady's slipper orchid is a very powerful herb of this type, as are skullcap and mistletoe.

74 As described in the works of modern psychologist CG Jung.

75 *Yoga Sutras IV.1.*

76 *Atharva Veda XI.6.15.*

77 Note appendix for the 'Search for the Original Soma Plant' and a further discussion of these details.

78 Soma is described in the *Rigveda* in various terms that indicate ecstasy, bliss or inebriation. These include *madhu* or honey, *madhumattama* or most honey like, *svādhu* or sweet, *mada* or intoxicating, *mastsara* or delightful, ananda or bliss, *nanda* or happiness, *sumnā* or happy minded, *muda* and *pramuda* or exhilarating. These reflect the yogic intoxication of Samadhi or the inner state of bliss, not any mere outer intoxicant, herb or drug.

79 *Om* is the seed mantra of the Shiva or cosmic masculine energy among its other connotations.

80 Parashakti is the Supreme Shakti. The bija of the prime Shakti energy is *Aim*.

81 Note Ayurvedic herbals like the author's Yoga of Herbs for more details on this type of herbs.

82 Note the book *Ayurveda and Pancha Karma* by Sunil Joshi.

83 Shadkarmas, *Hatha Yoga Pradipika II.22.*

84 *Hatha Yoga Pradipika II.21.*

85 What is called Purishadhara Kala or the membrane that holds the feces in Ayurvedic thought.

86 *Ama* is an Ayurvedic term for the mass of undigested or improperly digested food particles that ferments and promotes the disease process. It usually stands opposite Agni or the digestive fire that promotes positive health.

87 Note The *Serpent Power* of John Woodroofe, for the description of the thousand-petal lotus or crown chakra relative to the Moon and its nectar.

88 The *Yoga Sutras* reflects the older Samkhya-Yoga tradition that in turn is connected to various yogic teachings in the *Vedas*, *Upanishads* and *Bhagavad Gita*, including Vaishnava and Shaivite (Pashupata) traditions. The Hatha Yoga, Siddha Yoga and Tantric traditions are mainly a Shaivite tradition. The *Mahabharata* discusses the Samkhya-Yoga, Vaishnava and Shaivite Yogas prior to the time of Patanjali and connects them to Veda and Vedanta as well.

89 The first section of the *Yoga Sutras* is called *Samadhi Pada*, suggesting Soma or the samadhi flow of the mind as the essence of Yoga.

90 *Yoga Sutras*, Vyasa Commentary I.2.

91 *Yoga Sutras IV.29*, Dharma Megha Samadhi.

92 Soma and *Ṛtam Bṛhat*, *Rigveda IX.107.15* and *108.8* for some examples.

93 *Yoga Sutras I.48*, *Ṛtambhara Prajña* which reflects the highest Samadhi.

94 There are many Hindu Tantric texts from all regions of the country and covering many centuries, including Kashmiri, Bengali and Tamilian traditions. Most of Hinduism in the Middle Ages, including the manner of Hindu temple worship, was largely Tantric, such as we best see in the big temple cities of South India.

95 The *Hatha Yoga Pradipika* not only discusses the Kundalini but also the Amrit, nectar or Soma in some detail.

96 The three lower chakras starting with the root chakra are regarded as the region of fire or Agni in yogic thought, while the three higher chakras ending with the crown chakra are the region of the moon or Soma. The heart in between is the region of the Sun, which also includes the navel and the throat as transitional regions.

97 Note the author's books in this regard: *Inner Tantric Yoga: Working with the Universal Shakti*, and *Tantric Yoga and the Wisdom Goddesses: Spiritual Secrets of Ayurveda.*

98 Five koshas or layers of the Self, starting with *Taittiriya Upanishad 3;* a common teaching in the literature of Advaita Vedanta. The Anandamaya kosha or sheath of bliss can be connected with the Madhu kosha or sheath of honey with which Soma is closely associated in the *Rigveda.*

99 The subtle body complex or linga of Samkhya thought, is behind the chakra system, with its groups of the five elements, five tanmatras, five sense organs and five motor organs, which correspond to the powers of the lower five chakras, with buddhi and Purusha to the higher two chakras.

100 Note author's *Inner Tantric Yoga* for its discussion of relevant mantras like those of Sundari.

101 Soma is often called Pavamana or purifying throughout the *Rigveda.*

102 Note the author's *Ayurveda and the Mind* for a discussion of the three gunas.

103 Mahamudra is discussed in some detail in the *Hatha Yoga Pradipika III.10-18.*

104 *Yoga Sutras* I.12-13 for which the practice of Yoga overall is defined as the control of the mind and a development of discrimination and detachment (viveka and vairagya), through which the inner Self or Purusha withdraws from the outer material nature or Prakriti that is rooted in the physical body.

105 *Satapatha Brahmana XII.3.2.8.*

106 Note the author's *Neti: Yoga and Ayurveda* for a detailed discussion of this practice.

107 *Hatha Yoga Pradipika II.72-75,* the highest kumbhaka or pranayama that arouses the Kundalini but must be approached with caution as it rests upon wisdom and devotion, not merely physical effort.

108 *Aparokshanubhuti* of Shankara, in which he also outlines his Fifteenfold Raja Yoga that is a bit different than the Raja Yoga of Patanjali and more knowledge or Jnana based.

109 *Hatha Yoga Pradipika III.32-41* and following.

110 Note the Mantra Purusha mantras in the author's *Mantra Yoga and Primal Sound*, which are a subject of much discussion in the book.

111 Most Vedic texts ascribe the sex organs to the root chakra and the anus to the sex or water chakra. This is because the root of the sexual impulse lies in the root chakra, whereas the impulse to discharge it lies in the second chakra. Yet for common purposes, it makes more sense to relate the excretory system to the root chakra and the urogenital system to the second chakra as these more simply reflect the earth and water elements in the body.

112 *Neti: Healing Secrets of Yoga and Ayurveda.*

113 Touching the tips of the bent little and ring figure with the thumbs, with the other two fingers extended. There are other helpful mudras for the five vayus.

114 A number of these Yoga practices are discussed in the author's *Yoga and Ayurveda* and in *Ayurveda and Marma Therapy*.

115 Note the author's *Mantra Yoga and Primal Sound.*

116 Saumya and Raudra or Agneya in Sanskrit.

117 Bija mantra of Narasimha, the man-lion, the protective form of Lord Vishnu.

118 Along with *Saundarya Lahiri* are *Ananda Lahari*, and *Tripura Sundari Stotra* as important works of Shankaracharya to Sundari and Soma.

119 Sanskrit recognizes 16 vowels, 25 consonants, and 9 ushma (heat-producing) semivowels and sibilants. These also govern the petals of the chakras starting with the 16 vowels as the 16 petals of the throat chakra, the 25 consonants as starting with the 12 petals of the heart, the 10 petals of the navel and the first 3 of the 6 petals of the sex center; the 9 semivowels and sibilants are the second 3 of the 6 petals of the sex center, the 4 petals of the root chakra and the two petals of the Third Eye. Sometimes the 16 vowels, the first 16 of the consonants, the last 9 of the consonants and the first 7 of the semi-vowels and sibilants form three groups of 16.

120 Note author's *Mantra Yoga and Primal Sound*, for its discussion of Shakti mantras.

121 Most commonly used is the *Krishna Yajurveda* style of Vedic chanting used mainly in South India. Rigvedic style is slightly different. *Shukla Yajurveda* or Sanatani style of the north is yet very different. Arya Samaj and Gayatri Pariwar have some modern variations as well. Some Vedic verses like Gayatri or Mrityunjaya are chanted in the tonality of classical Sanskrit poems as well, which is yet different.

122 Note the author's book *Mantra Yoga and Primal Sound* for more details.

123 There are many audio CDs of such mantras including Yogini Shambhavi's *Yogini Bhava* that the reader can also consult.

124 *Yoga Sutras I.24-28.*

125 *Yoga Sutras, I.23.*

126 Note the Kalasha or water pitcher design motifs used in this book as examples.

127 *Rigveda IX.107.1.*

128 Sundari is discussed in the author's *Tantric Yoga and the Wisdom Goddess*, and in *Inner Tantric Yoga*: Working with the Universal Shakti. These books discuss the practices used in her worship, her mantra, and her place in inner yogic practices.

129 *Ka E Ī La Hrīm, Ha Sa Ka Ha La Hrīm, Sa Ka La Hrīm.* Note author's *Inner Tantric Yoga* for more information on this important Soma-Sundari mantra.

130 Tripura Sundari Gayatri: *Aim Vāgīśvari vidmahe, Klīm Kameśvari dhīmahi, Sauḥ Tan no Śakti pracodayāt.*

131 *Rigveda II.33.4,* Rudra as the best of all the doctors.

132 *Rigveda X.60.12* as reflecting the healing power of the hands.

133 Note the explanation of the Mrityunjaya Mantra in *Inner Tantric Yoga*.

134 This Madhu Vidya is highlighted in the *Upanishads* like the *Brihadaranyaka II.2.1-19*, and is rooted in several Vedic verses.

135 Gayatri mantra, *Rigveda III.62.10*, is the Tat Savitur mantra. Aditya Hridaya Stotra is the chant taught by sage Agastya to Lord Rama in the *Ramayana*, which allows him to defeat Ravana.

136 The ninth book or mandala of the *Rigveda* is dedicated exclusively to Soma and has 114 hymns, although a few Soma hymns and verses do occur elsewhere in the text (book I and VIII mainly). In addition Soma as a deity is commonly mentioned in the hymns to other Vedic deities, notably Indra, where Soma is a common topic as Indra is the drinker of the Soma.

137 Listening to the chanting of the ninth mandala of the *Rigveda* has been promoted by the TM (Transcendental Meditation) organization and audio versions of the ninth book of the *Rigveda* can be found available.

138 This mantra has its inspiration in the works of Brahmarshi Daivarata, one of the main disciples of Ganapati Muni and Ramana Maharshi, who Maharishi Mahesh Yogi brought to the West several times and drew his Vedic inspiration from. Unfortunately his great works like *Chandodarshana* and *Vak Sudha* are not in print.

139 This particular Soma Gayatri does not occur in the *Rigveda*, but derives from later Tantric works.

140 Note author's *Tantric Yoga and the Wisdom Goddesses*, which discusses these ten deities including relative to Agni and Soma.

141 Note ancient *Upanishads* like the *Kena*, *Katha* and *Mandukya*, Shankara's shorter works like *Vivekachudamani* or *Aparokshanubhuti* or any works related to Ramana Maharshi, particularly the Ramana Gita.

142 William Blake, Auguries of Innocence.

143 *Ashtavakra Gita*, a famous Advaitic text.

144 There are helpful mantra practices in this regard such as discussed in *Mantra Yoga and Primal Sound*.

145 Note discussion of Shambhavi Mudra in *Inner Tantric Yoga*.

146 Note particularly the *Aitareya Upanishad* which emphasizes the inquiry Who am I (Ko'ham).

147 The *Yoga Sutras* of Patanjali as one of the six schools of Vedic thought accepts the authority of the *Vedas* and *Upanishads* and should be viewed in the same background.

148 Note *Ramana Gita* in particular.

149 Like the works of Shankara or the *Yoga Vasishta*, or works of modern teachers like Ramana Maharshi, Swami Dayananda, Swami Chinmayananda, Swami Vivekananda.

150 *Brihadaranyaka Upanishad II.4.5.*

151 This amrita nadi is described by Ramana Maharshi and his disciple Ganapati Muni, as bringing us to the hridaya or spiritual heart.

152 What are called 'upachaya houses' in Vedic astrology. Sometimes the tenth house is included here as well.

153 Note author's book *Ayurvedic Astrology* for more information on this subject.

154 Note Yogini Shambhavi's *Jyotir Bhava* Vedic astrology mantra CD.

155 Note various books on the Nakshatras, like the book of Dennis Harness.

156 Notably through the Vimshottari Dasha system, which is based upon them.

157 To be more specific the fifth, tenth and eleventh tithis of the waxing Moon are usually the best.

158 Vedic astrology uses a sidereal zodiac of the fixed stars, whereas tropical astrology uses a tropical zodiac of the solstices and equinoxes. The Vedic planetary positions are more than twenty degrees less than those of western tropical astrology.

159 Note *Mantra Yoga and Primal Sound, Chapter 18.*

160 *Rigveda X.97.7.*

161 *Rigveda VII.49.4.*

162 *Sushruta Samhita Chikitsa Sthana XXIX.5-8.*

163 *Sushruta Samhita Chikitsa Sthana XXIX.27-31.*

164 *RigvedaVIII.7.29, Rigveda VIII.64.11.*

165 *Rigveda IX.65.22-3.*

166 *Jaiminiya Brahmana* for example.

167 *Rigveda VIII.91.1.*

168 *Rigveda IX.113.1.* Sharanyavat is mentioned several times in the text along with other Soma lands like Sushoma, Arjika and Pastyavat, though Somas are found in all lands and among all the five Vedic peoples.

169 Munjavat in *Rigveda X.34.1*, also mentioned in *Mahabharata.*

170 Notably the Ayurvedic tonic herb, vamsa rochana.

171 Bhagwan Singh is of this view in his book the *Vedic Harappans.*

172 *Atharva Veda XI.6.15*, The five great plants, of which Soma is the best, appear to be Soma, darbha (a kind of grass), bhanga (marijuana), yava (barley) and sahas (identity unknown). Apart from marijuana, the other plants do not seem to be narcotic in their properties.

173 Soma as tree or *vanaspati* in the *Rigveda IX.12.10* and *IX.12.7*, "Gaining eternal praise, the tree, hidden in our thoughts, yielding milk to all, moving through all the ages of mankind."

174 *Atharva Veda XIX.39.5, 6,* connects Soma with the herb kushta and the ashvattha tree.

175 The cluster or Udambara fig is the most commonly used of these rejuvenative fig plants in Ayurveda.

176 *Atharva Veda XIX. 39.5.* "Kushta which holds all medicines dwelled together with Soma."

177 *Vitality Strengthening Astavarga Plants*, Sharma and Bal Krishan.

178 *Rigveda II.42,7*, gavashira (cooked in milk), yavashira (cooked in grain or barley); *Rigveda IX.63.15* dadhyashira (cooked in curds or yogurt); also rasashira (cooked in its own plant juice).

179 *Kena Upanishad I.2.*

180 *Sushruta Samhita Chikitsa Sthana* XXIX.5-8; quoted earlier, includes Somas named after the prime Vedic meters of Gayatri, Trishtubh, Jagati and Pankti.

181 Note the authors *Wisdom of the Ancient Seers* for translations of many more Soma hymns and other hymns from the *Rigveda*.

182 *Bhagavad Gita* X.37, where Krishna identifies himself with Ushanas. Note that Krishna is another Soma figure, a veritable avatar of the Soma of devotion or bhakti.

183 As the other main seer family the Angirasas is more connected to Agni.

184 Note Indra as the seer (drashta) in the *Aitareya Upanishad I.3.*

INDEX